Atlas of Inflammatory Bowel Diseases

Won Ho Kim • Jae Hee Cheon
Editors

Atlas of Inflammatory Bowel Diseases

Springer

Editors
Won Ho Kim, MD, PhD
Department of Internal Medicine
and Institute of Gastroenterology
Yonsei University College of Medicine
Seoul
Korea

Jae Hee Cheon, MD, PhD
Department of Internal Medicine
and Institute of Gastroenterology
Yonsei University College of Medicine
Seoul
Korea

ISBN 978-3-642-39422-5 ISBN 978-3-642-39423-2 (eBook)
DOI 10.1007/978-3-642-39423-2
Springer Heidelberg New York Dordrecht London

Library of Congress Control Number: 2015930009

Printed on acid-free paper

Springer is part of Springer Science+Business Media (www.springer.com)

Preface

Inflammatory bowel diseases (IBD) are standing in the middle of growing attention and interest than ever in the field of gastroenterology based on highly increasing prevalence and achieving advanced knowledge in pathogenesis, diagnosis, and treatment. With the expansion of knowledge in IBD, a demand for the precise endoscopic diagnostic criteria and differential diagnoses has also been increased. In particular, the incidence and prevalence of IBD have recently been increasing throughout Asia. This trend in IBD epidemiology indicates the necessity of specific attention and education in this area. Additionally, many infectious enterocolitides or intestinal Behçet's disease that are prevalent in Asia should be differentiated from IBD, but it is often a difficult task.

While some excellent atlases have been published on other fields of gastroenterology, there have been no atlases of IBD to the best of the authors' knowledge. The present atlas attempts to fill this gap in response to the intense interest. We aimed to provide detailed guidance on endoscopic indices of disease activity, diagnosis, differential diagnosis, and complications of IBD.

This comprehensive atlas, containing more than 500 high-quality images, illustrates the complete spectrum of presentations of IBD. With detailed explanations of each endoscopic finding, it provides the most important differential diagnoses. Especially, it is focused on the most recent developments in the use of endoscopy in IBD as well as proper diagnosis using conventional endoscopy. In addition to ileocolonoscopy, small bowel endoscopy, and esophagogastroduodenoscopy, chapters are included on the role of both established radiological techniques, such as CT, MRI, and the newest approaches, including high-resolution endoscopy, narrow band imaging, and confocal laser endomicroscopy. The present volume also completes and extends the endoscopic characterization of other related intestinal diseases as well as IBD and incorporates original figures. Where possible, summarizing tables were placed for a better understanding of readers. To constitute this atlas, more informative and valuable extraintestinal manifestations and complications are also addressed in separate chapters, and it concludes by presenting surgical findings.

The authors are international authorities in the Asian-Pacific region with diverse expert knowledge who have collaborated to create an ideal tool for all who wish to master endoscopic evaluation in IBD. We anticipate that the illustrations and descriptions will increase knowledge as a practical text for both practitioners and trainees in gastroenterology. Through continuous improvement of knowledge and increasing practice experiences, we are sure this atlas will continue to develop.

Concluding the preface, we attentively hope this can be regarded as a best guideline for use in diagnostic and prognostic decisions and individualized therapeutic planning. Also we look forward to receiving any suggestions that may assist us in continuing to offer a top-quality atlas.

Seoul, South Korea

Jae Hee Cheon, MD, PhD
Won Ho Kim, MD, PhD

Contents

Contributors

Seung Hyuk Baik, MD, PhD Section of Colon and Rectal Surgery, Department of Surgery, Yonsei University College of Medicine, Seoul, South Korea

Dongsik Bang Department of Dermatology and Cutaneous Biology Research Institute, Yonsei University College of Medicine, Seoul, South Korea

Heyson Chi-hey Chan Department of Medicine and Therapeutics, Institute of Digestive Disease, The Chinese University of Hong Kong, Hong Kong, The People's Republic of China

Jae Hee Cheon, MD, PhD Department of Internal Medicine, Institute of Gastroenterology, Yonsei University College of Medicine, Seoul, South Korea

Suhyun Cho Department of Dermatology and Cutaneous Biology Research Institute, Yonsei University College of Medicine, Seoul, South Korea

Min Ju Choi Department of Dermatology and Cutaneous Biology Research Institute, Yonsei University College of Medicine, Seoul, South Korea

Fumihito Hirai Department of Gastroenterology, Fukuoka University Chikushi Hospital, Chikushino, Fukuoka, Japan

Sung Pil Hong Department of Internal Medicine and Institute of Gastroenterology, Yonsei University College of Medicine, Seoul, South Korea

Naoki Hosoe Center for Diagnostic and Therapeutic Endoscopy, School of Medicine, Keio University, Shinjuku, Tokyo, Japan

Do Young Kim Department of Dermatology and Cutaneous Biology Research Institute, Yonsei University College of Medicine, Seoul, South Korea

Duk Hwan Kim Digestive Disease Center, CHA Bundang Medical center, CHA University College of Medicine, Seongnam, South Korea

Won Ho Kim, MD, PhD Department of Internal Medicine, Institute of Gastroenterology, Yonsei University College of Medicine, Seoul, South Korea

Joon Seok Lim Department of Radiology, Yonsei University College of Medicine, Severance Hospital, Seoul, South Korea

Phillip Fai Ching Lung Department of Imaging and Interventional Radiology, The Chinese University of Hong Kong, Hong Kong, The People's Republic of China

Toshiyuki Matsui Department of Gastroenterology, Fukuoka University Chikushi Hospital, Chikushino, Fukuoka, Japan

Makoto Naganuma Center for Diagnostic and Therapeutic Endoscopy, School of Medicine, Keio University, Shinjuku, Tokyo, Japan

Siew Chien Ng, PhD Department of Medicine and Therapeutics, Institute of Digestive Disease, The Chinese University of Hong Kong, Hong Kong, The People's Republic of China

Haruhiko Ogata Center for Diagnostic and Therapeutic Endoscopy, School of Medicine, Keio University, Shinjuku, Tokyo, Japan

Dong Il Park Department of Internal Medicine, Kangbuk Samsung Hospital, Sungkyunkwan University, School of Medicine, Seoul, South Korea

Eun Jung Park Department of Surgery, Yonsei University College of Medicine, Seoul, South Korea

Jae Jun Park, MD, PhD Department of Internal Medicine, Institute of Gastroenterology, Yonsei University College of Medicine, Seoul, South Korea

Ileocolonoscopy in Inflammatory Bowel Diseases

1

Jae Hee Cheon and Won Ho Kim

Because of the similar gastrointestinal symptoms and extraintestinal manifestations among various inflammatory intestinal disorders, it is important, but not always easy, to make a correct diagnosis of IBD for proper treatment. Of note, in endemic areas of tuberculosis, it is not an easy task to differentiate between CD and intestinal tuberculosis either clinically or endoscopically [1]. Furthermore, a correct diagnosis of indeterminate colitis is a major concern in dealing with IBD patients. Indeterminate or intermediate colitis has broadened to include colonoscopic, radiographic, or histologic appearances that show an overlap of diagnostic criteria for UC and CD.

In this context, ileocolonoscopy can be a valuable component of the initial approaches to suspected IBD patients (Table 1.1). With this, a correct diagnosis can be obtained through direct visualization of intestinal lesions and pathologic and microbiologic evaluations. Ileocolonoscopy was found to be accurate in 80–90 % in differentiating UC from CD in a prospective study [2]. Moreover, histologic parameters using mucosal biopsy specimens combined with serologic testing, clinical manifestations, and microbiologic cultures from fecal or tissue specimens can be helpful to differentiate IBD from enteric infections or intestinal tuberculosis.

Ileocolonoscopy can be used in various areas other than the initial diagnosis with mucosal examination. An assessment of the disease activity and extension is the other indication for ileocolonoscopy in IBD. Endoscopic localization of disease aids in determining the prognosis and appropriateness of medical therapies, as well as helps in decision-making in those undergoing surgical therapy [1]. In particular, several studies of biological agents considered endoscopic mucosal healing as an important end point [3, 4]. Biological agents induce the significant healing of mucosal lesions. The mucosal healing is believed to improve the long-term prognosis by reducing hospital admission rate and risk of surgery. Therefore, it is expected to increase in the use rate of endoscopic follow-up for evaluating mucosal healing in patients with IBD [5].

Management of bleeding and balloon dilation with or without corticosteroid injection into the stricture are examples of therapeutic implications of ileocolonoscopy in IBD. In addition to an assessment of response to treatments and prediction of relapse, surveillance of dysplasia or cancer in patients with long-standing chronic colonic IBD is the other crucial indication for colonoscopy in IBD [6].

In this regard, conventional endoscopy is still essential in IBD treatment, but it is very time-consuming and laborious, not that well accepted by the patients. Moreover, it is not always easy to make a correct diagnosis only using conventional endoscopy. To overcome those problems, more rapid, convenient, and accurate diagnostic technologies have been developed and are still evolving. Various novel techniques including chromoendoscopy with or without magnification, fluorescence endoscopy, narrowband imaging, optical coherence tomography, and confocal laser endomicroscopy are recently used in the diagnosis and management of IBD [7–11].

Table 1.1 The roles of ileocolonoscopy in inflammatory bowel diseases

Indications of ileocolonoscopy for IBD
Correct diagnosis of IBD
Differential diagnosis of IBD
Assessment of disease extent and severity
Assessment of disease activity
Assessment of response to treatments (therapeutic monitoring)
Assessment of complications – strictures, fistulae, or bleeding
Prediction of relapse
Therapeutic implications
Surveillance of dysplasia and colorectal cancer
Contraindications of ileocolonoscopy for IBD
Acute severe or fulminant ileocolitis
Patient's refusal or poor compliance
Suspected or impending bowel perforation

J.H. Cheon, MD, PhD (✉) • W.H. Kim, MD, PhD
Department of Internal Medicine, Institute of Gastroenterology, Yonsei University College of Medicine,
50-1 Yonsei-ro, Seodaemun-gu, Seoul 120-752, South Korea
e-mail: geniushee@yuhs.ac

W.H. Kim, J.H. Cheon (eds.), *Atlas of Inflammatory Bowel Diseases*,
DOI 10.1007/978-3-642-39423-2_1, © Springer-Verlag Berlin Heidelberg 2015

1.1 Ulcerative Colitis

1.1.1 Introduction

Ulcerative colitis (UC) is a type of IBD confined to the colorectum, characterized by repeated episodes of relapse and remission. UC involves the rectum and colon affecting mainly mucosal and submucosal layers. The pathogenesis is unknown though theories exist. Patients with UC have abnormalities of the immune system, but whether these problems are a cause or a result of the disease is still unclear. The treatment differs according to the disease activity and extent. The most common symptoms are mucoid stool, blood or pus in diarrhea, abdominal pain, urgency, and tenesmus. Other symptoms include anemia, fever, nausea, weight loss, loss of body fluids and nutrients, skin lesions, growth failure in children, etc.

UC can be difficult to diagnose because its symptoms are similar to those of other intestinal disorders. Flexible sigmoidoscopy and colonoscopy are the most accurate methods for diagnosing UC and ruling out other possible conditions, such as Crohn's disease, diverticular disease, or cancer.

The diagnosis of UC relies on the presence of bloody diarrhea with negative stool cultures and endoscopic evidence of diffuse, continuous mucosal inflammation involving the rectum and extending to a point more proximal in the colon. Sulfasalazine or mesalamine agents with or without corticosteroids are prevalent options in UC treatment. Patients who do not respond to mesalamine-based therapy can be treated with immunomodulators or anti-TNF therapies. Failure or occurrence of adverse reactions to these medications leaves the patients with little choice other than colectomy. However, it is important to take patient's quality of life and possibility of pouchitis into account before surgery.

Most patients with UC never develop colorectal cancer, but the two major factors that increase the risk of colorectal cancer are the duration of the disease and how much of the colon is affected.

1.1.2 Clinical Features

1.1.2.1 Symptoms and Signs

UC typically with diarrhea, abdominal pain, gross or occult rectal bleeding, urgency to defecate, or weight loss. The presence of anemia, thrombocytosis, or hypoalbuminemia may suggest inflammatory bowel disease, but most patients with ulcerative colitis will not have those abnormalities. C-reactive protein (CRP) level and erythrocyte sedimentation rate (ESR) are relatively insensitive for detecting ulcerative colitis. Serologic tests such as ANCA or ASCA might be helpful in the differential diagnosis, but not confirmative or pathognomonic. At the time of diagnosis, infective (enteric pathogens such as Salmonella, Shigella, Yersinia, Campylobacter, E. Coli 0157:H7, or Clostridium difficile), ischemic, irradiation causes of colitis must be excluded. Endoscopic biopsy plays a key role in confirming the diagnosis of UC.

1.1.2.2 Disease Activity Assessment

UC patients can be categorized by the severity of their disease. The accurate assessment of disease activity and extent is essential to the appropriate selection of various treatment modalities. The assessment of UC activity is based on the combination of symptoms, clinical and laboratory examinations, and endoscopic findings. Truelove-Witts criteria, Mayo score, Baron score, modified Baron Score, Sutherland index, Powell-Tuck index (St. Marks index), and Rachmilewitz index (endoscopic clinical activity index, CAI) are the commonly used disease activity measuring instruments.

According to Truelove and Witts' classification (Table 1.2) [12], mild disease is characterized by stools up to 4 times in a day with or without blood; a normal ESR or CRP; and with no systemic signs of toxicity. Moderate disease correlates with 4–6 bloody stools per day but with minimal signs of toxicity. Patients with severe diseases have more than six bloody stools a day or observable massive and significant bloody bowel movement and evidence of toxicity such as fever, tachycardia, anemia, or an elevated ESR or CRP. Fulminant disease may manifest as abdominal tenderness or distension, continuous bleeding, and anemia with transfusion requirement or colonic dilatation [13–16].

With the importance of clinical severity assessment, endoscopy is a mainstay in the diagnosis of UC and also represents a valuable tool for assessing disease activity and extent of disease (Table 1.3). The original endoscopic grading of UC is Baron's index. Baron index was developed mainly based on the severity of bleeding. The ulceration was not assessed in this index [17]. Mayo endoscopic scoring system has been most widely used for the assessment of endoscopic activity for UC in both clinical practice and clinical investigational settings. Mayo score consists of a 4-point scale (0–3) of appearance of the rectal mucosa [18]. UCEIS (Ulcerative Colitis Endoscopic Index of Severity) [19], a newly developed index on a 100-point scale, began to be used in the diagnosis of UC recently. The UCEIS has been undergone independent validation with different videos and investigators, evaluating operating properties of the index (responsiveness and reliability).

Table 1.2 Severity of ulcerative colitis: Truelove and Witts' classification

	Stools per day (blood in stools)	Systemic toxicity	ESR or CRP	Temperature
Mild	<4 (+/–)	Absent	Normal	Normal
Moderate	4–6 (+)	Absent or minimal	Normal or elevated	Normal or intermediate
Severe	>6 (+)	Present	Elevated	>37.8
Fulminant	>10 (+)	Present	Elevated	>37.8

Modified from Adams and Bornemann [16]

Table 1.3 Severity of ulcerative colitis: endoscopic indices

Baron index (Modified from Osada et al. [17])

Score	Severity	Activity indices
0	Normal	Mat mucosa, ramifying vascular pattern clearly visible throughout, no spontaneous bleeding, no bleeding to light touch
1	Abnormal	Appearances between 0 and 2
2	Moderate	Bleeding to light touch, but no spontaneous bleeding seen ahead of instrument on initial inspection
3	Severe	Spontaneous bleeding seen ahead of instrument at initial inspection and bleeds to light touch

Mayo score (Modified from Lewis et al. [18])

Score	Severity	Activity indices
0	Normal	Normal or inactive disease
1	Mild	Erythema, decreased vascular pattern, mild friability
2	Moderate	Marked erythema, absent vascular pattern, friability, erosions
3	Severe	Spontaneous bleeding, ulceration

UCEIS [19]

Descriptor	Likert scale	Definition
Vascular pattern	Normal (1)	Normal vascular pattern with arborization of capillaries clearly defined or with blurring or patchy loss of capillary margins
	Patchy obliteration (2)	Patchy obliteration of vascular pattern
	Obliterated (3)	Complete obliteration of vascular pattern
Bleeding	None (1)	No visible blood
	Mucosal (2)	Some spots or streaks of coagulated blood on the surface of the mucosa ahead of the scope, which can be washed away
	Luminal mild (3)	Some free liquid blood in the lumen
	Luminal moderate (4)	Frank blood in the lumen ahead of endoscope or visible oozing from mucosa after washing intraluminal blood or visible oozing from a hemorrhagic mucosa
Erosions and ulcers	None (1)	Normal mucosa, no visible erosions or ulcers
	Erosions (2)	Tiny (≤5 mm) defects in the mucosa of a white or yellow color with a flat edge
	Superficial ulcer (3)	Larger (>5 mm) defects in the mucosa, which are discrete fibrin-covered ulcers in comparison with erosions, but remain superficial
	Deep ulcer (4)	Deeper excavated defects in the mucosa, with a slightly raised edge

1.1.3 Endoscopic Features

1.1.3.1 Indication for Endoscopy

The indications for endoscopy in UC are the following: initial diagnosis, follow-up in asymptomatic patients, surveillance of dysplasia and colorectal cancer, and at any time that symptoms worsen or new symptoms occur.

The diagnosis of UC can be made initially by sigmoidoscopy. Mucosal biopsies are used to confirm the diagnosis and indicate the initial therapy. Colonoscopy in UC plays an important role in assessing the extension and severity of disease as well. In addition to this, colonoscopy can be used in evaluating the response to the treatment. With regard to therapeutic applications, obstructive symptoms caused by benign fibrotic strictures can be treated adequately by endoscopic balloon dilation. Epidemiological studies have demonstrated an increased risk of colorectal cancer in patients with both UC and colonic Crohn's disease. Surveillance endoscopy is indicated for regularly obtaining multiple biopsies to exclude possible malignancy, especially in the setting of UC [1].

1.1.3.2 Extent of Disease

Continuous inflammation without skipped area and the involvement of rectum is a typical feature of UC. Inflammation or ulceration of mucosa initiates from the superjacent area of the anal canal and is distributed in a continuous and symmetrical manner. Some exceptional cases include appendiceal orifice inflammation, proximal colon involvement only, and rectal sparing after local therapy, which will be described later in this chapter. The extent of UC can be classified as proctitis, left-sided colitis, and extensive colitis (Table 1.4) [20].

For approximately one third of patients with UC is classified as having proctitis. Proctitis is limited to the rectum, especially involves up to 15 cm from the anal verge (Fig. 1.1). Because of its limited extent of colitis, it is regarded as a milder form of UC. It is associated with fewer complications and offers a better prognosis than more extensive disease. Because of its location, ulcerative proctitis can be misdiagnosed as a hemorrhoid unless careful observation is performed.

Left-sided UC includes inflammation that begins from the rectum, involving up to the colon near the splenic flexure. When inflammation is located in the rectum and sigmoid colon, it specifically refers to proctosigmoiditis (Fig. 1.2). Typically, it presents bloody diarrhea, cramps, or tenesmus. Moderate pain on the lower left side of the abdomen may occur in active disease.

The extensive colitis is an inflammation involving more proximal area to splenic flexure. Extensive colitis may begin in the rectum and spread to the transverse or more proximal colon (Fig. 1.3). In particular, inflammation of the whole colonic mucosa from the rectum to cecum is referred to as pancolitis (Fig. 1.4). Patients with extensive colitis show more frequent complications, extraintestinal manifestations, and systemic symptoms. They are also at a higher risk of colorectal cancer and are likely to receive more immunosuppressive and surgical therapies [21]. Lesions usually get more severe towards the rectum, but sometimes it is less severe inversely. Moreover, normal mucosa is usually clearly distinguishable from inflamed mucosa in UC, but sometimes, lesions are scattered around the margin, making it difficult to diagnose.

Cecal patch is the presence of flat periappendiceal lesions, and it has been recognized mostly in patients with left-sided UC or proctitis. This cecal patch or appendiceal orifice inflammation (AOI) (Fig. 1.5) is observed with reddish and friable mucosa in the cecum, especially around the appendiceal orifice. It is more frequently observed in patients with less extensive UC and is unlikely the result of patchy improvement due to treatments. Segmental ulcerative colitis (Fig. 1.6) is a term designated for cases not involving the rectum, but involving the colon focally and segmentally. Rectal sparing also can occur after local therapies such as rectal mesalamine suppositories or enema (Fig. 1.7). These are often misdiagnosed as having Crohn's disease of the colon. Inflammation of the proximal colon and distal area such as the rectum with grossly normal skipped areas between proximal and distal areas is also considered as one of the endoscopic features of UC. Rarely, atypical inflammatory mucosal change characteristic for UC in various colonic segments without continuity can also be observed, and they are suggested to be one of the features of UC as well (Fig. 1.8).

Sometimes, nonspecific mucosal inflammation in the terminal ileum is observed in patients with UC although, by definition, UC is restricted to the colon. Involvement of the terminal ileum in UC is termed backwash ileitis. It is characterized by the presence of active enteritis involving the terminal ileum in a contiguous pattern from the cecum (Fig. 1.9) [22].

Table 1.4 Montreal classification of extent of ulcerative colitis [20]

Extent		Anatomy
E1	Ulcerative proctitis	Involvement limited to the rectum (i.e., proximal extent of inflammation is distal to the rectosigmoid junction)
E2	Left-sided UC (distal UC)	Involvement limited to a proportion of the colorectum distal to the splenic flexure
E3	Extensive UC (pancolitis)	Involvement extends proximal to the splenic flexure

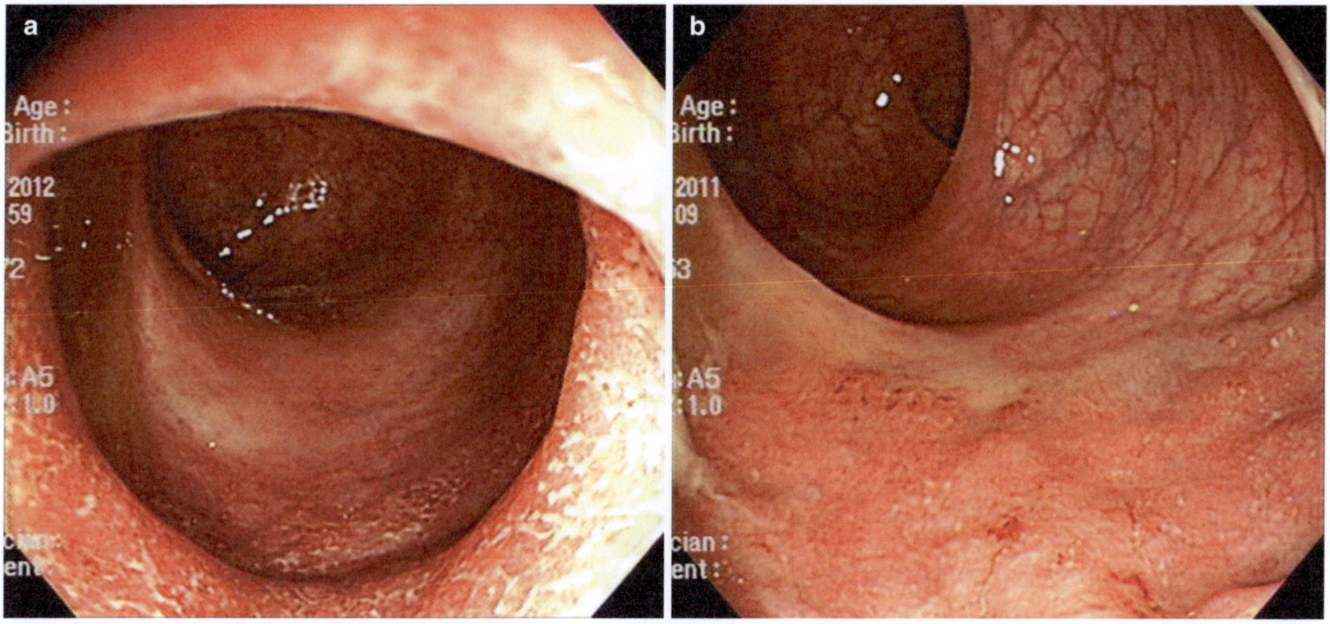

Fig. 1.1 (**a**) Ulcerative colitis limited to the rectum. (**b**) Mild UC involves the superjacent area of anal verge

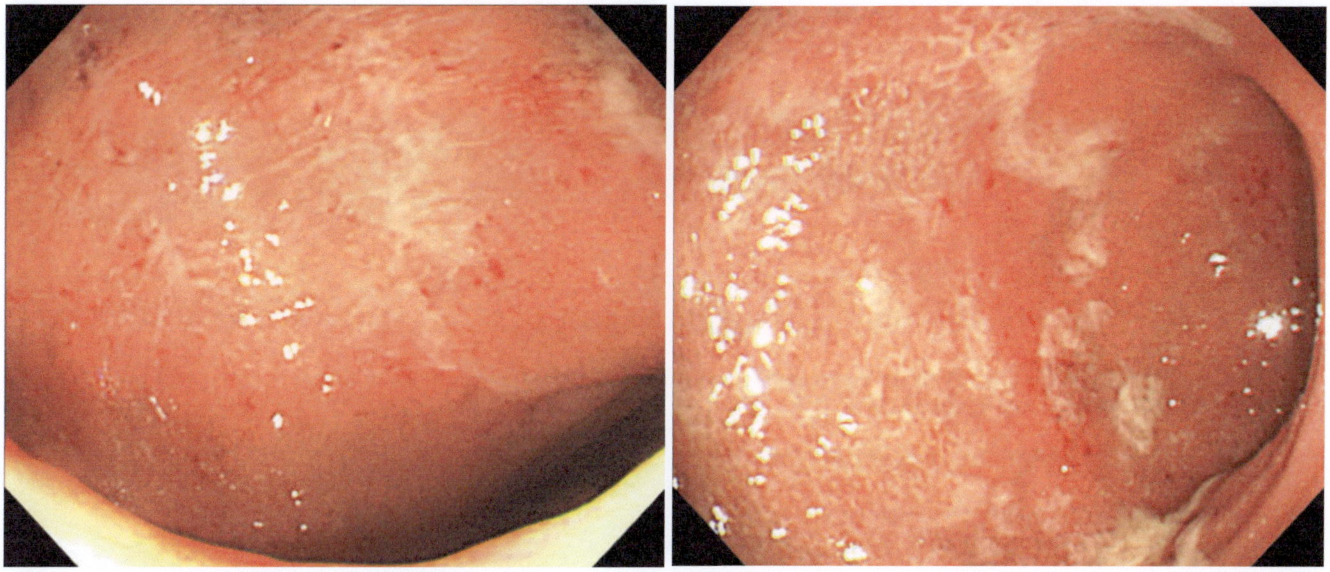

Fig. 1.2 Left-sided ulcerative colitis. Ulcerative colitis up to the sigmoid colon. The border between colitic and normal mucosa is clearly seen in the sigmoid colon

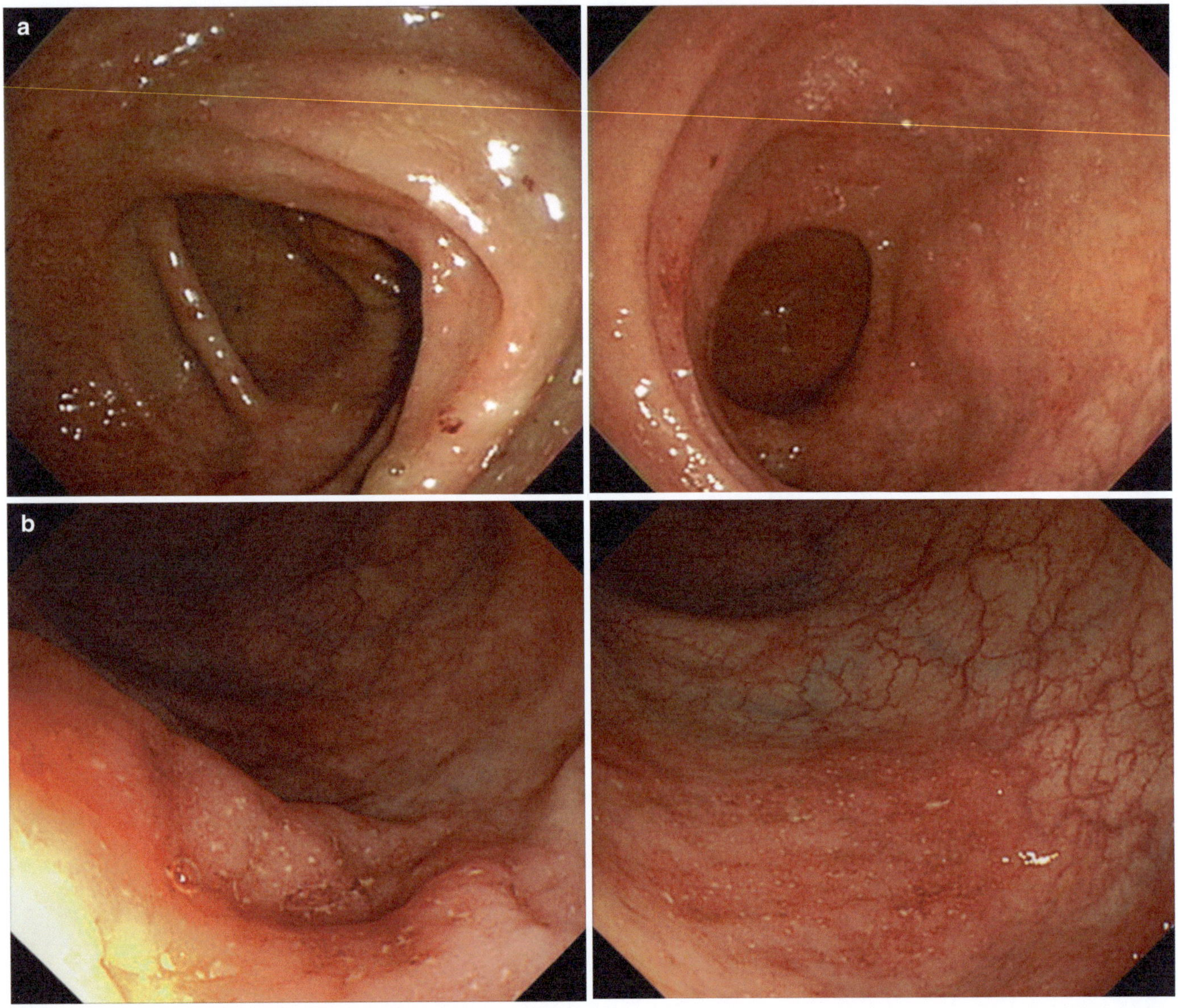

Fig. 1.3 Extensive ulcerative colitis. (**a**) The inflammation is seen up to the transverse colon. (**b**) Clear distinct margin is seen between normal mucosa and inflamed mucosa in the transverse colon

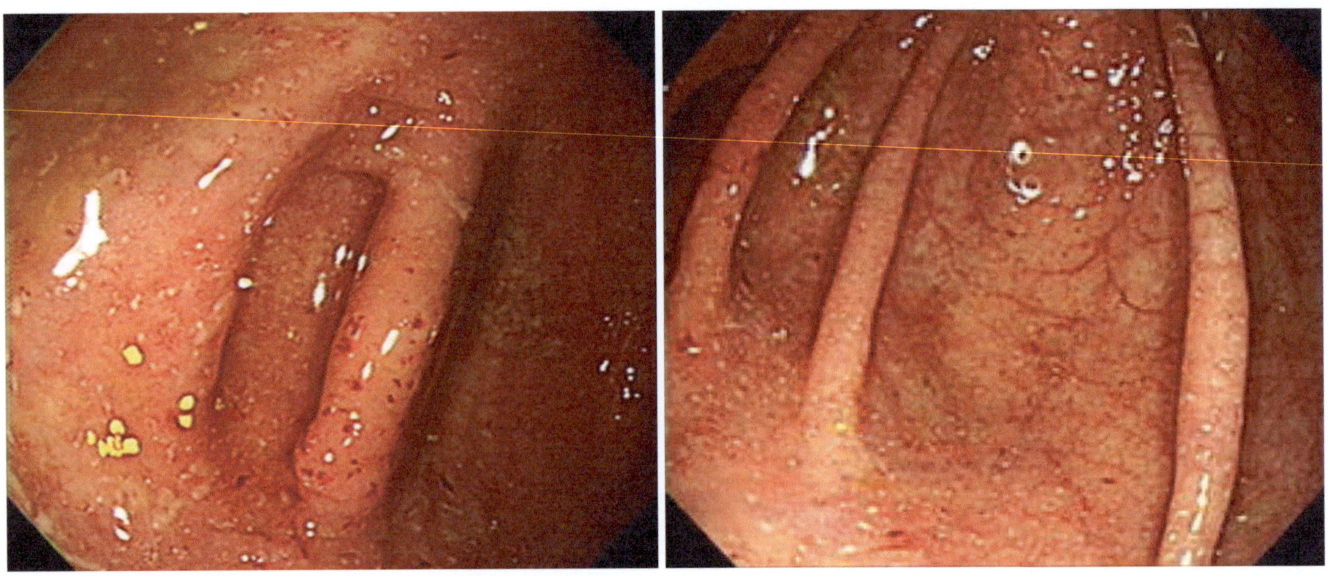

Fig. 1.4 Pancolitis. Colitis extends to the cecum and ascending colon

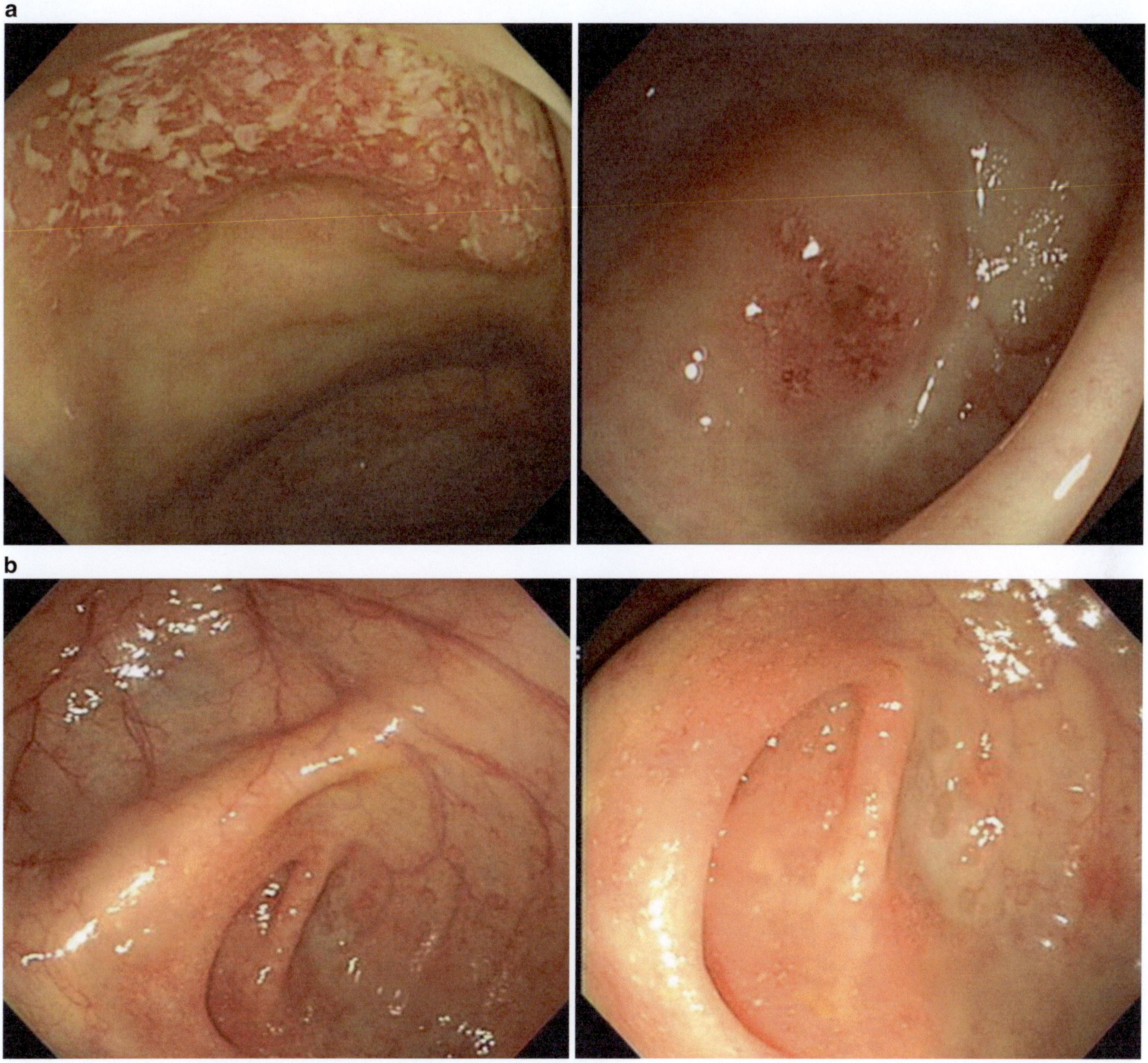

Fig. 1.5 Cecal patch or appendiceal orifice inflammation in ulcerative colitis. It is basically a similar mucosal finding to inflamed mucosa in the distal area of ulcerative colitis. (**a**) AOI confined to appendiceal orifice. (**b**) It often extends to the cecum

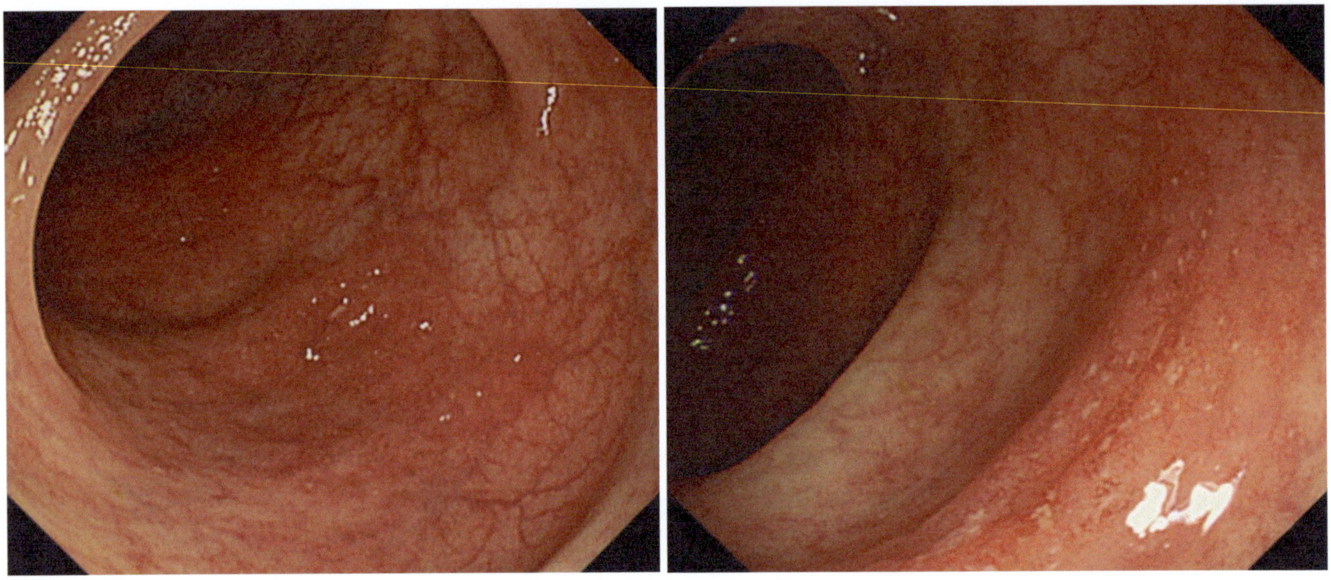

Fig. 1.6 Segmental ulcerative colitis. Inflammation involves the colon segmentally with the normal-looking intervening mucosa

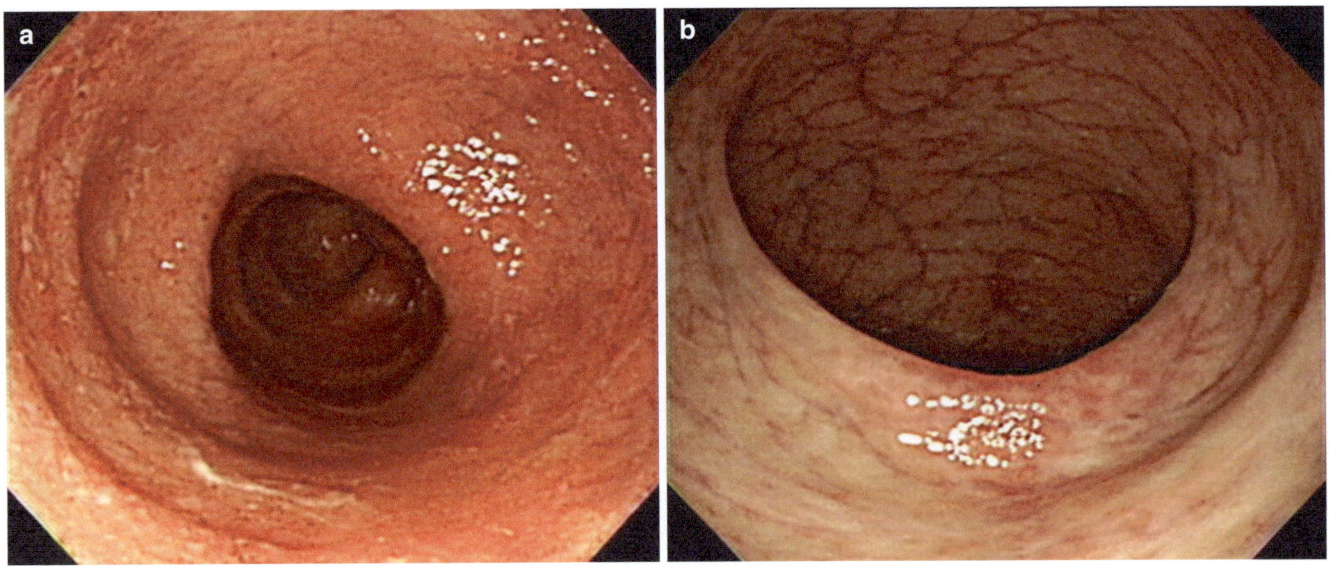

Fig. 1.7 Rectal sparing in a patient with ulcerative colitis. The patient was receiving a mesalazine suppository therapy at the time of colonoscopy. (**a**) Active inflammation is seen in the sigmoid colon. (**b**) Whitish scar change remains, but there is no evidence of inflammation in the rectum

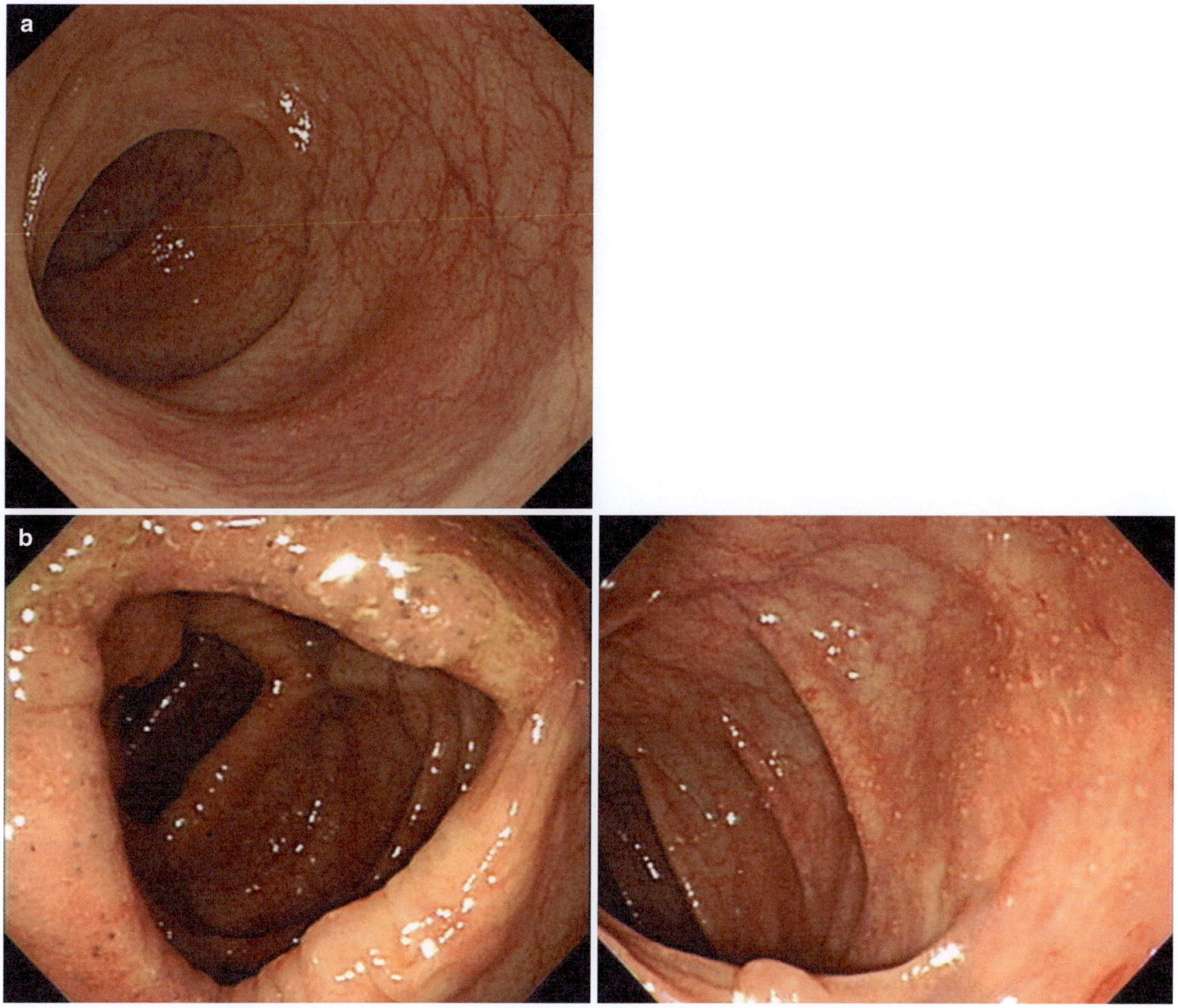

Fig. 1.8 Skipped pattern of mucosal inflammation in ulcerative colitis. (**a**) Focal segmental inflamed mucosal patches with skipped normal area are seen in the sigmoid colon. (**b**) Active inflammation is observed in the ascending colon. With the skipped normally looking mucosa in the proximal transverse colon, another focal inflamed mucosa is observed in the distal transverse colon

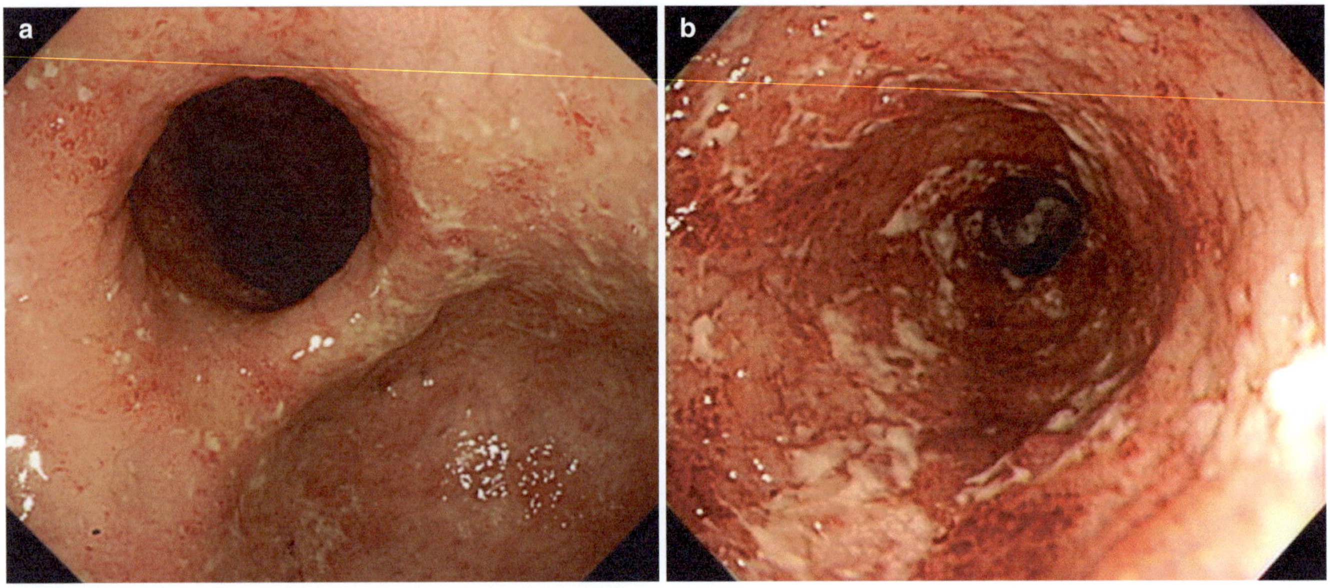

Fig. 1.9 Backwash ileitis. (**a**) The patulous ileocecal valve is seen. (**b**) When the colonoscope passed through the ileocecal valve, active inflammation was observed in the terminal ileum

1.1.3.3 Characteristics of Endoscopic Features According to Disease Status

Active UC

Active disease in UC is characterized by the endoscopic appearance of superficial ulcerations, friability, distorted mucosal vascular pattern, and exudates (Table 1.5). Erythema, erosions, and blurring of the normal vascular and mucosal patterns are the signs of low or mild activity. Severe active disease is characterized by edema, ulcerations, and mucopurulent exudates, as well as pseudopolyps and friable mucosa with spontaneous bleeding. Treatment of the condition depends on the extent of disease and the degree of inflammation.

Blurring of vascularity in UC patients is observed from the early stage of inflammation, and normal vascularity completely disappears in severe inflammation (Fig. 1.10).

Mucosal edema is defined as thick and swollen mucosa which is pooled with fluid. Edematous mucosal change develops, and it gets more severe with the progression of inflammation. With severe edema, colonic lumen shows narrowed appearance (Fig. 1.11).

Erythema is red coloration of the membrane composed of dilated veins. It is observed in mild or moderate UC rather than severe UC (Fig. 1.12). Mucopurulent exudates are frequently observed in UC, and mucinous exudates are exudates composed of the mixture of blood and pus (Fig. 1.13). Mucosal inflammation lends a granular appearance to the surface of the bowel (Fig. 1.14). As inflammation increases, the bowel wall and haustra thicken. Progression of inflammation might induce spontaneous bleeding, and it is a major feature of severe UC. Spontaneous bleeding after luminal inflation, easy touch bleeding, and even without any physical stimuli can be observed due to severe inflammation (Fig. 1.15).

Typically, the ulcers of UC are superficial and small in cases of mild to moderate inflammation (Fig. 1.16). In severe cases of UC, larger and deeper ulcers are observed (Fig. 1.17). Severe ulcerative changes include various shapes of ulcers including wide mucosal defects (Fig. 1.18), punched-out ulcers, deep and longitudinal ulcers (Fig. 1.19), irregular ulcers, geographic ulcers (Fig. 1.20), and cobblestone-like appearance (Fig. 1.21). Deep geographic and serpiginous (snakelike) ulcers are also common endoscopic findings in Crohn's disease, which thus often makes it difficult to differentiate between the two diseases.

Symptoms of diarrhea and abdominal pain are common to both infectious colitis and IBD. The endoscopic findings of infectious colitis and UC are often alike in the acute phase. In this case, clinical manifestations are occasionally helpful in the differential diagnosis (Table 1.6). Statistically, major symptoms of infectious colitis are acute onset, early fever, and frequent bowel movements. Fever is a usual symptom of infectious colitis and occurs within the first week at onset. Bowel movements are more than 12 times a day. Severe abdominal pain and vomiting at an early time point are the other symptoms of infectious colitis. In contrast, the symptoms of IBD onset are more gradual and insidious. The fever is rare and typically does not appear within the first week at onset.

In patients with UC, risk for reactivation of latent cytomegalovirus (CMV) infection is increased and is significantly higher than in CD (10–56.7 % vs. 0–29.6 %) [23]. The risk of CMV reactivation depends on the type of immunomodulators used and is higher in steroid-refractory than in steroid-responding patients. CMV reactivation should be routinely sought for in cases of disease flares or unresponsiveness to treatment (Fig. 1.22). The colonoscopic findings of UC patients infected with CMV are complicated, because inflammatory changes due to UC itself in the colonic mucosa exist prior to CMV infection [24]. Colonoscopic features include various types of lesions, a mucosal erythema, mucosa erosions and wide mucosal defects, solitary ulcer or ulcerations, and even perforation. The most common feature is multiple ulcers with at least one large ulcer from the persistent inflammation and fibrotic changes [25–27].

Although *Clostridium difficile* (*C. difficile*) colonizes the colon, it is not usually invasive, and tissue injury and inflammation are mediated by exotoxin (toxin A or toxin B) generated by the bacteria (Fig. 1.23). The incidence of *C. difficile* infection in IBD has recently been increased, and it appears to predict recurrent flares. Especially, UC patients with *C. difficile* infection had significantly higher morbidity and surgery rates [28]. The typical visualized endoscopic features of UC patients infected with *C. difficile* do not exist. However, nonspecific mucopus and pseudomembrane can be observed endoscopically. Pseudomembranous colitis is presented as the ulcerated colon mucosa covered by fibrinoid exudate. Rectal ulcers with bleeding and oozing polypoid lesions are also observed [29]. The pseudomembranes on the colonic mucosa usually are presented in the right colon and may therefore be missed by a sigmoidoscopy [30]. *C. difficile* infection also can occur in the small bowel and specifically in patients who had undergone a colectomy and an ileal pouch-anal anastomosis [31].

Quiescent UC

Clinical remission refers to the absence of symptoms such as diarrhea, bloody stool, and abdominal pain for more than a month, whereas endoscopic remission refers to the absence of signs such as ulceration, contact or spontaneous bleeding, and visible vascular patterns on the colonic mucosa. Although clinical symptoms of active UC, such as abdominal pain, diarrhea, and bloody stool, may disappear, it is often observed that endoscopic findings of active UC remain.

The major endoscopic aspect of patients with UC in its quiescent phase is the alteration or distortion of vascular markings. The regenerated vascularity can be observed in sparse and irregular appearance with white scar changes as a result of sequelae after inflammation disappearance (Fig. 1.24).

Between extensive scars, diverticular structures are usually observed and called pseudodiverticula (Fig. 1.25). Pseudodiverticulum and the classical cobblestone appearance result from deep transverse and longitudinal ulcers separated by residual areas of edematous mucosa. It is commonly associated with skip lesions, stricturing, and relative rectal sparing.

Patients with severely active disease can have deep ulcers and friability that result in spontaneous bleeding; meanwhile, inflammatory polyps may occur in quiescent UC (Fig. 1.26), and most of the polyps are located within an area of established colitis. Chronic inflammation in the colon results in inflammatory polyps. It is also known as pseudopolyps because they are different from the other typical forms of polyps and noncancerous nature. Inflammatory polyps can show various sizes, shapes, number, and surface changes. Sometimes, hyperplastic polyps are difficult to distinguish from small elevated polypoid areas of dysplasia (Fig. 1.27).

Severe inflammation can lead to luminal narrowing and bowel wall thickening with or without prestenotic dilatation. Strictures are classified as benign or malignant on the basis of histopathology obtained at endoscopy or surgery (Fig. 1.28). As the duration of the disease increases, the proportion of malignant strictures increases sharply [32].

The rigid and featureless appearance of the colon in chronic ulcerative colitis is called lead pipe appearance (Fig. 1.29), and this is derived from long-standing severe inflammation. The sign is a complete loss of haustral markings and usually a degree of uniform luminal narrowing due to chronic bowel wall thickening. In this case, the colon is typically shortened.

Table 1.5 Endoscopic characteristics of active UC

Severity	Characteristics
Low activities	Erythema, erosions, blurring, and decreased vascular and mucosal patterns
Severe activities	Edema, ulcerations, mucopurulent exudates, pseudopolyps, friable mucosa with spontaneous bleeding

Long-Standing UC

In case of long-standing UC patients, the colonic mucosa shows signs of chronic, recurrent inflammation and healing. It has various colonoscopic appearances ranging from normal colonic appearance to severe inflammation and from scarring to multiple postinflammatory polyps. A featureless colon with complete loss of haustration, a shortened or tubular colon indicative feature of chronicity of the disease, total blurring of the normal vascular pattern, a granular-like mucosa, colonic strictures, and postinflammatory polyps are common colonoscopic features of long-standing UC patients.

Friable mucosa or ulceration is a typical endoscopic evidence of active inflammation, and tubular colonic appearance or strictures usually represent an ongoing inflammation or sequelae of chronic inflammatory process. Chronic endoscopic changes, such as scarring and postinflammatory polyps, are not always related to current disease activity, but it signifies previous significant inflammation [33].

A shortened or tubular colon indicates chronically active colitis and is associated with ongoing inflammatory process and higher neoplasia risk. Especially, stricture formation should be regarded as a highly suspicious sign of malignancy and is considered the strongest indication for colectomy (Fig. 1.30) [32]. However, it is not easy to detect dysplastic lesions especially in the scarred colon with many pseudopolyps. Therefore, multiple biopsies from all different segments are usually performed during colonoscopy for the surveillance of colorectal cancer in long-standing UC patients. In a similar point of view, it is possible that flat neoplastic polyps could be missed at endoscopy with random biopsy since it does not present dysplasia endoscopically. Therefore, more effective and advanced techniques in detecting flat dysplasia are recommended, for instance, dye-based chromoendoscopy or high-resolution electronic video endoscopy [34, 35]. Furthermore, careful and detailed considerations including histologic and radiologic assessment are needed to rule out dysplasia and malignancy in all cases of long-standing UC patients.

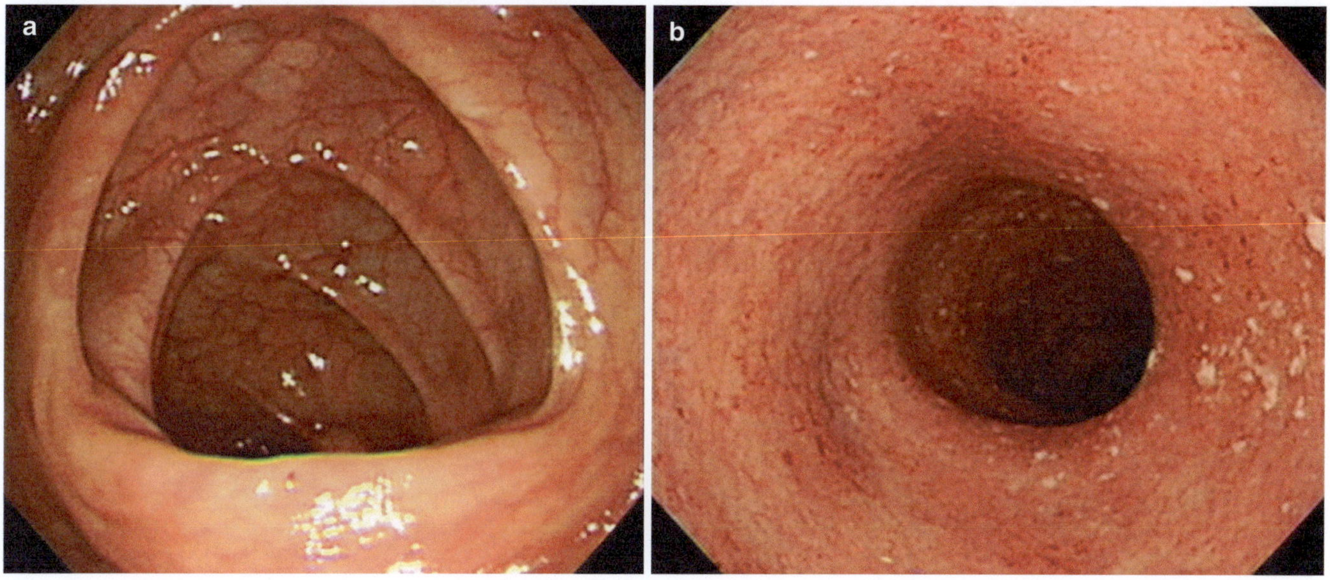

Fig. 1.10 Blurring or loss of vascularity in UC. (**a**) Normal mucosal vascularity. (**b**) Near complete loss of mucosal vascularity is observed in moderate UC

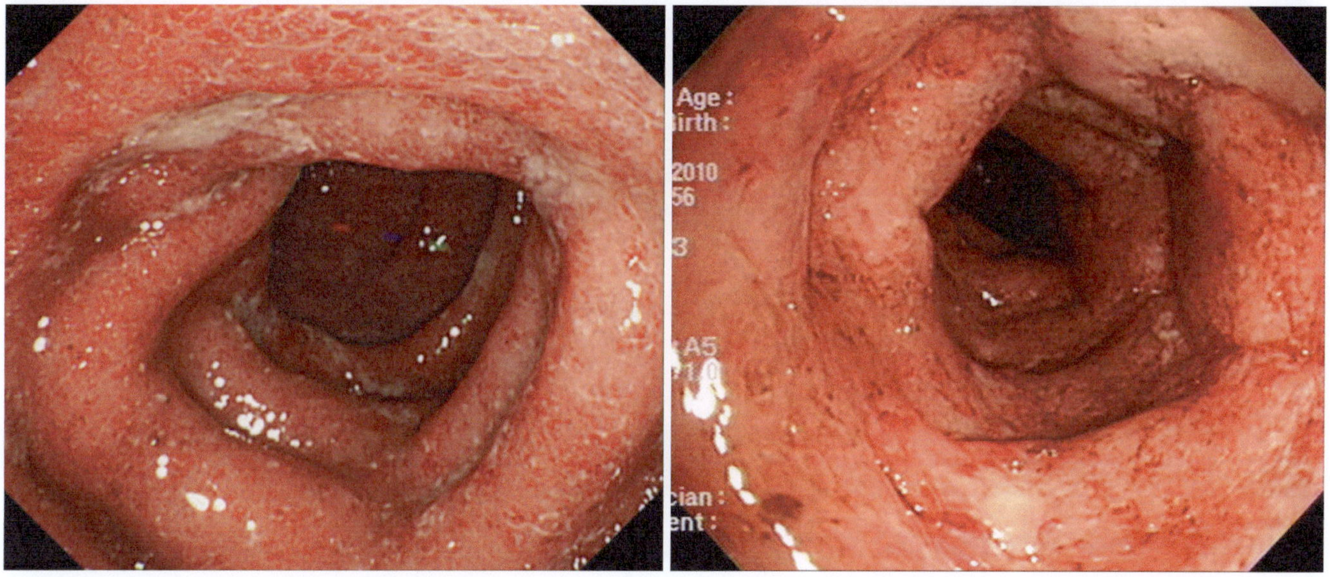

Fig. 1.11 Mucosal edema. The swollen mucosa and thickened haustral folds are observed. In severe edema, mucosal narrowing can be shown

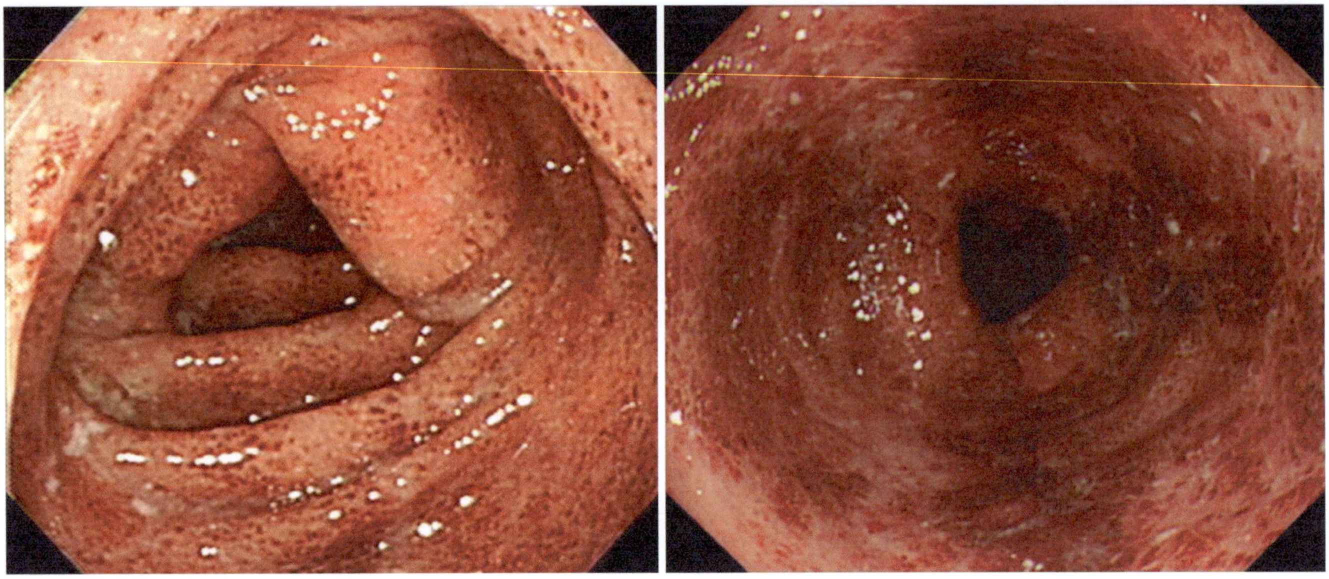

Fig. 1.12 Erythema in ulcerative colitis

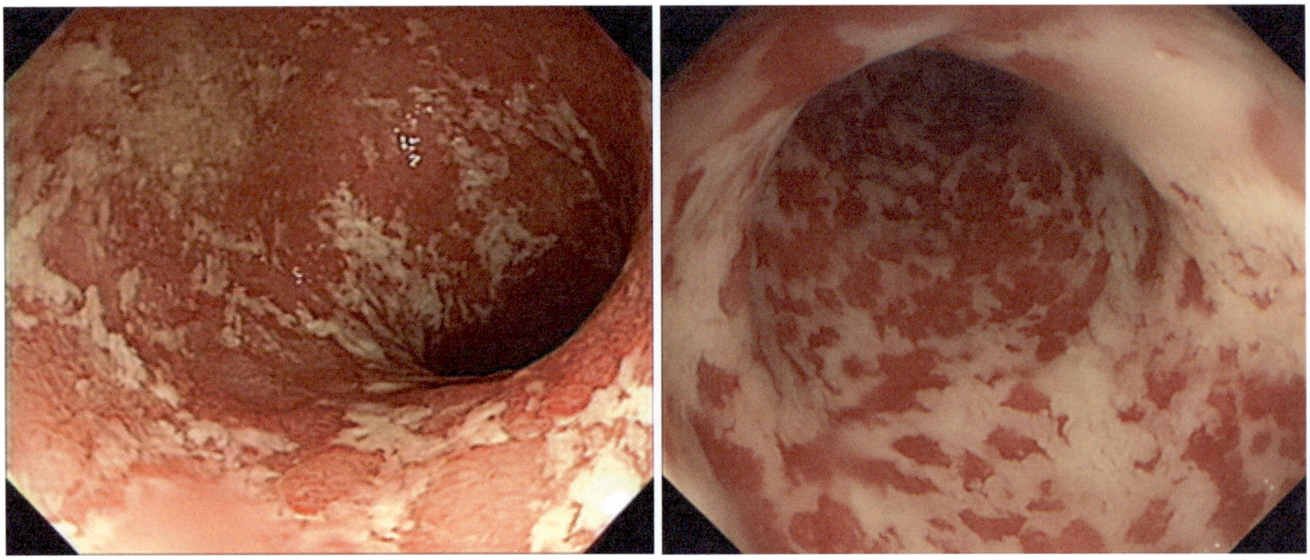

Fig. 1.13 Exudates in ulcerative colitis

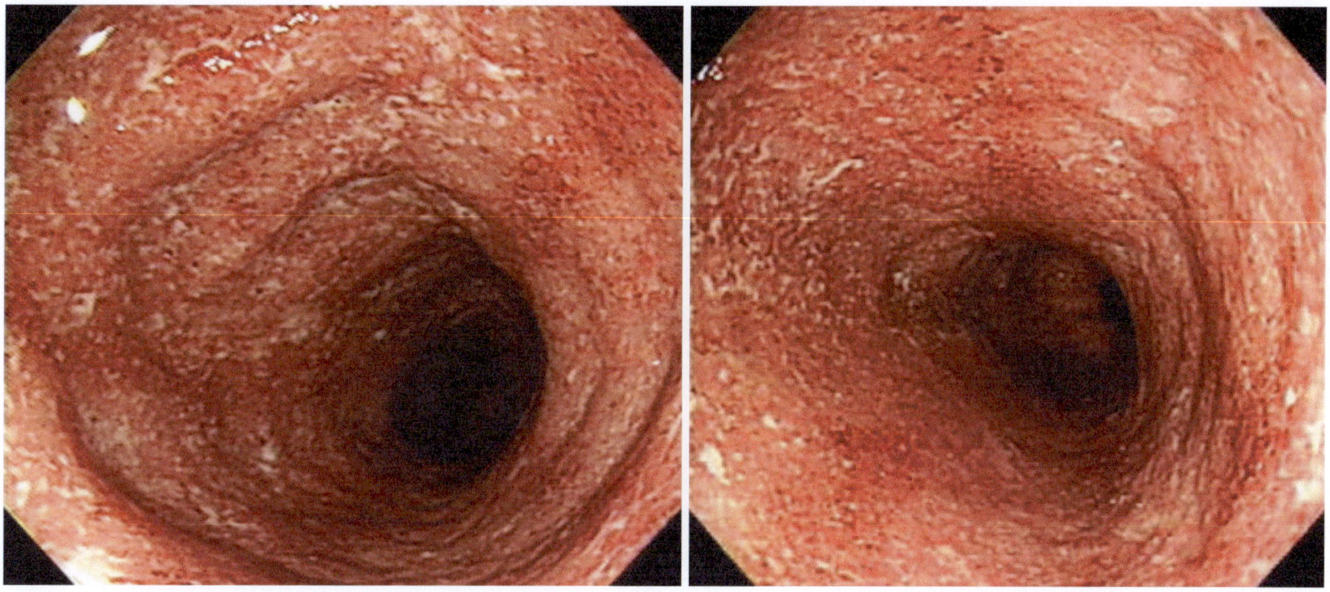

Fig. 1.14 Granular appearance in ulcerative colitis

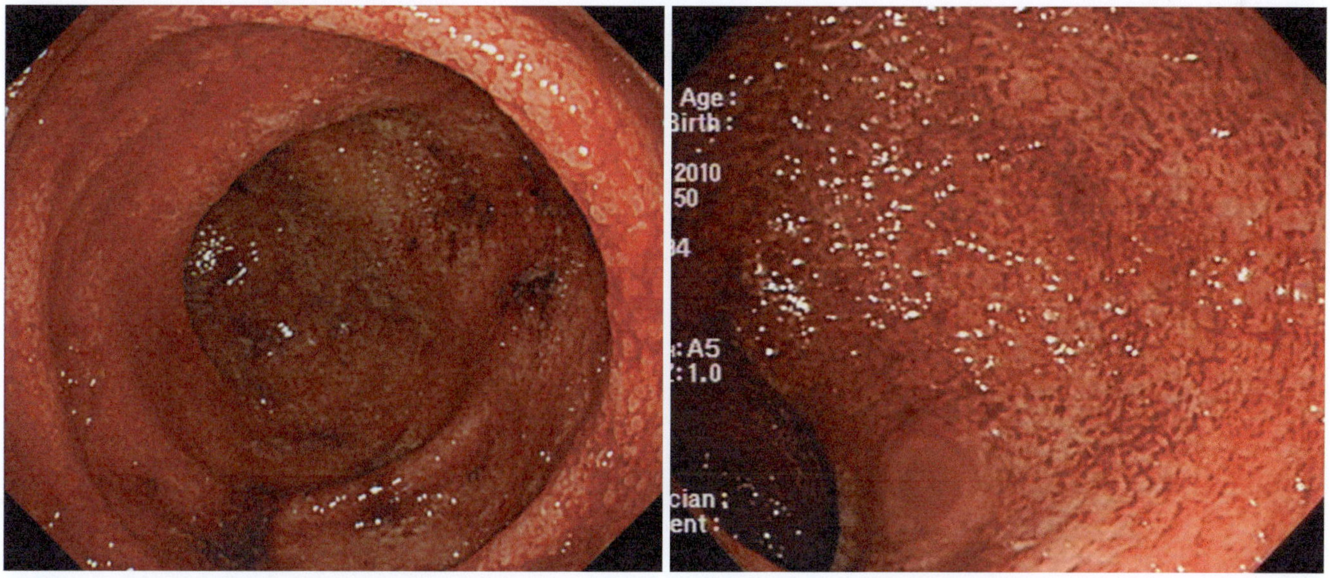

Fig. 1.15 Spontaneous hemorrhage in ulcerative colitis

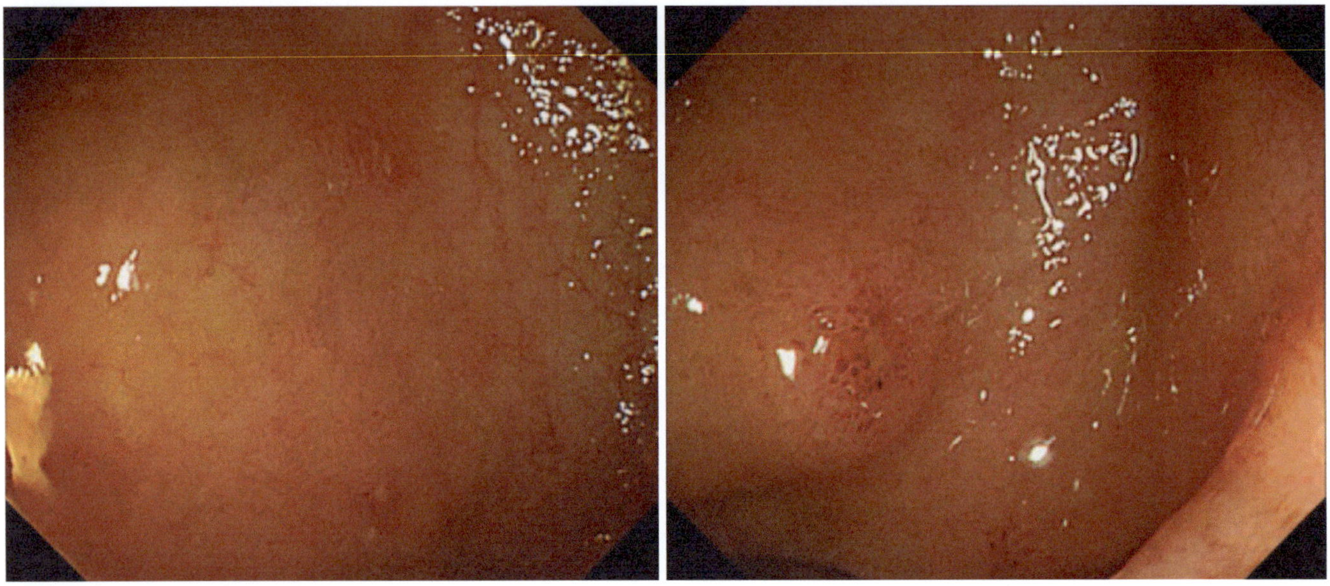

Fig. 1.16 Small ulcers in ulcerative colitis

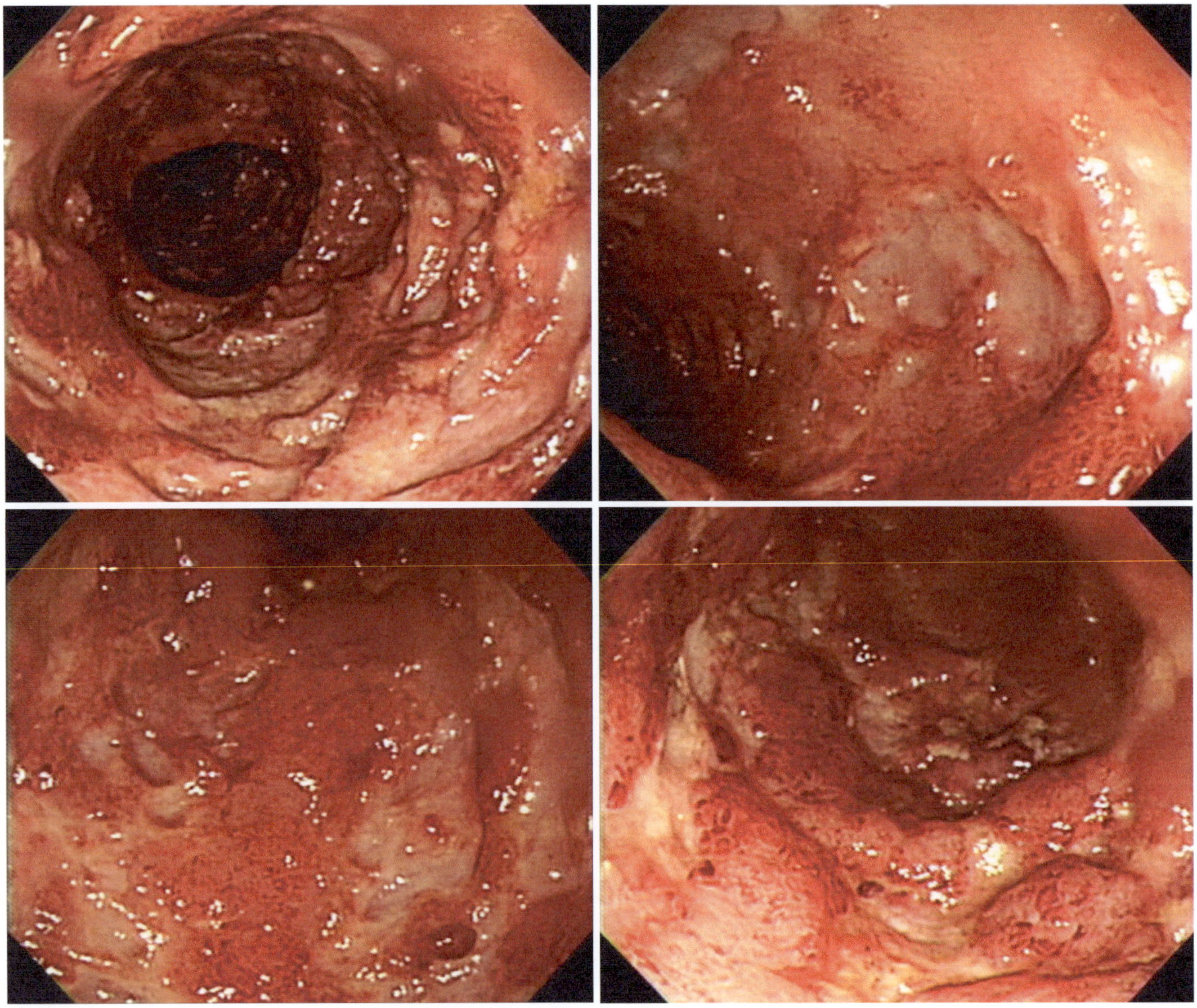

Fig. 1.17 Various shapes of ulcers in severe ulcerative colitis

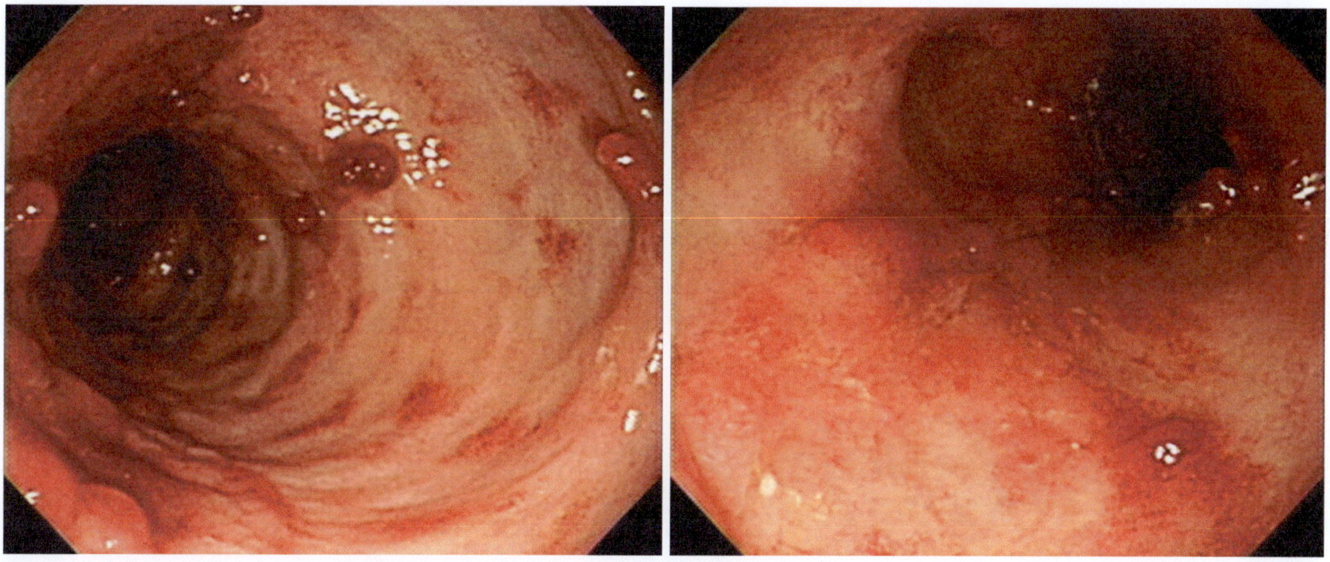

Fig. 1.18 Wide mucosal defects in ulcerative colitis. The remnant mucosa shapes pseudopolyps

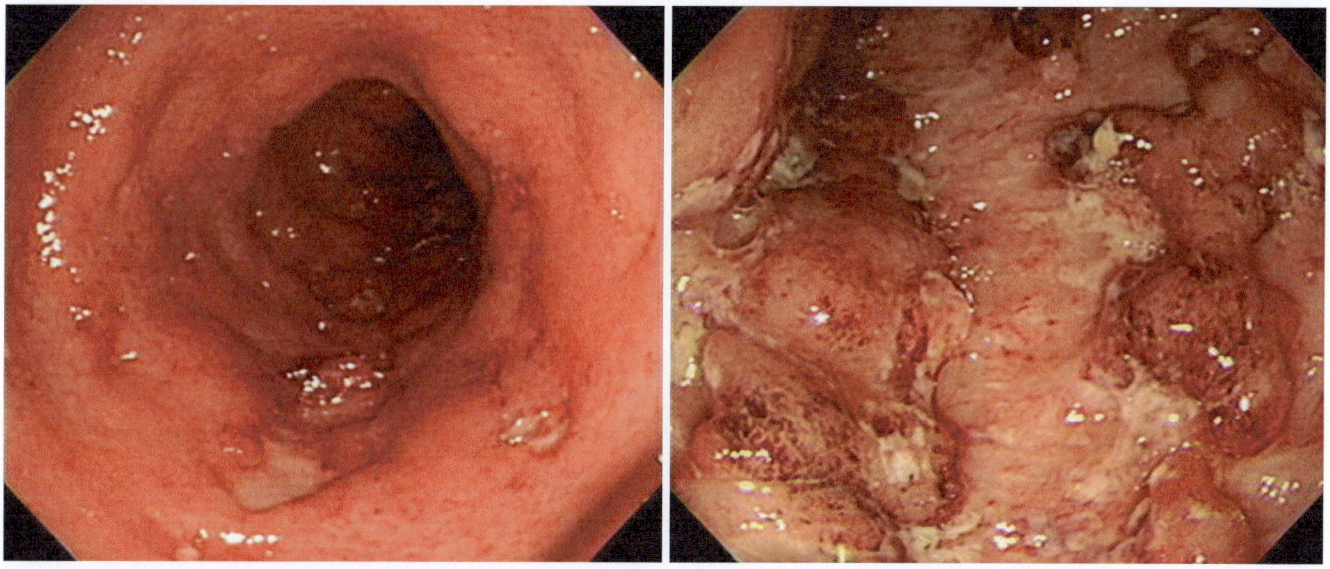

Fig. 1.19 Deep, longitudinal ulcers in ulcerative colitis. They are often misdiagnosed as ulcers in Crohn's disease

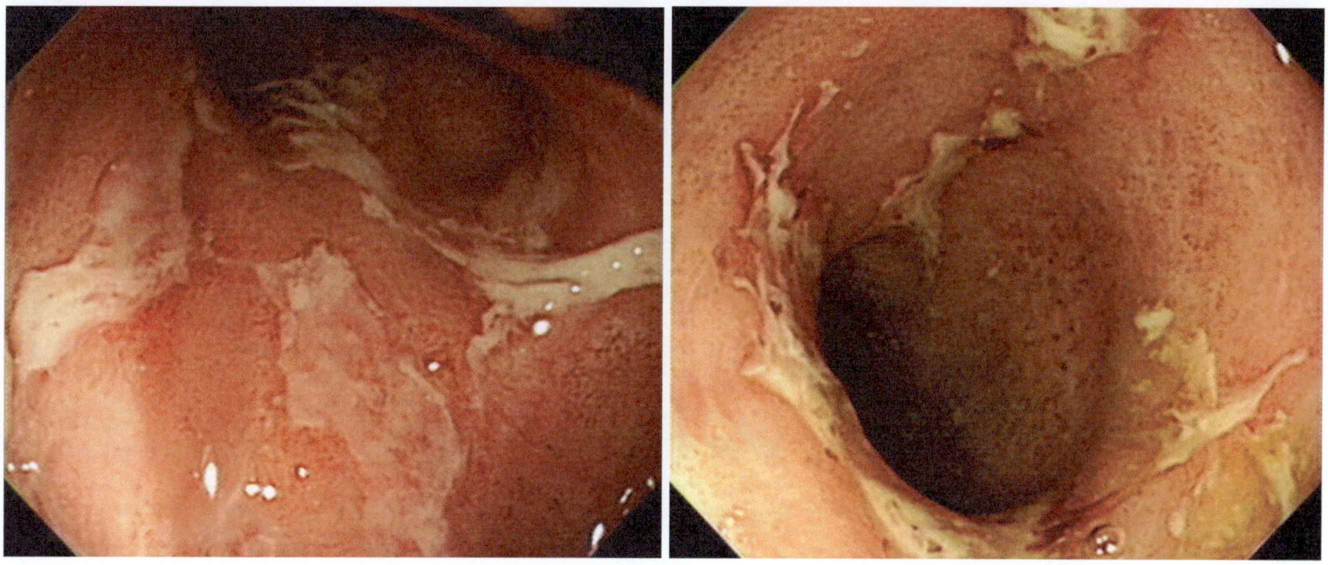

Fig. 1.20 Irregular and geographic ulcers in ulcerative colitis

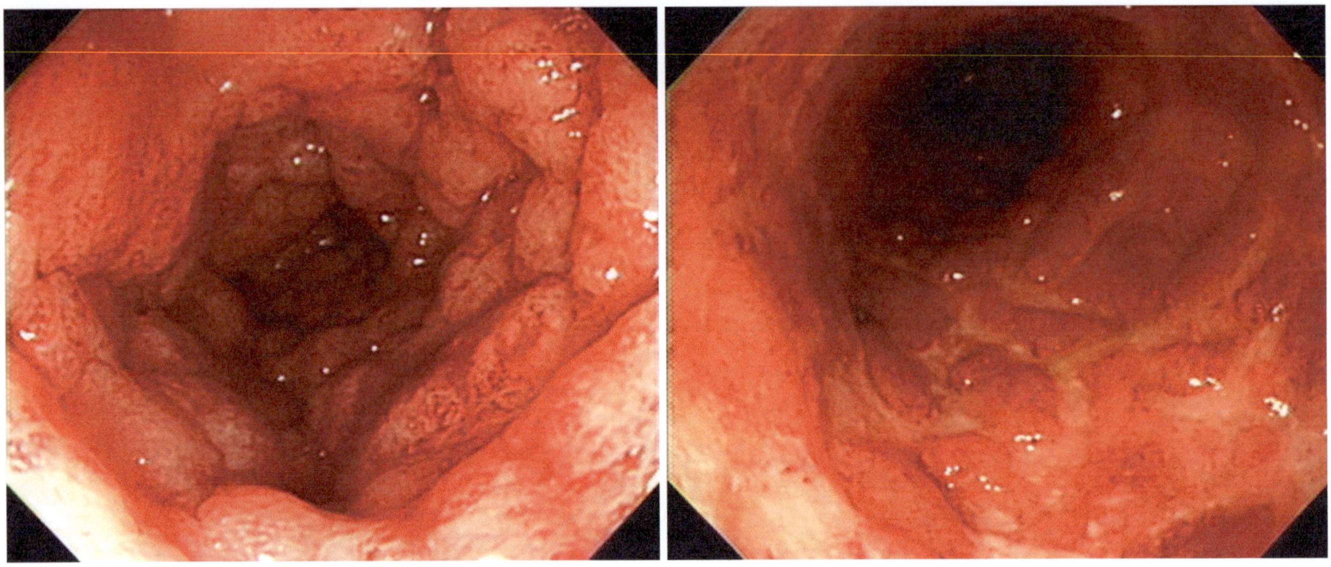

Fig. 1.21 Cobblestone appearance in ulcerative colitis

Table 1.6 Clinical features of infectious colitis and IBD

Clinical features	Infectious colitis	IBD
Onset	Acute	Usually insidious
Fever	Usual early (within 1st week)	Rare late (after 1st week)
Bowel frequency	>12/day at onset	<4/day at onset
Other symptoms	Severe abdominal pain, vomiting	Acute deterioration, previous mild symptoms

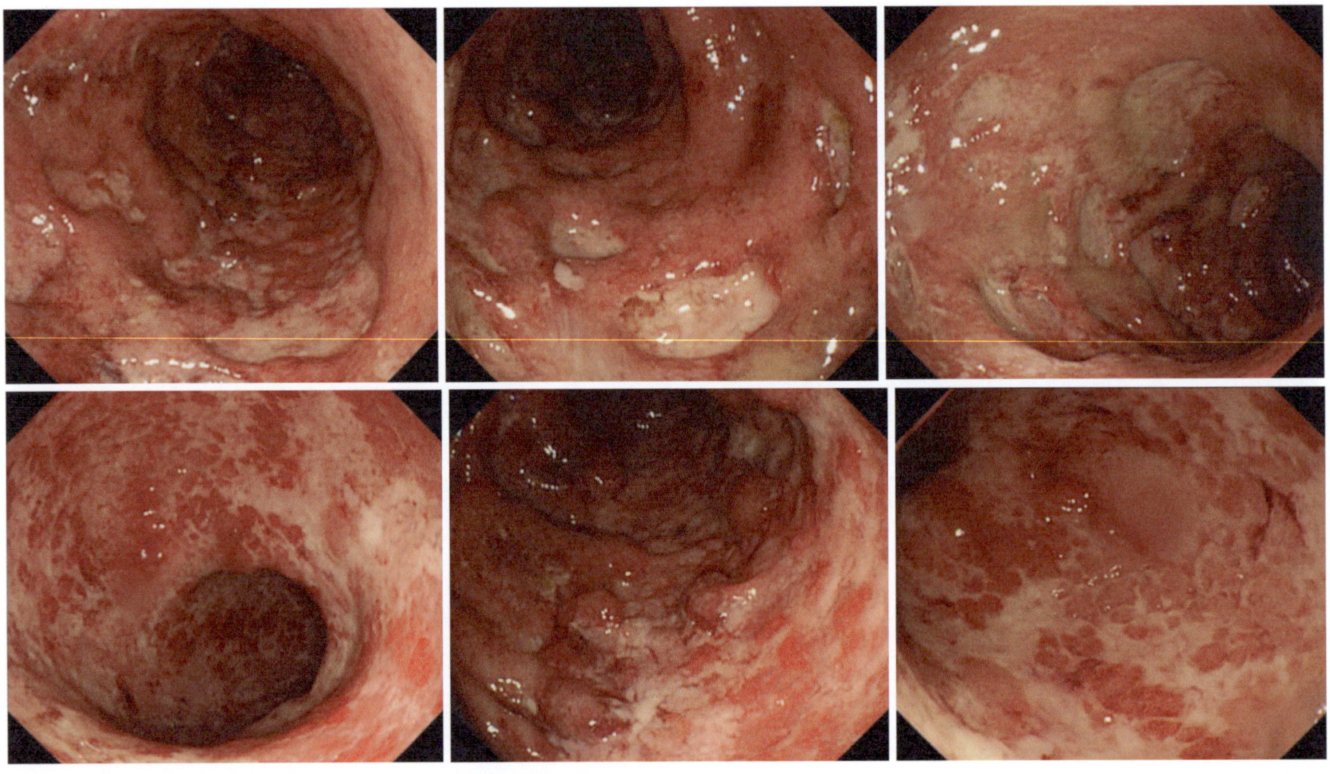

Fig. 1.22 CMV colitis in patients with ulcerative colitis. Variable sized and shaped ulcers are observed accompanying inflammation due to ulcerative colitis in the colon

Fig. 1.23 Pseudomembranous colitis accompanying ulcerative colitis. Multiple yellowish pseudomembranes overlie the inflamed mucosa caused by ulcerative colitis

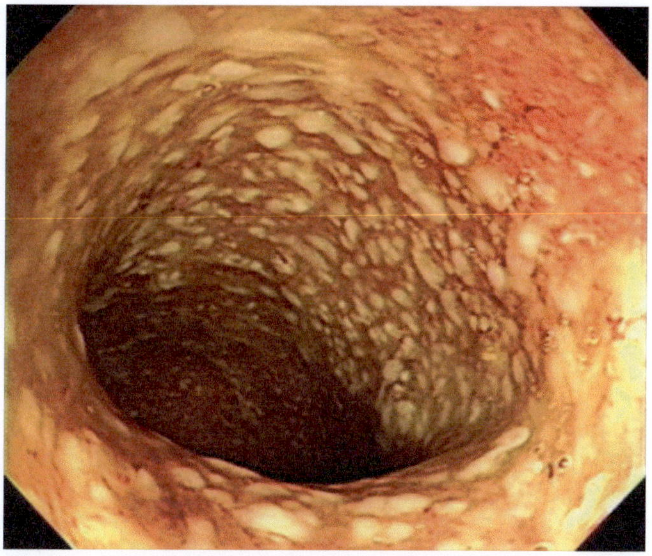

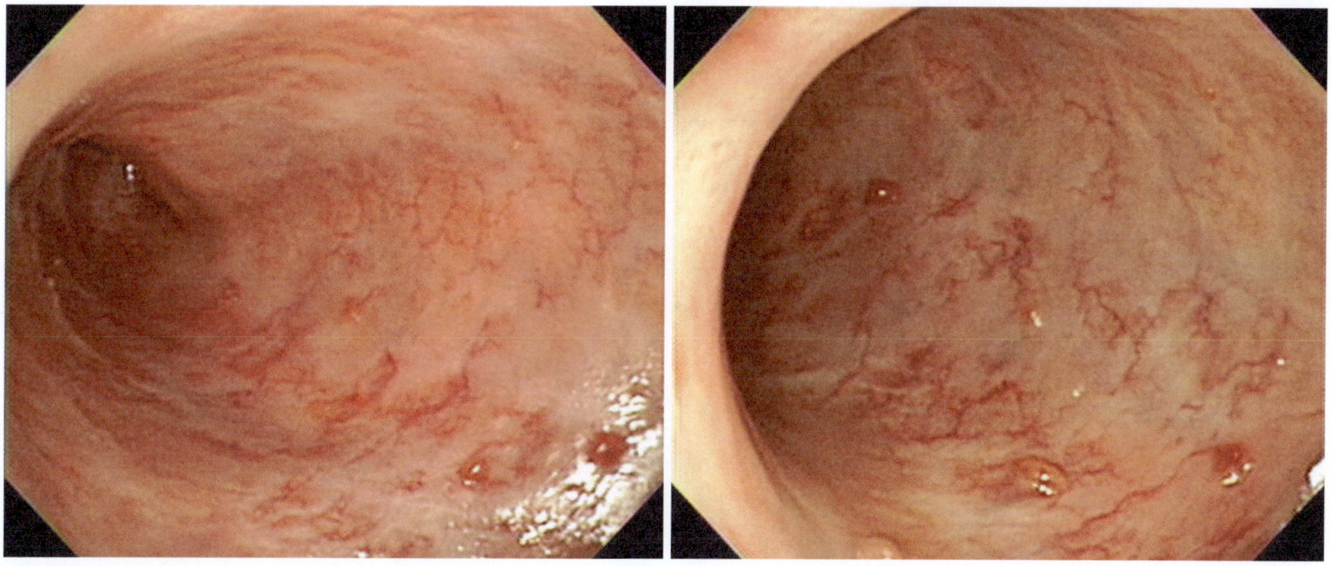

Fig. 1.24 Quiescent ulcerative colitis with distortion of vascular markings and whitish scar changes

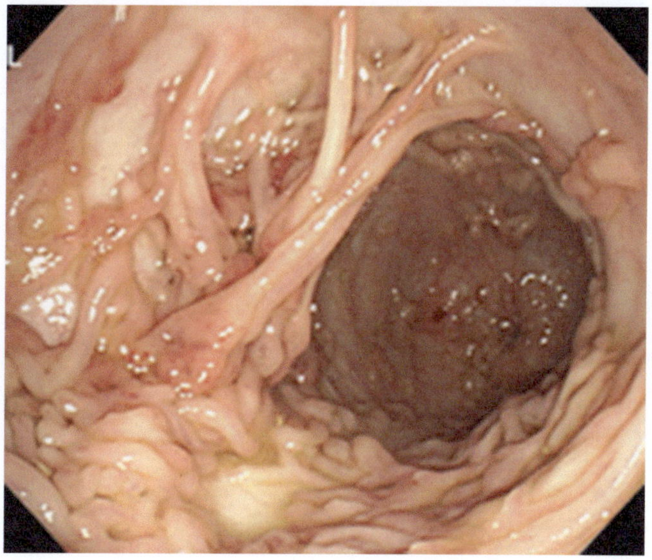

Fig. 1.25 Pseudodiverticula in quiescent ulcerative colitis

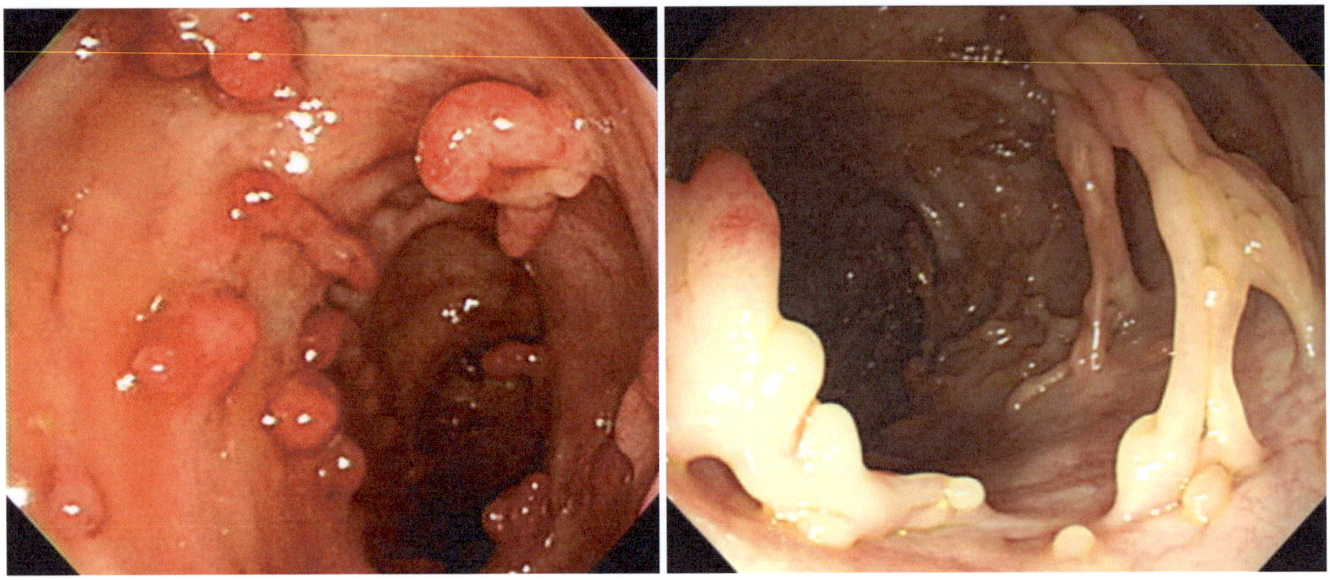

Fig. 1.26 Inflammatory polyps in quiescent ulcerative colitis. Some of them form mucosal bridges

Fig. 1.27 Hyperplastic polyp in a patient with ulcerative colitis

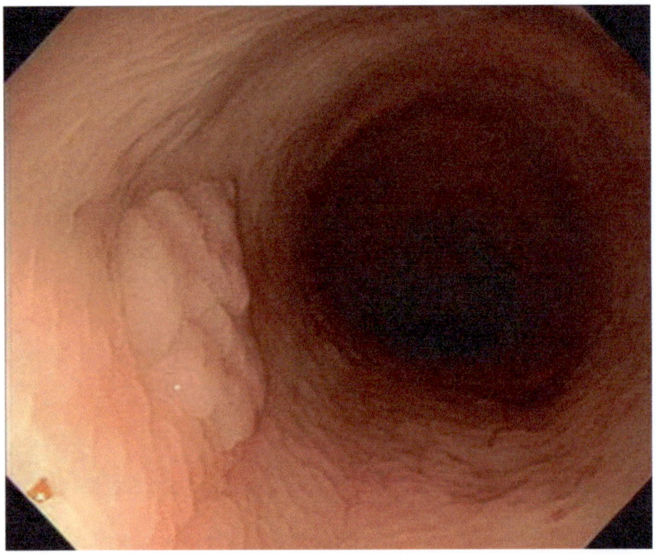

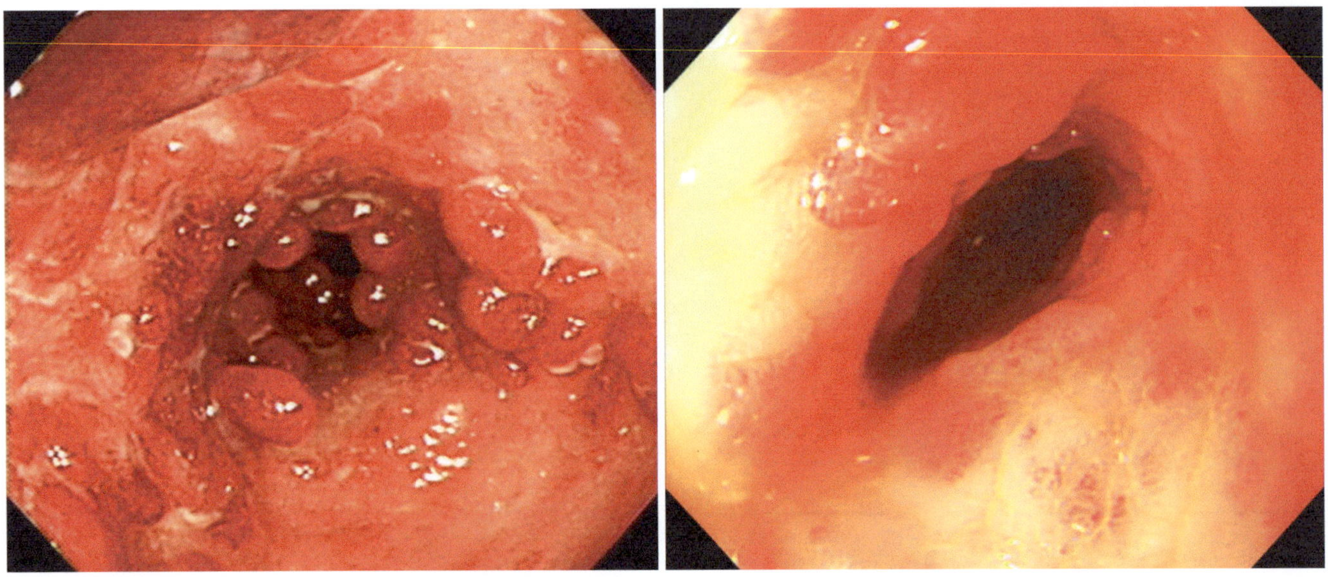

Fig. 1.28 Stricture in long-standing ulcerative colitis

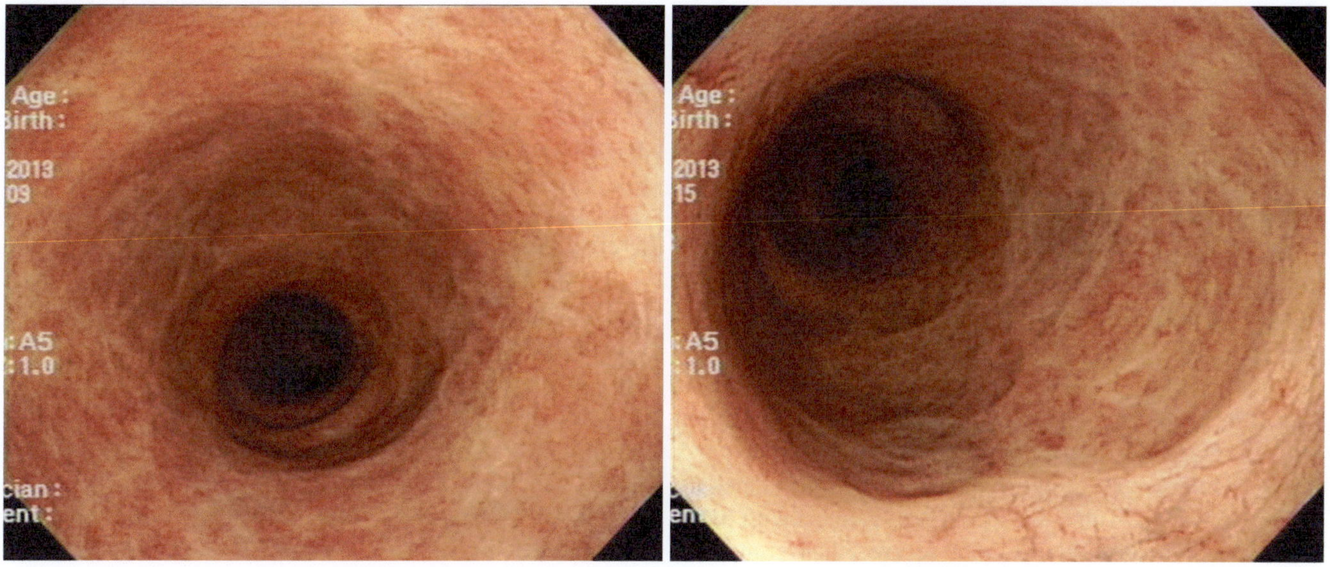

Fig. 1.29 Loss of haustral markings with lead pipe appearance in long-standing quiescent ulcerative colitis

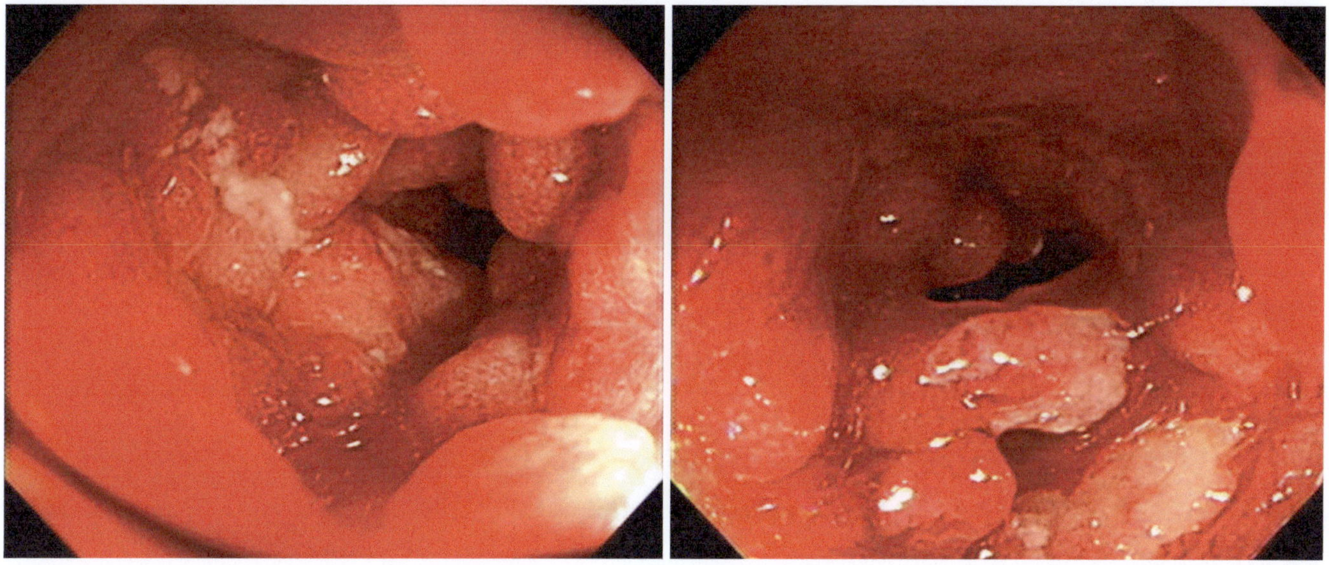

Fig. 1.30 Stricture with active inflammation in long-standing ulcerative colitis

1.1.3.4 Differential Diagnostic Considerations

Despite the importance of precise diagnosis of IBD in order to make proper therapy and follow-up procedures, difficulties in diagnosis arise usually when inflammation is confined to the colon. Indeterminate colitis is a disease with clear evidence of IBD, but with insufficient evidence to allow a specific diagnosis of either Crohn's disease or UC. Commonly accepted catalogue of well-defined criteria or a point score for classification of UC does not currently exist. Approximately 4–5 % of cases in IBD cannot be characterized definitively as either Crohn's disease or UC; these patients are regarded to have indeterminate colitis (Fig. 1.31) [36]. It is usually considered as a temporary or tentative diagnosis. In this regard, follow-up endoscopy and multiple colorectal biopsies should be performed to make a precise diagnosis. The clinical course of patients with indeterminate colitis is usually more severe when compared with UC. Endoscopic diagnostic difficulty comes along with overlapping of clinical and pathologic features of UC and Crohn's disease.

Challenging and underestimated diagnostic problems are diagnosis of indeterminate colitis and differentiation of IBD from other intestinal disorders (Table 1.7) [14]. In this context, radiology, serologic testing (ASCA, anti-Saccharomyces *cerevisiae* and ANCA, antineutrophil cytoplasmic antibody), and upper endoscopy combined with random biopsies for evaluating granuloma are recommended. Novel diagnostic tools as well as conventional endoscopy are needed to positively identify this group [1]. Although endoscopic ultrasonography had been initially recognized to be effective in differentiating between CD and UC, it is now considered to have a limited function in this setting. Instead, other radiologic evaluations such as CT enterography or MR enterography are more commonly used to evaluate small bowel involvement [37].

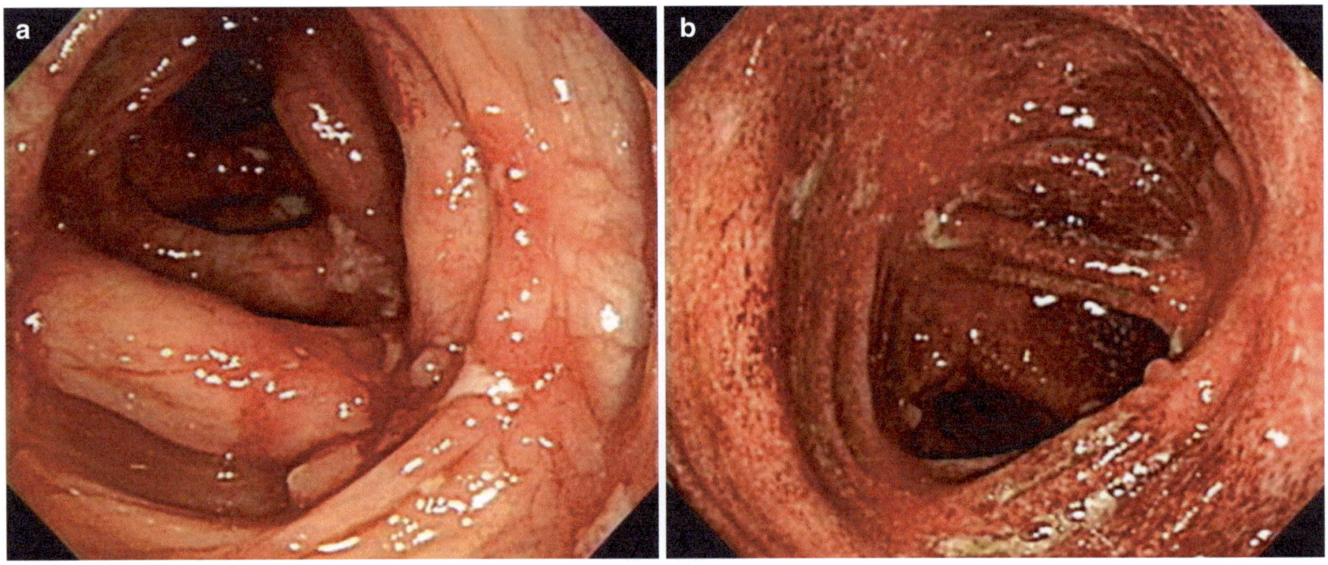

Fig. 1.31 Indeterminate colitis. On the initial colonoscopy, a longitudinal ulcer was observed (**a**), but 1 year later, endoscopic features were of ulcerative colitis (**b**)

Table 1.7 Differential diagnosis of ulcerative colitis and Crohn's disease

	Ulcerative colitis	Crohn's disease
Symmetricity	Symmetric	Asymmetric
Continuity	Continuous inflammation extends proximally from the rectum	Skip lesions with intervening normal mucosa
Involvement	Colon only	Panintestinal
Depth of involvement	Mucosal inflammation	Transmural inflammation
Pathology	No granulomas	Noncaseating granulomas
Serologic test	Perinuclear ANCA (pANCA) positive	ASCA positive
Clinical presentations	Bleeding (common)	Bleeding (uncommon)
	Fistulae (rare)	Fistulae (common)
	Weight loss (uncommon)	Weight loss (common)
	Perianal disease (rare)	Perianal disease (common)

1.1.4 Histologic Features

The inflammation may be confined to the mucosa or spread into the superficial part of the submucosa. Histologically, UC is characterized by diffuse inflammatory cell infiltration of the mucosa with basal plasmacytosis, crypt architectural change, and a reduction of mucus-secreting goblet cells.

The pathologic finding in UC typically involves widespread cryptitis (Fig. 1.32), crypt distortion (Fig. 1.33), crypt abscess (Fig. 1.34), and crypt atrophy; heavy, diffuse lamina propria cell infiltration (Fig. 1.35); and basal plasmacytosis. Crypt distortion is used to differentiate between UC and other acute colitides and is considered the strongest indicator of chronicity of the inflammation. The inflammatory infiltrate, composed of lymphocytes, plasma cells, and neutrophils, leads to cryptitis and crypt abscesses, which is defined as the presence of neutrophils within crypt epithelium and the presence of neutrophils within crypt lumen. Crypt abscesses are more commonly observed in patients with UC (41 %) than those with CD (19 %) [38, 39].

Fig. 1.32 Widespread cryptitis

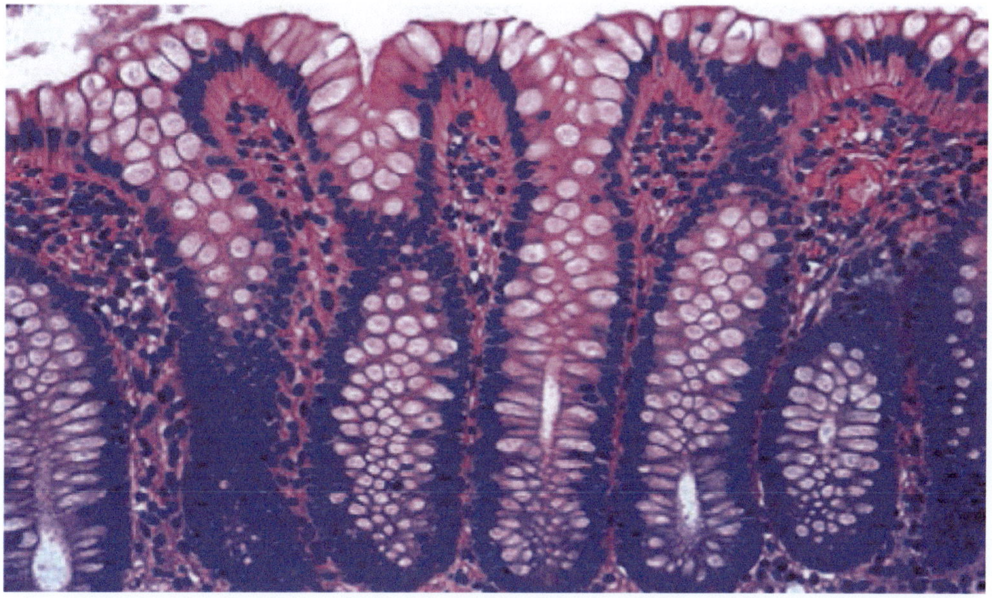

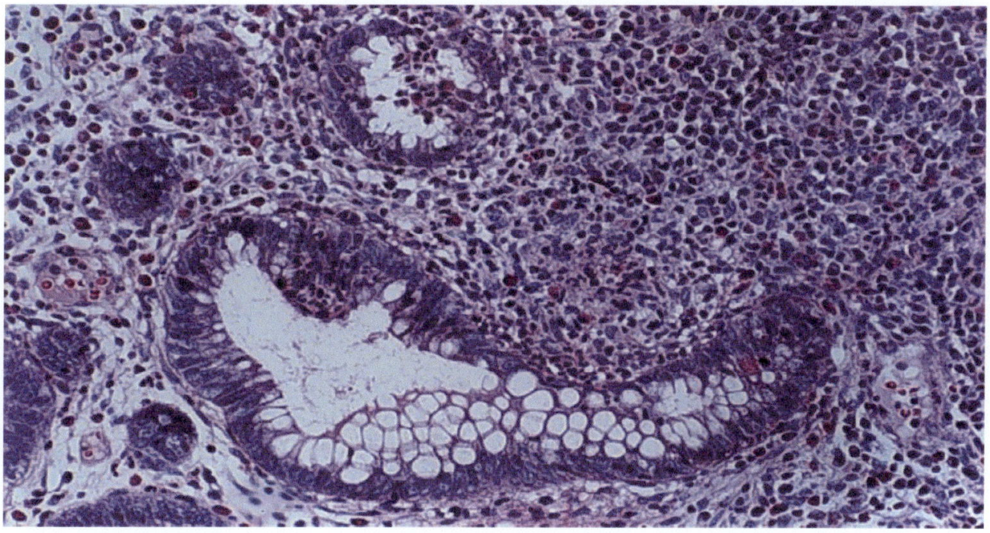

Fig. 1.33 Crypt distortion

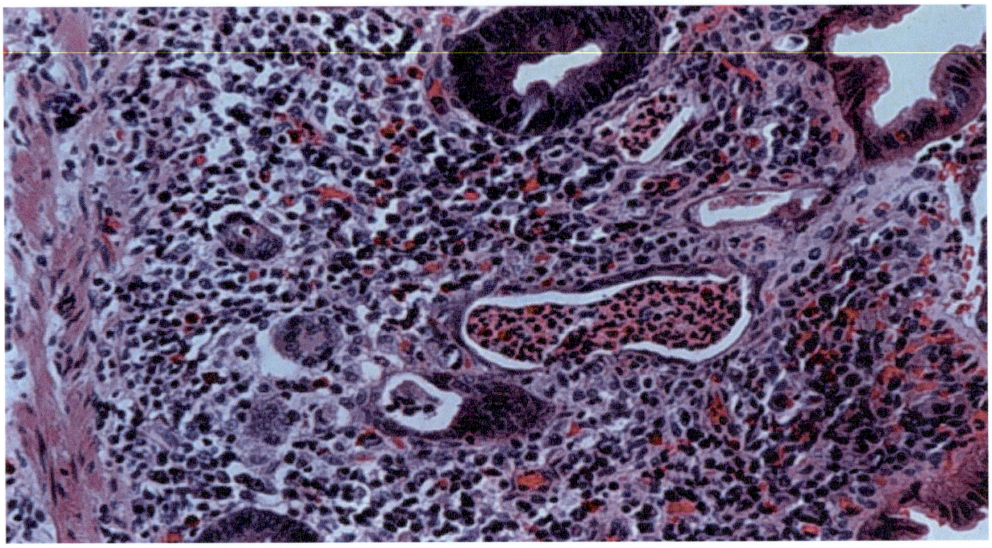

Fig. 1.34 Crypt abscess

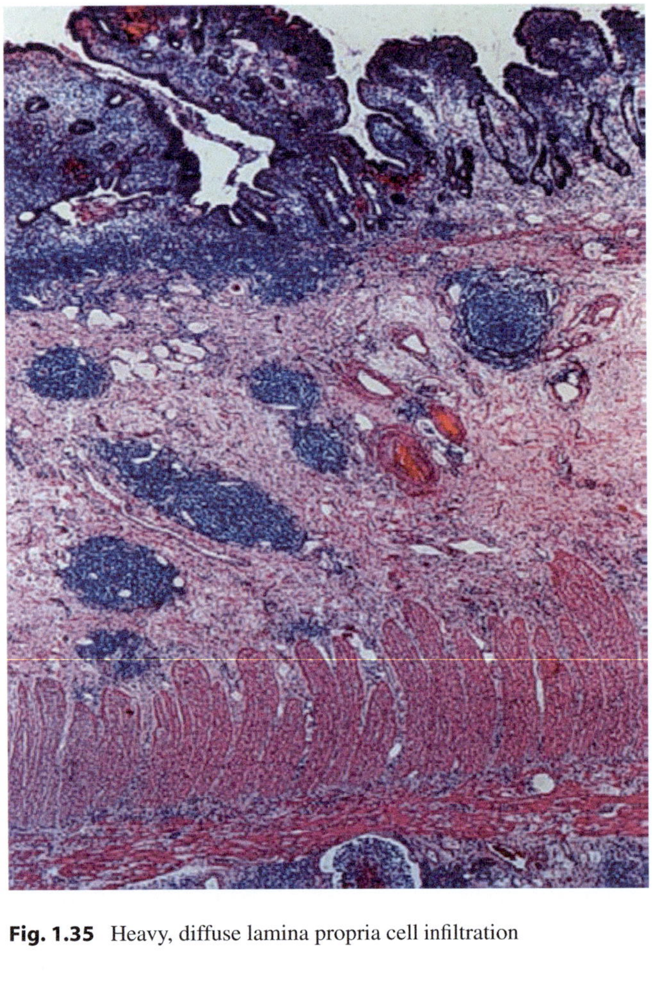

Fig. 1.35 Heavy, diffuse lamina propria cell infiltration

1.1.5 Pouchitis

The most common long-term complication after proctocolectomy with ileal pouch-anal anastomosis (IPAA) for UC is pouchitis. Patients who develop pouchitis frequently suffer from symptoms such as increased stool frequency, fecal urgency, abdominal cramping, and pelvic discomfort, although these symptoms may be caused by inflammation of the rectal cuff. Pouchitis resembles recurrence of UC, irritable bowel syndrome, jejunoileal bacterial overgrowth, Crohn's disease, and pouch-outlet obstruction [40]. The etiology of pouchitis is currently unknown [41, 42].

To obtain the accuracy of a pouchitis diagnosis, clinical symptoms and endoscopic findings should be associated. Normal pouch shows ringlike folds, staple lines, mild redness near an afferent loop, and a normal vascular pattern (Fig. 1.36). Various endoscopic findings of pouchitis are as follows: edema, erosion, ulcer, friability, purulent mucous, spotty erythema, and granularity (Fig. 1.37). In many cases with distinct edema, ringlike folds are not clear, and erosions can be observed frequently against a background of remarkable edema and redness. Ulcerations in pouchitis have various features. A large ulcer or multiple ulcers and linear or irregular shapes are also observed. Friable mucosa often bleeds easily with endoscope insertion. Otherwise, the surface is oozing with blood against a background of red mucosa. Purulent mucus adhering to the mucosal surface is presented against a background of edematous and granular mucosa. Staple lines are usually found running from the anus side to the oral side.

According to the severity of inflammation, the endoscopic appearance can be categorized as follows. Mild inflammation of pouch shows redness, slight edema, and aphthoid lesions without erosion or ulcerations. Moderate pouchitis presents disappearance of mucosal vascular pattern with edema, solitary or regional ulcerations. Aphthoid lesions are frequent, and an irregular pattern of erosion can be found. Diffuse, spotty redness and linear erosion and exudation of purulent yellow mucus are also observed. Compared to moderate inflammation, extensive or multiple ulcers can be observed in severe pouchitis. Diffuse erythema, spontaneous bleeding, and erosions are the other endoscopic findings of severe pouchitis. Clean-bordered ulcers accompanied by upheaval at the circumference are present with various shapes in extremely severe inflammation.

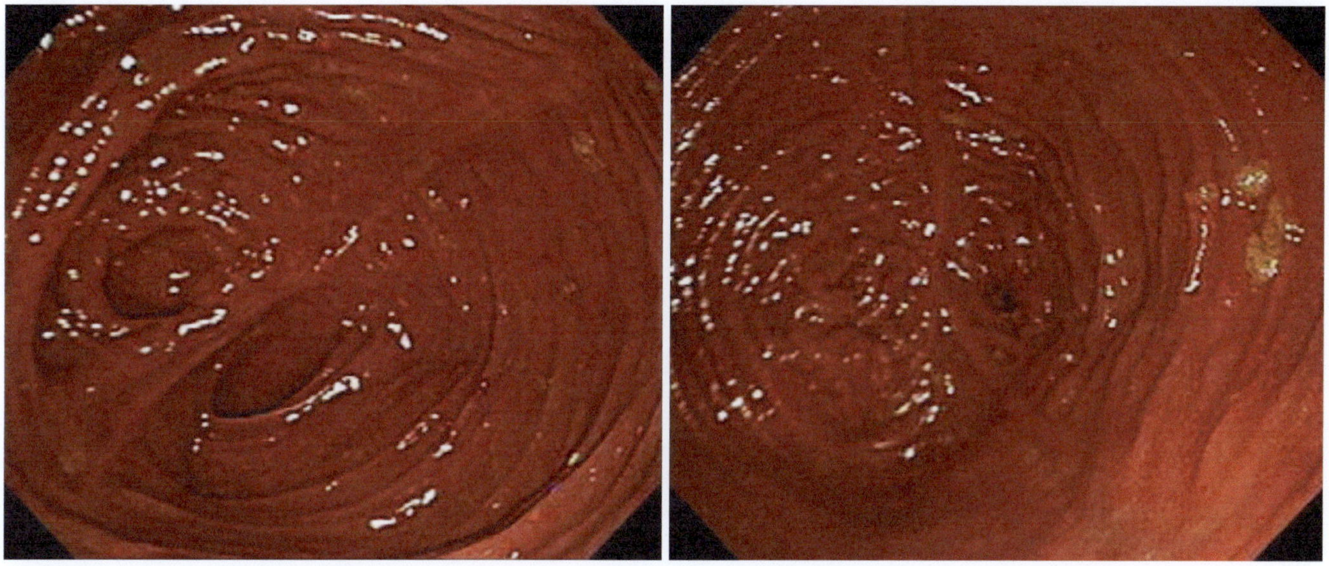

Fig. 1.36 Endoscopic findings of normal ileoanal pouch after ileal pouch-anal anastomosis

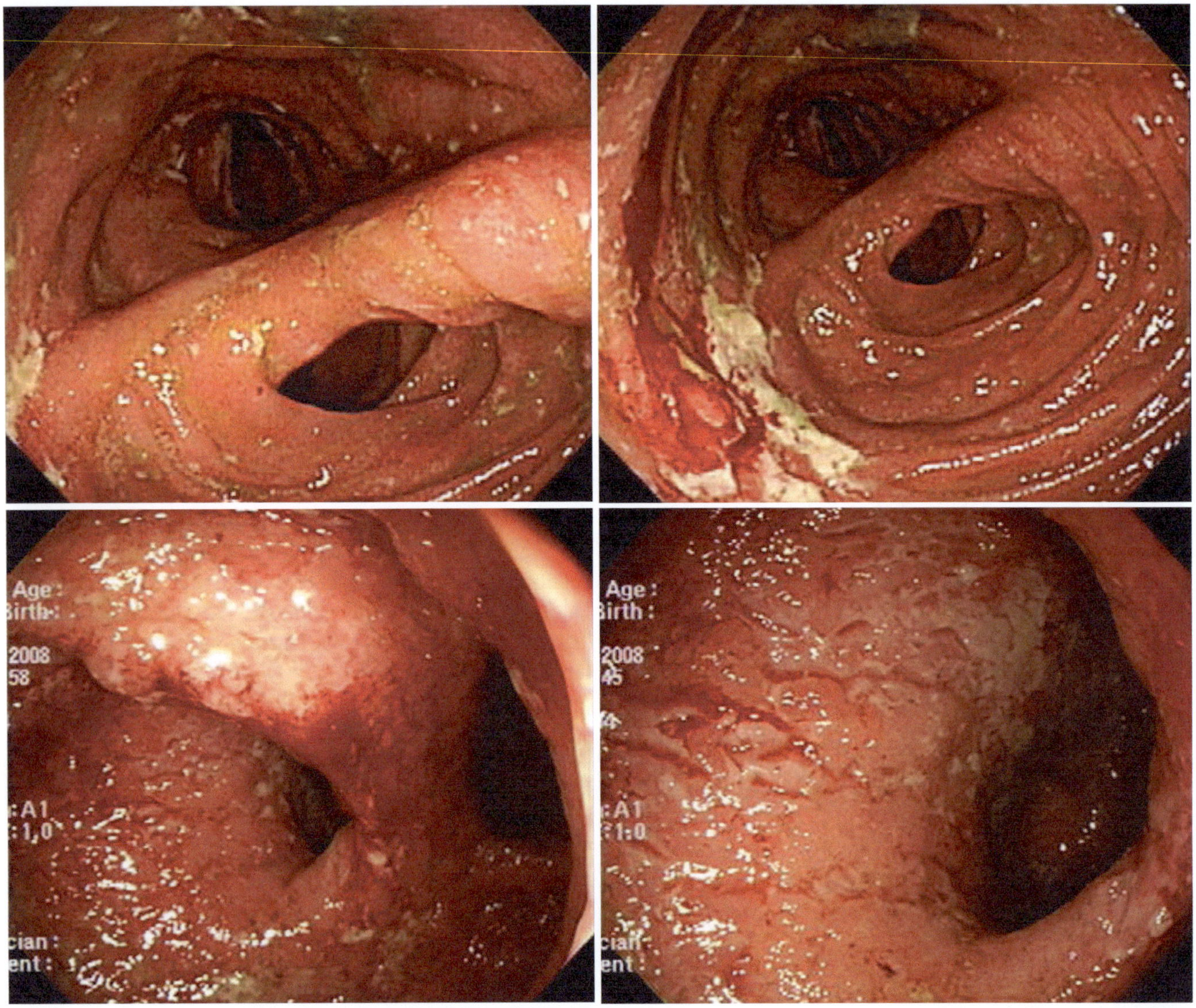

Fig. 1.37 Pouchitis after ileal pouch-anal anastomosis

1.1.6 Extraintestinal Manifestations

Approximately one third of patients with UC have extraintestinal manifestations, which may be present even when the disease is inactive [43] Arthritis, aphthous stomatitis, primary sclerosing cholangitis, uveitis, erythema nodosum, ankylosing spondylitis, pyoderma gangrenosum, and/or psoriasis are the generally observed extraintestinal manifestations.

Primary sclerosing cholangitis (PSC) (Fig. 1.38) is one of the most important extraintestinal manifestations in UC. PSC is a potentially severe associated condition resulting in cholestatic jaundice and liver failure. Therefore, it requires transplantation occasionally. Approximately 5 % of patients with UC have cholestatic liver disease, and 40 % of those have PSC [44, 45]. Also, Patients with UC and PSC have higher incidence of colorectal neoplastic disease compared to patients with UC only [46].

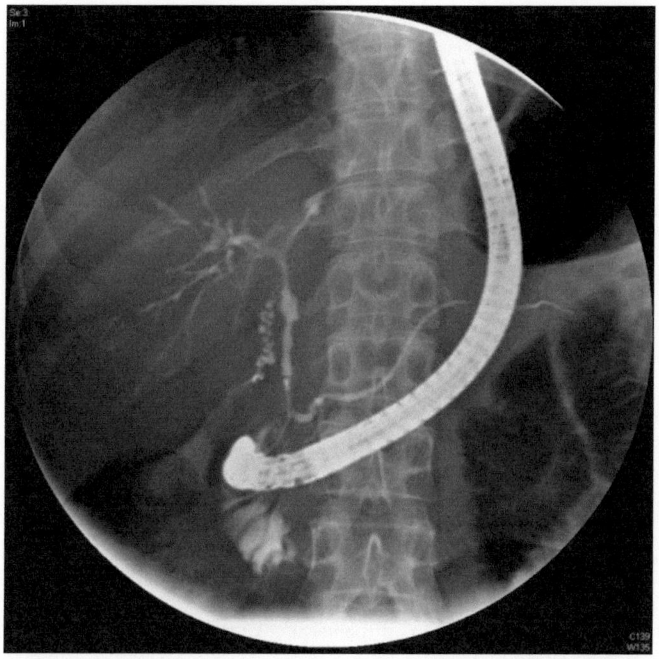

Fig. 1.38 ERCP finding of primary sclerosing cholangitis in a patient with UC. The whole intra- and extrahepatic bile ducts are irregularly narrowed

1.1.7 Gastroduodenal Lesions in Ulcerative Colitis

These lesions of the upper gastrointestinal tract associated with UC are very rare, and the characteristic clinical features of UC patients and the mechanisms still remain unresolved. The gastroduodenal lesions of UC patients extended between the stomach and the duodenum or involved the duodenum alone. Continuous granular mucosa and erosions are observed as in the case of colonic lesions. In addition, mucosal friability and bleeding, ulcers, and thickening of the Kerckring's folds are observed among patients with ulcerative colitis complicated by gastroduodenal lesions [47].

References

1. Cheon JH, Kim WH. Recent advances of endoscopy in inflammatory bowel diseases. Gut Liver. 2007;1(2):118–25. doi:10.5009/gnl.2007.1.2.118.
2. Pera A, Bellando P, Caldera D, Ponti V, Astegiano M, Barletti C, David E, Arrigoni A, Rocca G, Verme G. Colonoscopy in inflammatory bowel disease. Diagnostic accuracy and proposal of an endoscopic score. Gastroenterology. 1987;92(1):181–5.
3. Rutgeerts P, Feagan BG, Lichtenstein GR, Mayer LF, Schreiber S, Colombel JF, Rachmilewitz D, Wolf DC, Olson A, Bao W, Hanauer SB. Comparison of scheduled and episodic treatment strategies of infliximab in Crohn's disease. Gastroenterology. 2004;126(2):402–13.
4. Colombel JF, Rutgeerts P, Reinisch W, Esser D, Wang Y, Lang Y, Marano CW, Strauss R, Oddens BJ, Feagan BG, Hanauer SB, Lichtenstein GR, Present D, Sands BE, Sandborn WJ. Early mucosal healing with infliximab is associated with improved long-term clinical outcomes in ulcerative colitis. Gastroenterology. 2011;141(4):1194–201. doi:10.1053/j.gastro.2011.06.054.
5. Neurath MF, Travis SP. Mucosal healing in inflammatory bowel diseases: a systematic review. Gut. 2012;61(11):1619–35. doi:10.1136/gutjnl-2012-302830.
6. Leighton JA, Shen B, Baron TH, Adler DG, Davila R, Egan JV, Faigel DO, Gan SI, Hirota WK, Lichtenstein D, Qureshi WA, Rajan E, Zuckerman MJ, VanGuilder T, Fanelli RD. ASGE guideline: endoscopy in the diagnosis and treatment of inflammatory bowel disease. Gastrointest Endosc. 2006;63(4):558–65. doi:10.1016/j.gie.2006.02.005.
7. Kiesslich R, Neurath MF. Chromoendoscopy and other novel imaging techniques. Gastroenterol Clin North Am. 2006;35(3):605–19. doi:10.1016/j.gtc.2006.07.004.
8. Ochsenkuhn T, Tillack C, Stepp H, Diebold J, Ott SJ, Baumgartner R, Brand S, Goke B, Sackmann M. Low frequency of colorectal dysplasia in patients with long-standing inflammatory bowel disease colitis: detection by fluorescence endoscopy. Endoscopy. 2006;38(5):477–82. doi:10.1055/s-2006-925165.
9. Kuznetsov K, Lambert R, Rey JF. Narrow-band imaging: potential and limitations. Endoscopy. 2006;38(1):76–81. doi:10.1055/s-2005-921114.
10. Brand S, Poneros JM, Bouma BE, Tearney GJ, Compton CC, Nishioka NS. Optical coherence tomography in the gastrointestinal tract. Endoscopy. 2000;32(10):796–803. doi:10.1055/s-2000-7714.
11. Kiesslich R, Burg J, Vieth M, Gnaendiger J, Enders M, Delaney P, Polglase A, McLaren W, Janell D, Thomas S, Nafe B, Galle PR, Neurath MF. Confocal laser endoscopy for diagnosing intraepithelial neoplasias and colorectal cancer in vivo. Gastroenterology. 2004;127(3):706–13.
12. Truelove SC, Witts LJ. Cortisone in ulcerative colitis; final report on a therapeutic trial. Br Med J. 1955;2(4947):1041–8.
13. Kornbluth A, Sachar DB. Ulcerative colitis practice guidelines in adults (update): American College of Gastroenterology, Practice Parameters Committee. Am J Gastroenterol. 2004;99(7):1371–85. doi:10.1111/j.1572-0241.2004.40036.x.
14. Kornbluth A, Sachar DB. Ulcerative colitis practice guidelines in adults: American College Of Gastroenterology, Practice Parameters Committee. Am J Gastroenterol. 2010;105(3):501–23; quiz 524. doi:10.1038/ajg.2009.727.
15. Seo M, Okada M, Yao T, Okabe N, Maeda K, Oh K. Evaluation of disease activity in patients with moderately active ulcerative colitis: comparisons between a new activity index and Truelove and Witts' classification. Am J Gastroenterol. 1995;90(10):1759–63.
16. Adams SM, Bornemann PH. Ulcerative colitis. Am Fam Physician. 2013;87(10):699–705.
17. Osada T, Ohkusa T, Yokoyama T, Shibuya T, Sakamoto N, Beppu K, Nagahara A, Otaka M, Ogihara T, Watanabe S. Comparison of several activity indices for the evaluation of endoscopic activity in UC: inter- and intraobserver consistency. Inflamm Bowel Dis. 2010;16(2):192–7. doi:10.1002/ibd.21000.
18. Lewis JD, Chuai S, Nessel L, Lichtenstein GR, Aberra FN, Ellenberg JH. Use of the noninvasive components of the Mayo score to assess clinical response in ulcerative colitis. Inflamm Bowel Dis. 2008;14(12):1660–6. doi:10.1002/ibd.20520.
19. Travis SP, Schnell D, Krzeski P, Abreu MT, Altman DG, Colombel JF, Feagan BG, Hanauer SB, Lemann M, Lichtenstein GR, Marteau PR, Reinisch W, Sands BE, Yacyshyn BR, Bernhardt CA, Mary JY, Sandborn WJ. Developing an instrument to assess the endoscopic severity of ulcerative colitis: the Ulcerative Colitis Endoscopic Index of Severity (UCEIS). Gut. 2012;61(4):535–42. doi:10.1136/gutjnl-2011-300486.
20. Satsangi J, Silverberg MS, Vermeire S, Colombel JF. The Montreal classification of inflammatory bowel disease: controversies, consensus, and implications. Gut. 2006;55(6):749–53. doi:10.1136/gut.2005.082909.
21. Katz J. The course of inflammatory bowel disease. Med Clin North Am. 1994;78(6):1275–80.
22. Navaneethan U, Jegadeesan R, Gutierrez NG, Venkatesh PG, Arrossi AV, Bennett AE, Rai T, Remzi FH, Shen B, Kiran RP. Backwash ileitis and the risk of colon neoplasia in ulcerative colitis patients undergoing restorative proctocolectomy. Dig Dis Sci. 2013;58(7):2019–27. doi:10.1007/s10620-013-2571-7.
23. Pillet S, Pozzetto B, Jarlot C, Paul S, Roblin X. Management of cytomegalovirus infection in inflammatory bowel diseases. Dig Liver Dis. 2012;44(7):541–8. doi:10.1016/j.dld.2012.03.018.
24. Suzuki H, Kato J, Kuriyama M, Hiraoka S, Kuwaki K, Yamamoto K. Specific endoscopic features of ulcerative colitis complicated by cytomegalovirus infection. World J Gastroenterol. 2010;16(10):1245–51.
25. Kojima T, Watanabe T, Hata K, Shinozaki M, Yokoyama T, Nagawa H. Cytomegalovirus infection in ulcerative colitis. Scand J Gastroenterol. 2006;41(6):706–11. doi:10.1080/00365520500408584.
26. Agaimy A, Mudter J, Markl B, Chetty R. Cytomegalovirus infection presenting as isolated inflammatory polyps of the gastrointestinal tract. Pathology. 2011;43(5):440–6. doi:10.1097/PAT.0b013e3283485e51.
27. Kambham N, Vij R, Cartwright CA, Longacre T. Cytomegalovirus infection in steroid-refractory ulcerative colitis: a case-control study. Am J Surg Pathol. 2004;28(3):365–73.
28. Saidel-Odes L, Borer A, Odes S. *Clostridium difficile* infection in patients with inflammatory bowel disease. Ann Gastroenterol. 2011;24(4):263–70.
29. Navaneethan U, Venkatesh PG, Shen B. Clostridium difficile infection and inflammatory bowel disease: understanding the evolving relationship. World J Gastroenterol. 2010;16(39):4892–904.
30. Ben-Horin S, Margalit M, Bossuyt P, Maul J, Shapira Y, Bojic D, Chermesh I, Al-Rifai A, Schoepfer A, Bosani M, Allez M, Lakatos PL, Bossa F, Eser A, Stefanelli T, Carbonnel F, Katsanos K, Checchin D, de Miera IS, Reinisch W, Chowers Y, Moran GW. Prevalence and clinical impact of endoscopic pseudomembranes in patients with inflammatory bowel disease and Clostridium difficile infection. J Crohns Colitis. 2010;4(2):194–8. doi:10.1016/j.crohns.2009.11.001.
31. Berg AM, Kelly CP, Farraye FA. Clostridium difficile infection in the inflammatory bowel disease patient. Inflamm Bowel Dis. 2013;19(1):194–204. doi:10.1002/ibd.22964.
32. Gumaste V, Sachar DB, Greenstein AJ. Benign and malignant colorectal strictures in ulcerative colitis. Gut. 1992;33(7):938–41.
33. Rutter MD, Saunders BP, Wilkinson KH, Rumbles S, Schofield G, Kamm MA, Williams CB, Price AB, Talbot IC, Forbes A. Cancer surveillance in longstanding ulcerative colitis: endoscopic appearances help predict cancer risk. Gut. 2004;53(12):1813–6. doi:10.1136/gut.2003.038505.

34. Jaramillo E, Watanabe M, Befrits R, Ponce de Leon E, Rubio C, Slezak P. Small, flat colorectal neoplasias in long-standing ulcerative colitis detected by high-resolution electronic video endoscopy. Gastrointest Endosc. 1996;44(1):15–22.
35. Thorlacius H, Toth E. Role of chromoendoscopy in colon cancer surveillance in inflammatory bowel disease. Inflamm Bowel Dis. 2007;13(7):911–7. doi:10.1002/ibd.20118.
36. Herrinton LJ, Liu L, Lewis JD, Griffin PM, Allison J. Incidence and prevalence of inflammatory bowel disease in a Northern California managed care organization, 1996–2002. Am J Gastroenterol. 2008;103(8):1998–2006. doi:10.1111/j.1572-0241.2008.01960.x.
37. Patel NS, Pola S, Muralimohan R, Zou GY, Santillan C, Patel D, Levesque BG, Sandborn WJ. Outcomes of computed tomography and magnetic resonance enterography in clinical practice of inflammatory bowel disease. Dig Dis Sci. 2014;59(4):838–49. doi:10.1007/s10620-013-2964-7.
38. Magro F, Langner C, Driessen A, Ensari A, Geboes K, Mantzaris GJ, Villanacci V, Becheanu G, Borralho Nunes P, Cathomas G, Fries W, Jouret-Mourin A, Mescoli C, de Petris G, Rubio CA, Shepherd NA, Vieth M, Eliakim R. European consensus on the histopathology of inflammatory bowel disease. J Crohns Colitis. 2013;7(10):827–51. doi:10.1016/j.crohns.2013.06.001.
39. Jenkins D, Balsitis M, Gallivan S, Dixon MF, Gilmour HM, Shepherd NA, Theodossi A, Williams GT. Guidelines for the initial biopsy diagnosis of suspected chronic idiopathic inflammatory bowel disease. The British Society of Gastroenterology Initiative. J Clin Pathol. 1997;50(2):93–105.
40. Shen B, Fazio VW, Remzi FH, Lashner BA. Clinical approach to diseases of ileal pouch-anal anastomosis. Am J Gastroenterol. 2005;100(12):2796–807. doi:10.1111/j.1572-0241.2005.00278.x.
41. Madden MV, Farthing MJ, Nicholls RJ. Inflammation in ileal reservoirs: 'pouchitis'. Gut. 1990;31(3):247–9.
42. Jarvinen HJ, Makitie A, Sivula A. Long-term results of continent ileostomy. Int J Colorectal Dis. 1986;1(1):40–3.
43. Vavricka SR, Brun L, Ballabeni P, Pittet V, Prinz Vavricka BM, Zeitz J, Rogler G, Schoepfer AM. Frequency and risk factors for extraintestinal manifestations in the Swiss inflammatory bowel disease cohort. Am J Gastroenterol. 2011;106(1):110–9. doi:10.1038/ajg.2010.343.
44. Marchesa P, Lashner BA, Lavery IC, Milsom J, Hull TL, Strong SA, Church JM, Navarro G, Fazio VW. The risk of cancer and dysplasia among ulcerative colitis patients with primary sclerosing cholangitis. Am J Gastroenterol. 1997;92(8):1285–8.
45. Cox KL, Cox KM. Oral vancomycin: treatment of primary sclerosing cholangitis in children with inflammatory bowel disease. J Pediatr Gastroenterol Nutr. 1998;27(5):580–3.
46. Moayyeri A, Daryani NE, Bahrami H, Haghpanah B, Nayyer-Habibi A, Sadatsafavi M. Clinical course of ulcerative colitis in patients with and without primary sclerosing cholangitis. J Gastroenterol Hepatol. 2005;20(3):366–70.
47. Hisabe T, Matsui T, Miyaoka M, Ninomiya K, Ishihara H, Nagahama T, Takaki Y, Hirai F, Ikeda K, Iwashita A, Higashi D, Futami K. Diagnosis and clinical course of ulcerative gastroduodenal lesion associated with ulcerative colitis: possible relationship with pouchitis. Dig Endosc. 2010;22(4):268–74. doi:10.1111/j.1443-1661.2010.01006.x.

Ileocolonoscopy in Crohn's Disease

2

Duk Hwan Kim, Heyson Chi-hey Chan,
Phillip Fai Ching Lung, Siew Chien Ng,
and Jae Hee Cheon

2.1 Background

Crohn's disease (CD) is a chronic inflammatory disease of unknown etiology with a variety of symptoms including abdominal pain, diarrhea, rectal bleeding, weight loss, and anemia. CD was firstly described as regional ileitis with chronic granulomatous inflammation of the terminal ileum in 1932 [3]. However, it is widely known to involve any part of the gastrointestinal tract from mouth to anus. The most common site of gastrointestinal involvement in CD is the ileocecal area, in which around 30 % of CD patients having disease located in this area [5]. Isolated colonic disease occurs in another 30 % of patients and 10 % may have upper gastrointestinal involvement, while around one-third of patients may have perianal disease during their course of disease.

Because there is no single gold standard test and pathognomonic symptoms or signs that can be used to definitively diagnose or determine the severity of CD, ileocolonoscopy is of pivotal importance in CD patients for the diagnosis, assessment of disease activity and extent, and cancer surveillance. It provides direct visual assessment and enables performing biopsy of the colonic and terminal ileal mucosa. Especially, biopsy of ileal mucosa can be achieved in at least 85 % of colonoscopies and increases the diagnostic yield of CD [7]. Moreover, ileocolonoscopy has been shown to be superior for the diagnosis of CD in the terminal ileum when compared with small bowel follow-through examination [12]. Therefore, achieving full colonoscopic evaluation including inspection of the terminal ileum has a critical value in assessing CD and has been accepted as the first-line procedure to establish the diagnosis of CD [24]. In the presence of severe and active, however, the value of full colonoscopy is limited by a higher risk of bowel perforation and flexible sigmoidoscopy or a radiologic imaging study may be safer in these circumstances. Ileocolonoscopy can be postponed until the clinical condition improves.

It is sometimes difficult to distinguish CD from other severe colitis because regenerative hyperplasia caused by heavy inflammation frequently conceals typical findings of CD. Therefore, accurate knowledge of endoscopic features with CD is mightily important for gastroenterologists to obtain optimal information about the disease.

D.H. Kim
Digestive Disease Center, CHA Bundang Medical center,
CHA University College of Medicine,
Seongnam, South Korea

H.C.-h. Chan • S.C. Ng, PhD (✉)
Department of Medicine and Therapeutics,
Institute of Digestive Disease,
The Chinese University of Hong Kong,
Hong Kong, The People's Republic of China
e-mail: siewchienng@cuhk.edu.hk

P.F.C. Lung
Department of Imaging and Interventional Radiology,
The Chinese University of Hong Kong,
Hong Kong, The People's Republic of China

J.H. Cheon, MD, PhD (✉)
Department of Internal Medicine, Institute of Gastroenterology,
Yonsei University College of Medicine,
50 Yonsei-ro, Seodaemun–gu, Seoul 120-752, South Korea
e-mail: geniushee@yuhs.ac

W.H. Kim, J.H. Cheon (eds.), *Atlas of Inflammatory Bowel Diseases*,
DOI 10.1007/978-3-642-39423-2_2, © Springer-Verlag Berlin Heidelberg 2015

2.2 Clinical Manifestations of Crohn's Disease

The clinical manifestations of CD are more varied than those of ulcerative colitis. Signs and symptoms of CD can range from mild to severe and may develop gradually or abruptly. Similar with ulcerative colitis, symptoms including diarrhea, abdominal pain, weight loss, fever, and rectal bleeding clinically reflect the underlying inflammatory process. Perianal fissures, fistulae, abscess, abdominal mass or tenderness, cachexia, and pallor can be observed as signs of CD patients (Table 2.1). Because of the transmural nature of the inflammation, fistulae, abscess, and perianal lesion favor the diagnosis of CD. Extraintestinal symptoms can include cutaneous manifestations, ocular inflammations, peripheral arthritis, spondylarthritis, and primary sclerosing cholangitis, and it will be described specifically in the following chapter.

Onset of CD is generally insidious, but it can also be presented with a fulminate onset or toxic megacolon. Recurrent abdominal pain usually occurs in ileal or ileocolic diseases, while diarrhea and rectal bleeding are observed significantly more often in colonic CD. Fistula complicates ileocolic disease more often than isolated colon involvement [10]. Predominant involvement of the mouth and gastroduodenal, jejunal, or perianal area can also be presented in CD patients but occurs in relatively fewer patients. Perianal manifestations are common and may precede the onset of bowel symptoms, particularly in the East Asian countries. CD limited to the appendix may mimic appendicitis [8].

It is sometimes difficult to distinguish CD from ulcerative colitis, jejunoileitis complicated by multifocal stenoses, bacterial overgrowth syndrome, intestinal tuberculosis, other chronic infectious enterocolitis, intestinal Behcet's disease, or protein-losing enteropathy.

Because CD is a multifactorial polygenic disease with various aspect of phenotype, accurate classification of the disease might have potential advantages with respect to choosing medications, predicting prognosis, and deciding surgery. Especially, behavior of disease is strongly associated with indication for surgery; therefore, some investigators tried to clarify dominating features of CD. However, behavioral features such as penetrating type and fibrostenotic type often coexist, and classification by only disease behavior revealed to be unsuitable for reproducing it. In 1998, the World Congress of Gastroenterology in Vienna proposed a new classification of CD considering age of onset (A), disease location (L), and disease behavior (B) as the predominant phenotypic elements [6]. This classification seems easy to apply and relatively stable through time. However, some clinicians use Montreal revision of Vienna classification because of recent attentions such as early age of onset or perianal issues [19] (Table 2.2).

Table 2.1 Clinical symptoms and signs of Crohn's disease [8]

General clinical features	
Symptoms	Chronic or nocturnal diarrhea
	Abdominal pain
	Weight loss
	Fever
	Rectal bleeding
Signs	Pallor
	Cachexia
	Abdominal mass or tenderness
	Perianal fissure
	Fistulae
	Abscess
Specific clinical features according to inflammatory area	
Ileum and colon	Intestinal obstruction
	Inflammatory mass
	Abscess
	Fistulae
Colon	Cramping abdominal pain
	Rectal bleeding and bloody diarrhea
	Hemorrhage
	Perianal complications
	Extraintestinal complications involving the skin or joints
Upper gastrointestinal involvement	Epigastric pain
	Nausea
	Vomiting
	Gastric outlet obstruction

Table 2.2 Vienna and Montreal classification for Crohn's disease

	Vienna	Montreal
Age at diagnosis	A1: below 40 years	A1: below 16 years
	A2: above 40 years	A2: between 17 and 40 years
		A3: above 40 years
Location	L1: terminal ileum	L1: ileal
	L2: colonic	L2: colonic
	L3: ileocolonic	L3: ileocolonic
	L4: upper[a]	L4: isolated upper disease[b]
Behavior	B1: non-stricturing, non-penetrating	B1: non-stricturing, non-penetrating
	B2: stricturing	B2: stricturing
	B3: penetrating	B3: penetrating
		p: perianal disease modifier[c]

[a]Any disease location proximal to the terminal ileum regardless of additional involvement of the terminal ileum or colon

[b]L4 is a modifier that can be added to L1–L3 when concomitant upper gastrointestinal disease is present

[c]"p" is added to B1`B3 and then concomitant perianal disease is present

2.3 Endoscopic Findings for Initial Diagnosis

2.3.1 Gross Findings

Classical endoscopic findings of CD in colonoscopic examination include discontinuous chronic mucosal inflammation, aphthoid ulcerations, longitudinal ulcerations, and cobblestone appearance with normal surrounding mucosa. Skipped inflammatory lesions with normal intervening bowel segment are one of the key findings that differentiate CD from ulcerative colitis. Strictures, both fibrotic and inflammatory, may also be present. More than two-thirds of CD patients have colonic involvement which is divided into pan-colonic and segmental colitis. Approximately 40 % patients with colonic CD show rectal sparing from inflammation, while whole rectal involvement is usually observed in ulcerative colitis [13].

Relatively initial characteristic finding of CD is aphthoid ulcer (Fig. 2.1). It shows as a small (less than 5 mm sized), covered with exudates (whitish or yellowish), and superficial (flat or slightly raised) punched-out ulceration with reddish border. Other colitis which needs to be distinguished from CD such as intestinal Behcet's disease, intestinal tuberculosis, and infectious colitis can also present this aphthoid ulcer. Thus, aphthoid ulcer itself is a nonspecific finding. Multiple presentations of aphthoid ulcers are more specific findings when diagnosing CD. Aphthoid ulcerations are developed over lymphoid follicles and frequently arranged along longitudinal axis of the colon in patients with early or mild CD (Fig. 2.2). Typical longitudinal ulcers of CD are thought to arise from these aphthoid ulcers in a longitudinal direction. Not only in the early stage can these aphthoid ulcers also be seen in the advanced stage of CD, especially around the main ulcerative lesions. Spotty erythematous lesions with localized edema (Fig. 2.3) of mucosa which are considered as beginning stages of CD also can be seen in the early state of CD.

As CD progresses, ulcers tend to be bigger and deeper. Adjacent mucosa shows grossly normal appearance. The shape of ulcers varies from round (Fig. 2.4) to irregular (Fig. 2.5). These types of ulcerations often present in a way of extensive irregular geographic borders or appearance of annular ulcers (Fig. 2.6) around intestinal lumen in CD. Therefore, in this case, it is difficult to differentiate from intestinal tuberculosis. However, the typical progress directions of the ulcerations are usually parallel to the axis of the colon (Fig. 2.7). Classic deep linear ulcerations with discrete margin are seen. Longitudinal alignment of ulceration might also be seen as a railroad track appearance (Fig. 2.8). In addition to linear mucosal features, serpentine mucosal lesion also can be observed by endoscopy in patients with CD, which may be accompanied by multiple geographic ulcers (Fig. 2.9).

As the ulcerations deteriorate, they coalesce into large network of lesions. Therefore, in active CD, the colonic mucosa may be thickened and swollen because of the intermittent pattern of diseased and healthy tissues. It is called as a "cobblestone" appearance, which is a highly specific finding of CD (Fig. 2.10). Remnant mucosal islands surrounded by ulcerations show edematous hyperplastic changes and look like multiple raised lesions. It is seen usually in the distal area of stenotic colon due to inflammation (Fig. 2.11); however, the small bowel near the terminal ileum is also able to show cobblestoning.

Long-standing CD with or without acute inflammation may be characterized by the presence of various mucosal changes including mucosal bridges, scars, fistulas, inflammatory polyps, and stenosis. As a result of fibrosis or scar arising from deep undermining ulceration (Fig. 2.12) and fissures, it can lead to mucosal bridge in the colonic mucosa (Fig. 2.13). During improvement of ulcerations, scars can be found by endoscopy (Fig. 2.14). Severe scarring change of the intestinal mucosa is sometimes indistinguishable from healed ulcerative colitis or infectious colitis such as salmonellosis. Inflammatory polyps also can be seen in patients with CD. These polyps are known as benign lesions caused by long-standing erosive inflammation of the intestine. Usually they are longer in dimension than are wide (Fig. 2.15).

As a result of repeated development and healing of ulcers, cicatricial contraction of bowel wall can be formed. Excessive contraction becomes severe stricture formation with ischemic damages (Fig. 2.16). Strictures can occur in the colon or small intestine and present single or multiple lesions. Sometimes, surrounding normal mucosa nearby stricture sticks together and makes diverticulum like structure, which is called pseudodiverticulum (Fig. 2.17). Most of the severe stricture can be managed by segmental resection and anastomosis; however, noninvasive intervention such as endoscopic balloon dilation can be applied in selected cases with short (<6 cm), moderately active lesions in generally good conditioned patients [9].

Recurrent severe transmural inflammation can lead to a resultant fistula (Fig. 2.18). Primary colonic fistulae are complications of CD, and sometimes the colon is secondarily involved due to small bowel Crohn's disease [13]. Fistula formation can develop not only bowel to bowel but to the any part of the adjacent organs. Detailed materials will be discussed in "Complication" chapter.

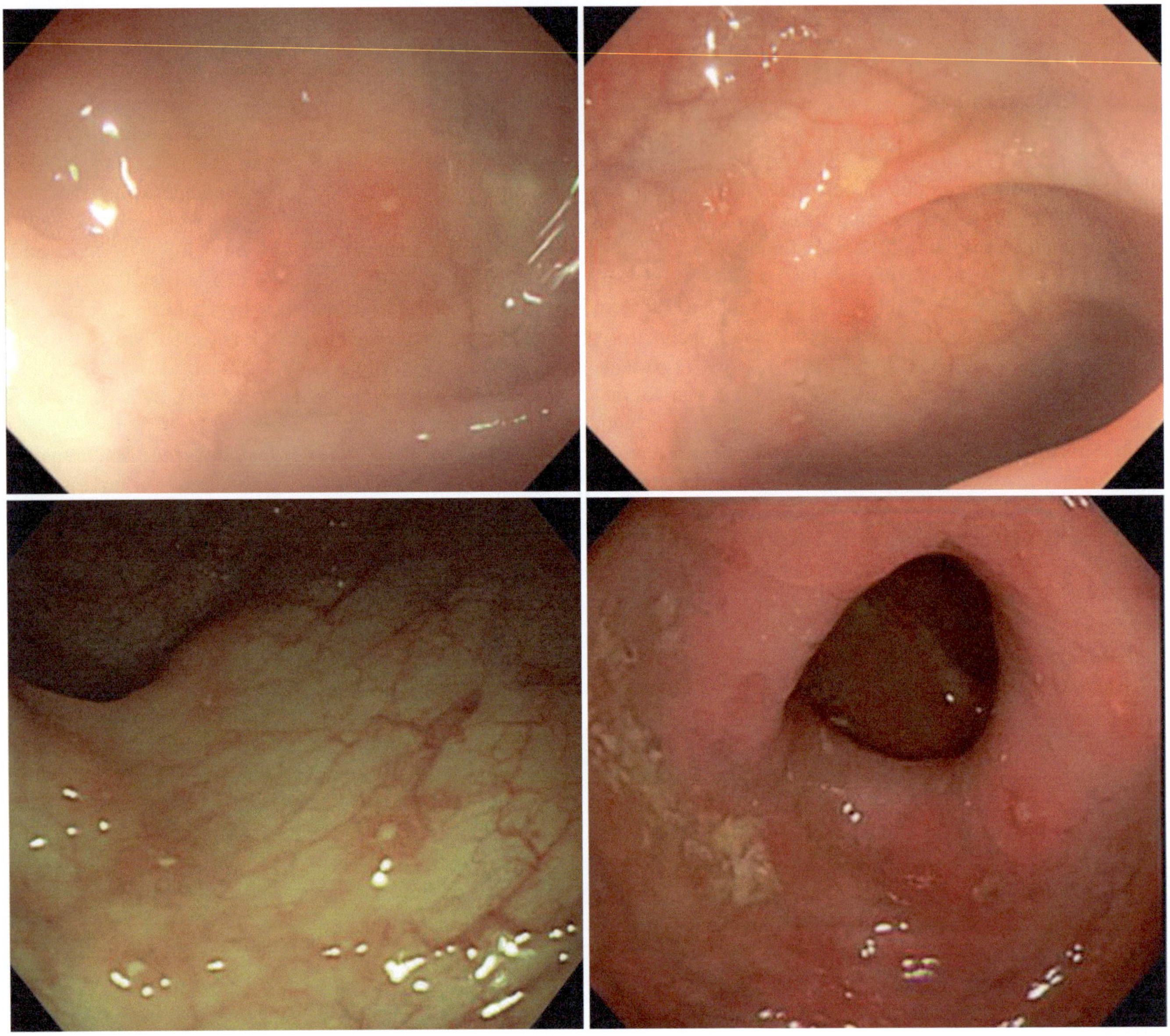

Fig. 2.1 Aphthoid ulcers

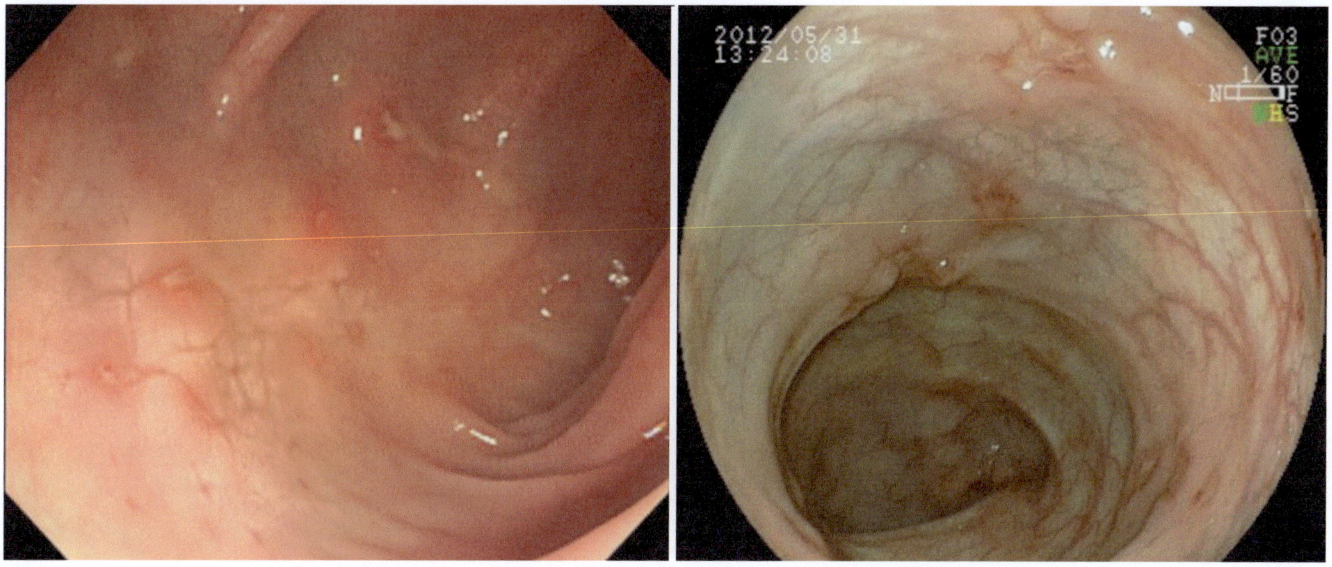

Fig. 2.2 Multiple aphthoid ulcers arranged in a longitudinal direction

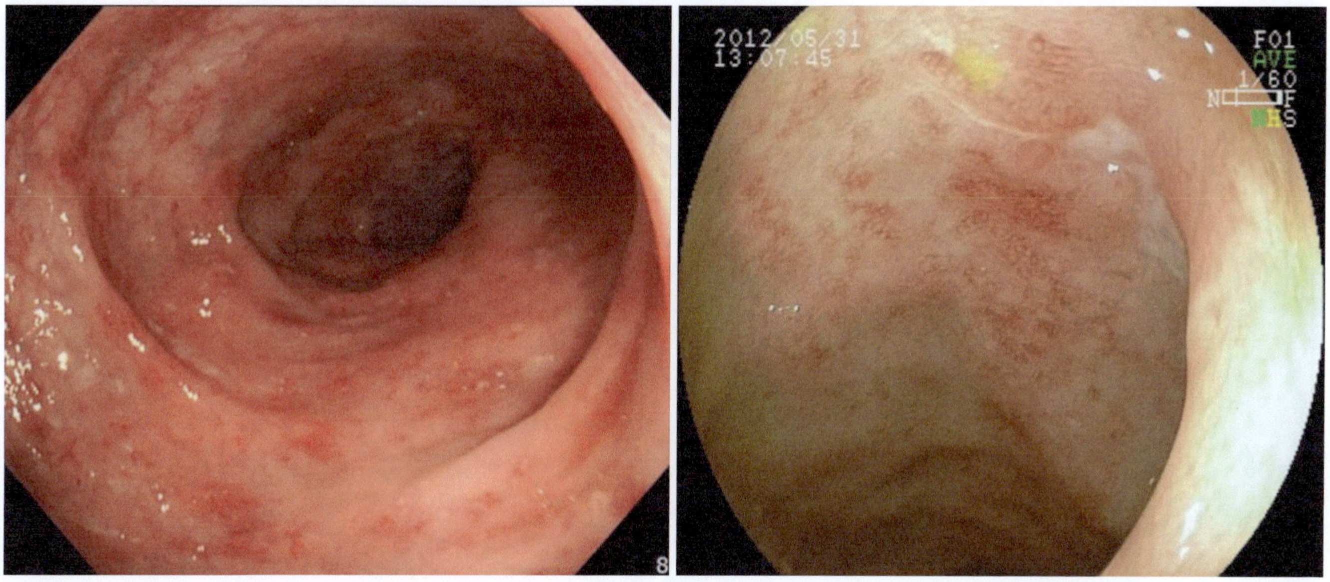

Fig. 2.3 Spotty erythematous lesions with localized edema

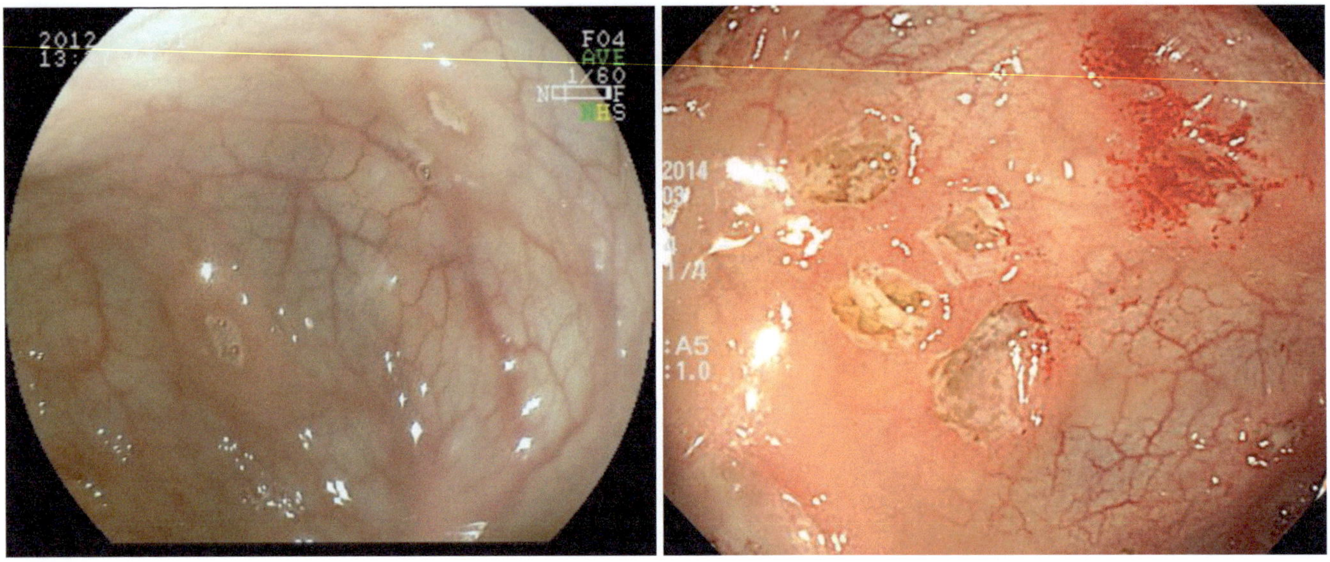

Fig. 2.4 Round ulcerations

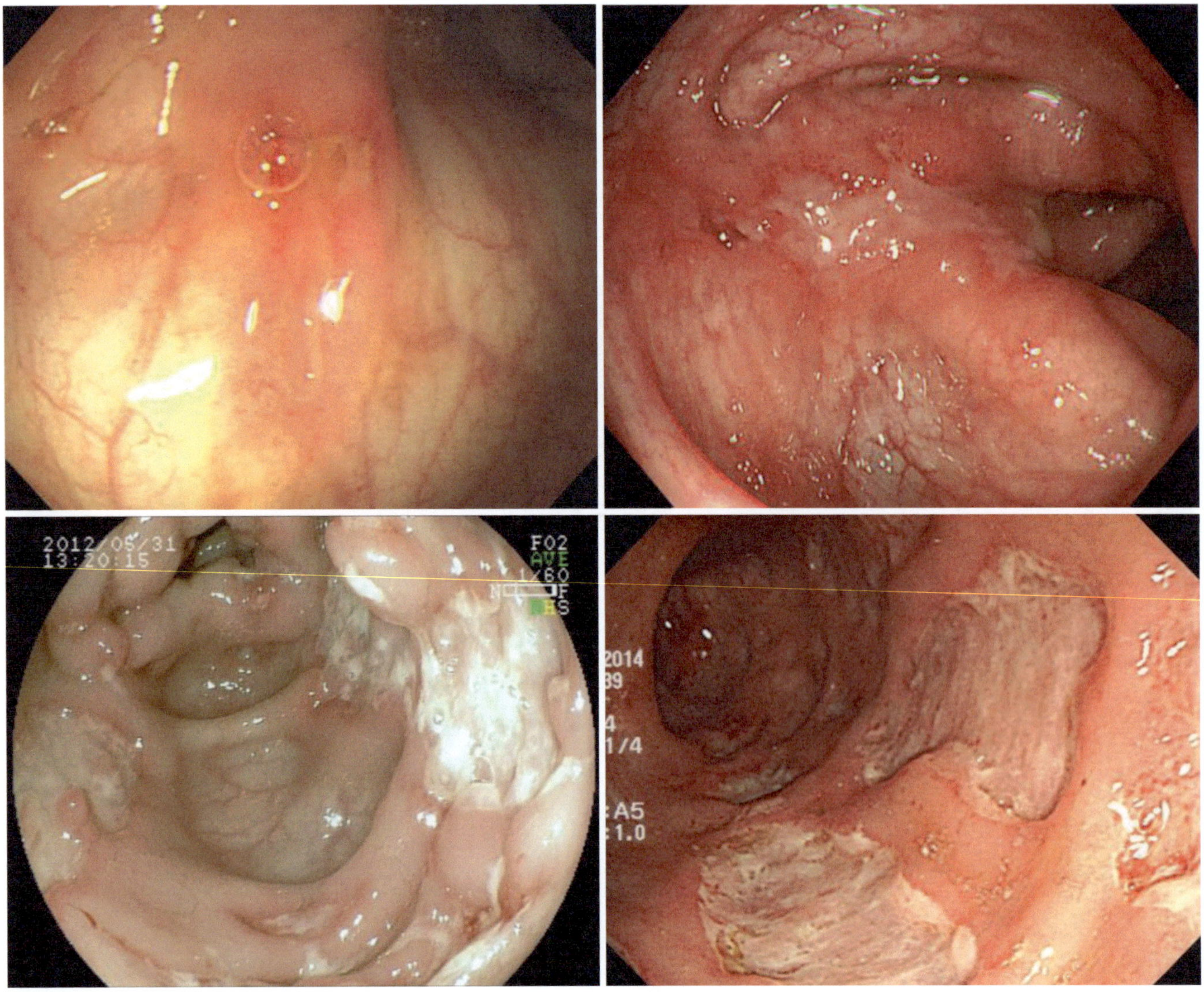

Fig. 2.5 Irregular ulcerations

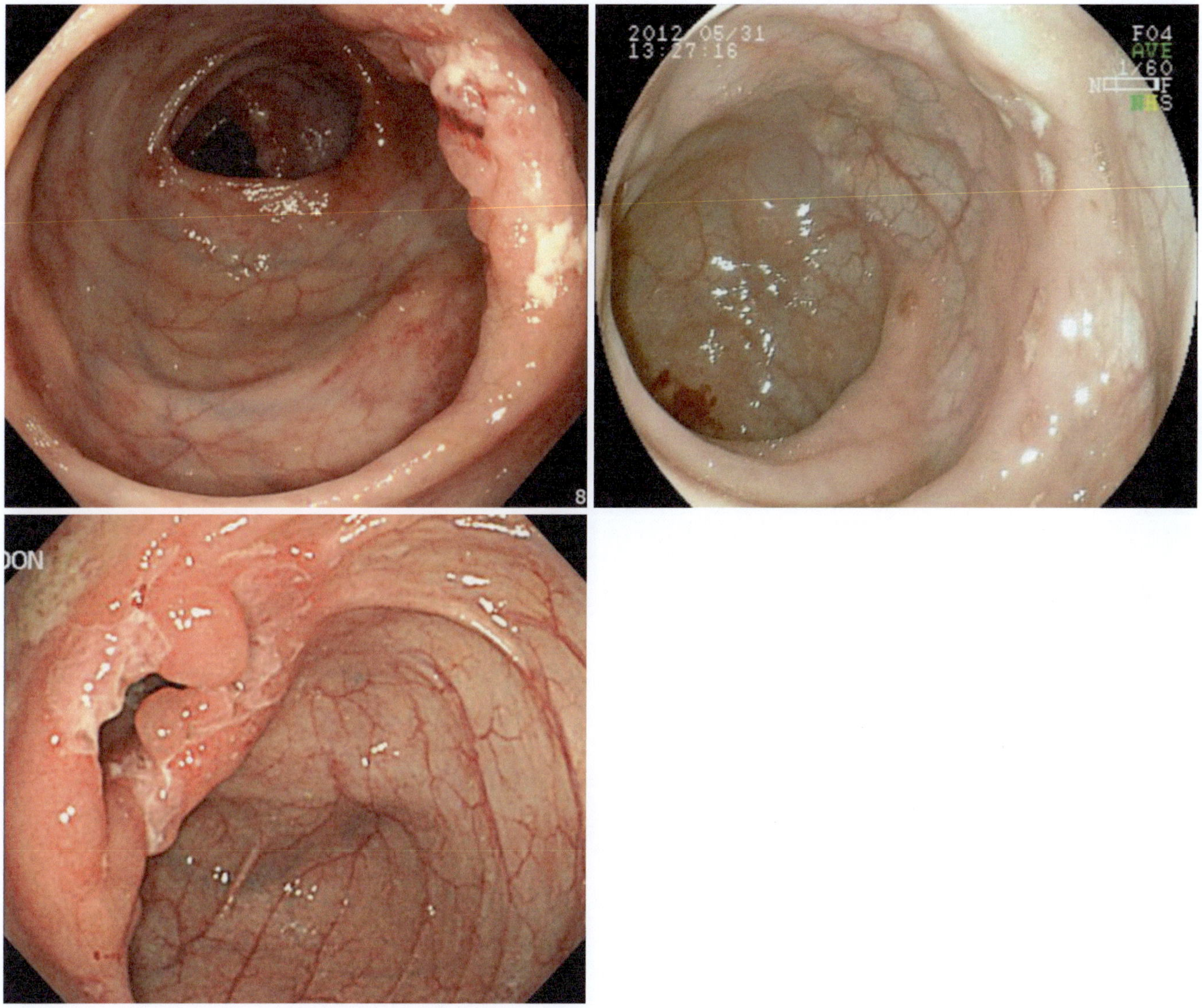

Fig. 2.6 Annular ulcerations which mimic intestinal tuberculosis

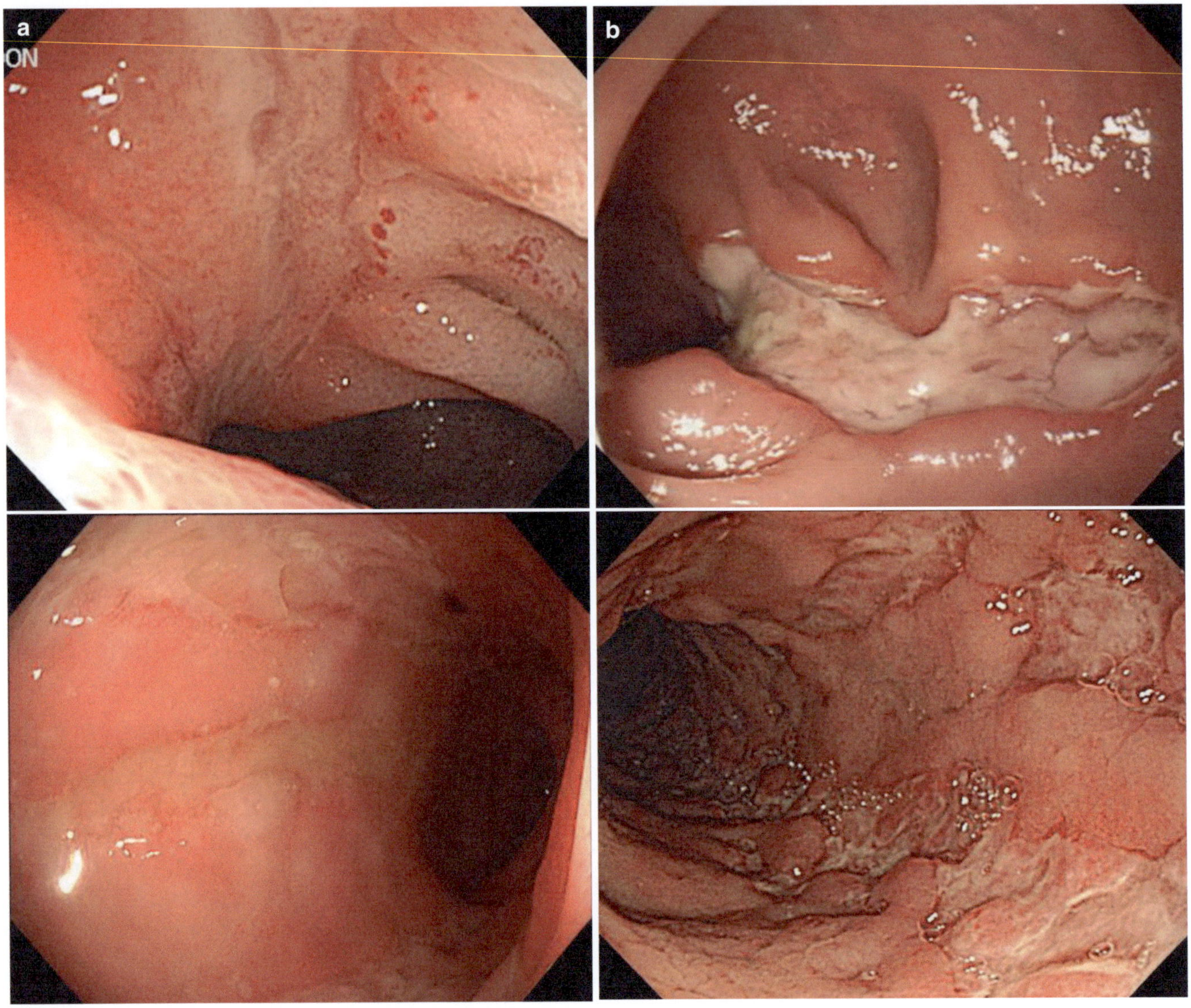

Fig. 2.7 Longitudinal ulcerations (**a** terminal ileum, **b** colon)

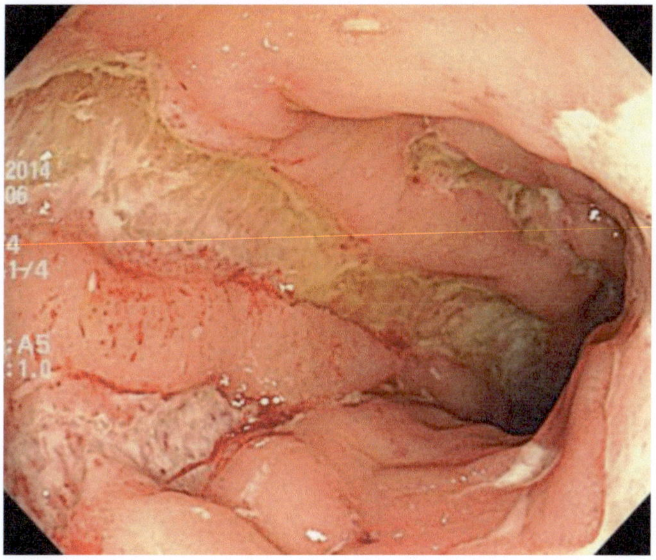

Fig. 2.8 Railroad track appearance

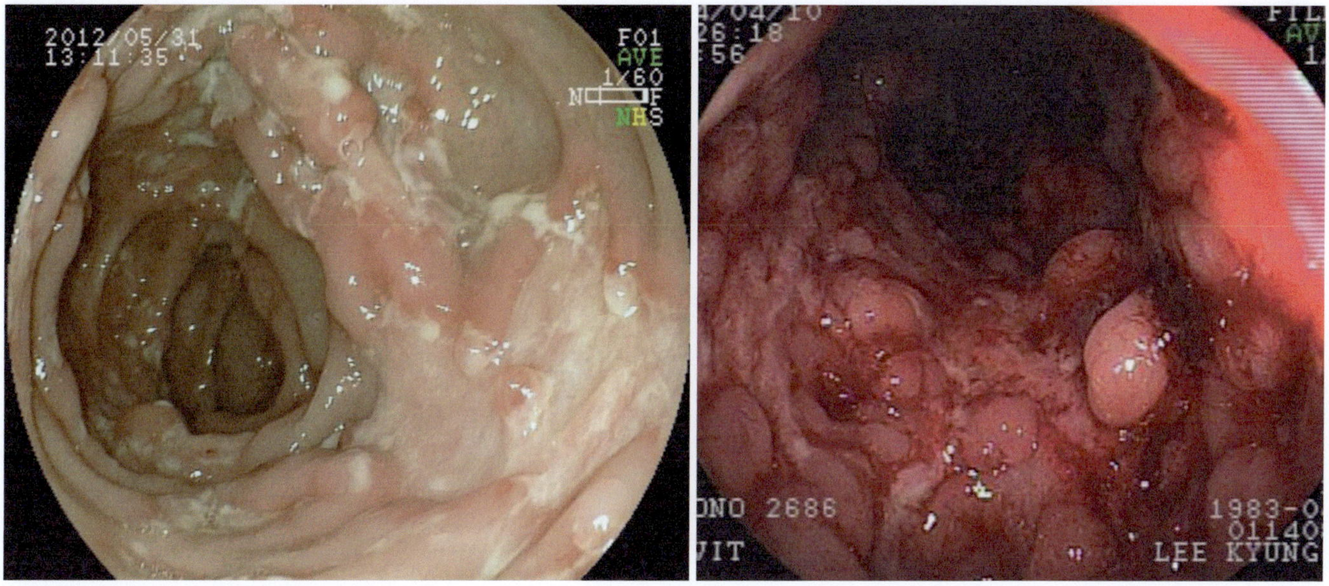

Fig. 2.9 Geographic ulcerations

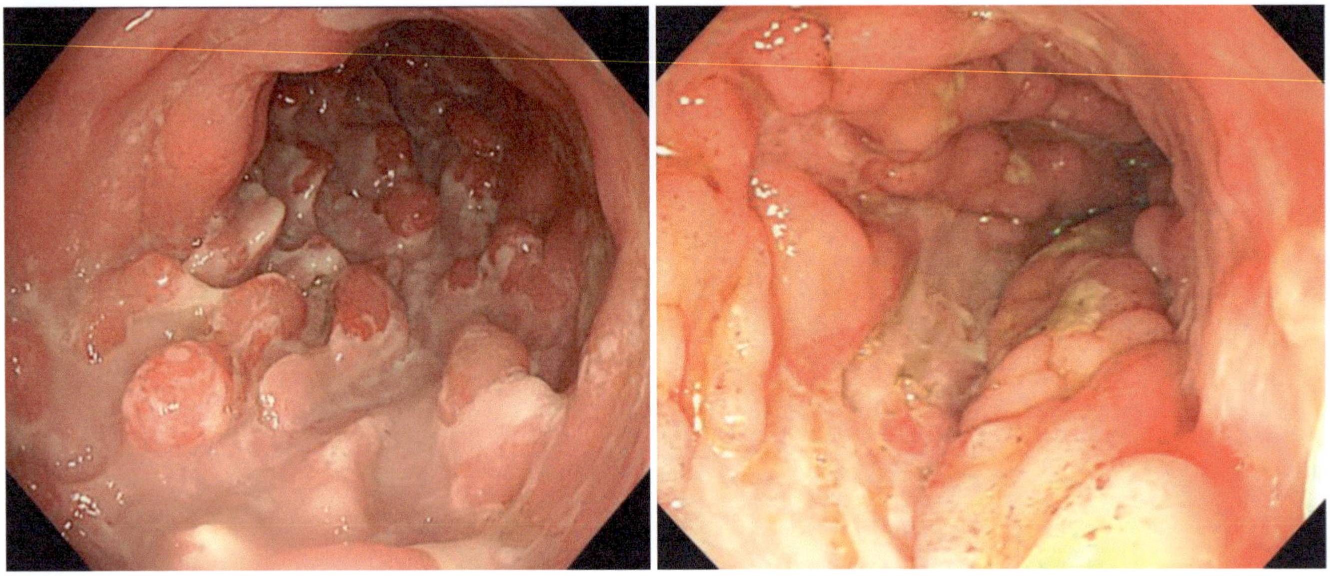

Fig. 2.10 Cobblestone appearance

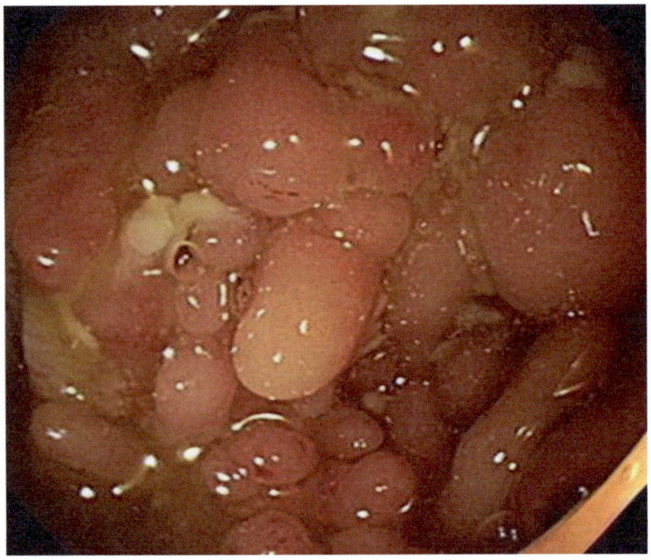

Fig. 2.11 Cobblestoning in front of the mildly stenotic ascending colon

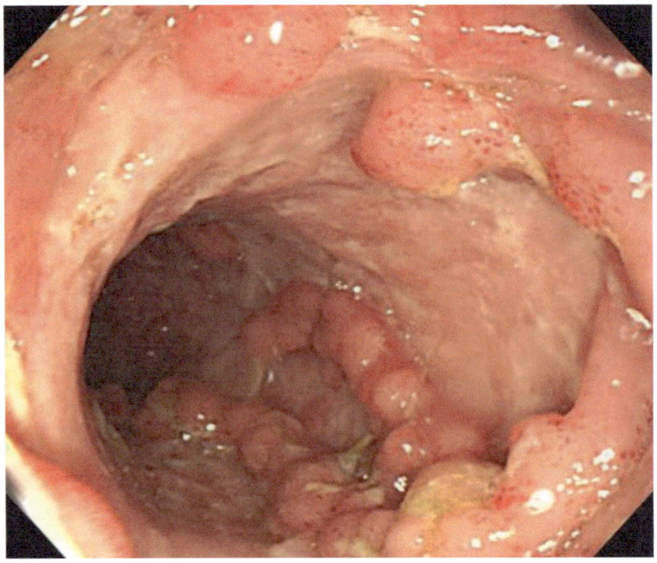

Fig. 2.12 Undermining ulcers

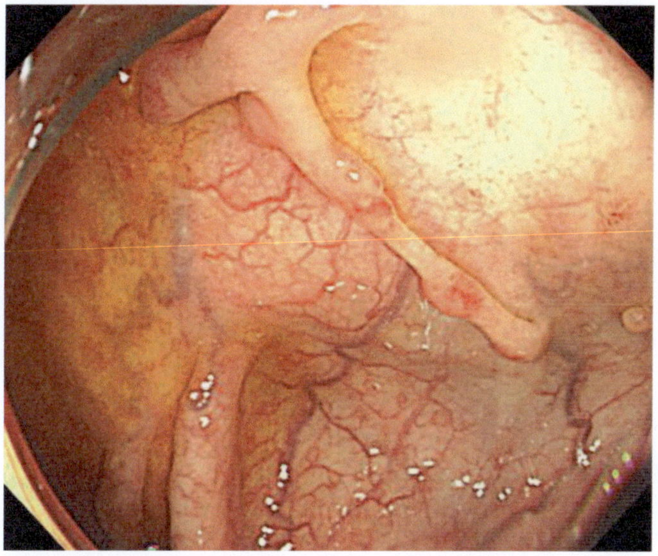

Fig. 2.13 Mucosal bridges

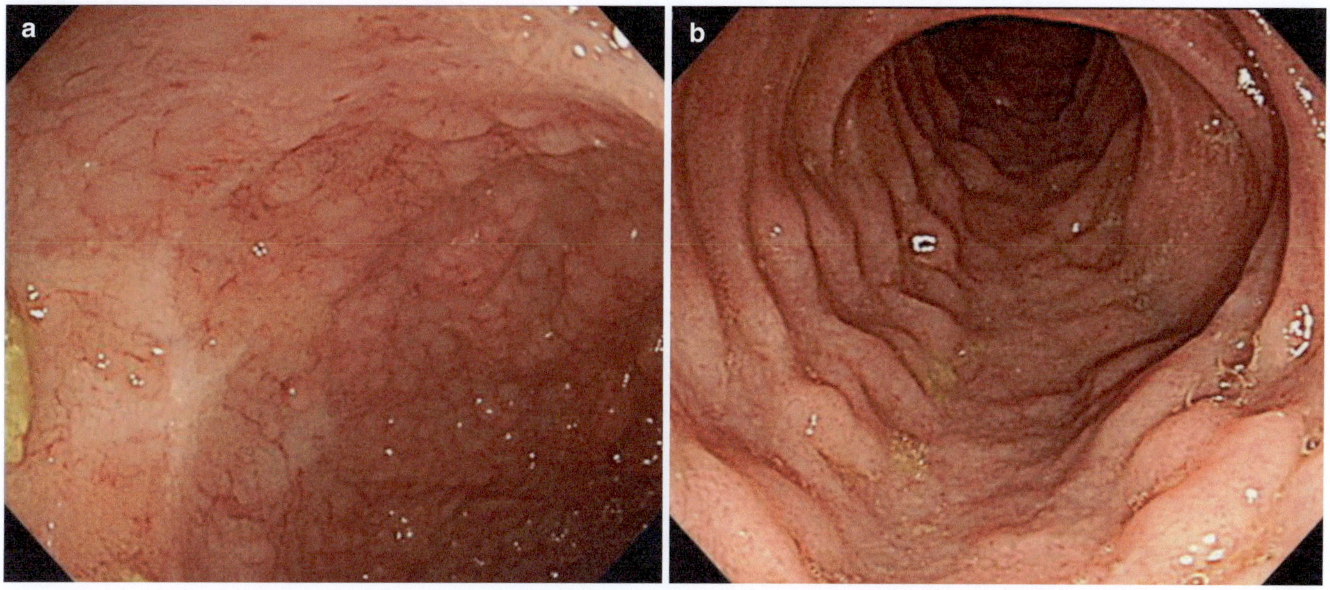

Fig. 2.14 Scars. (**a**) A star-shaped scar. (**b**) Longitudinal ulcer scars in the terminal ileum

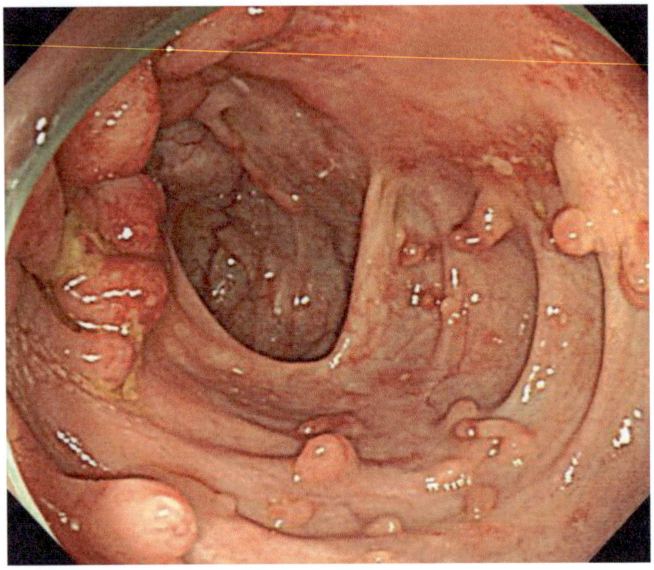

Fig. 2.15 Inflammatory polyps

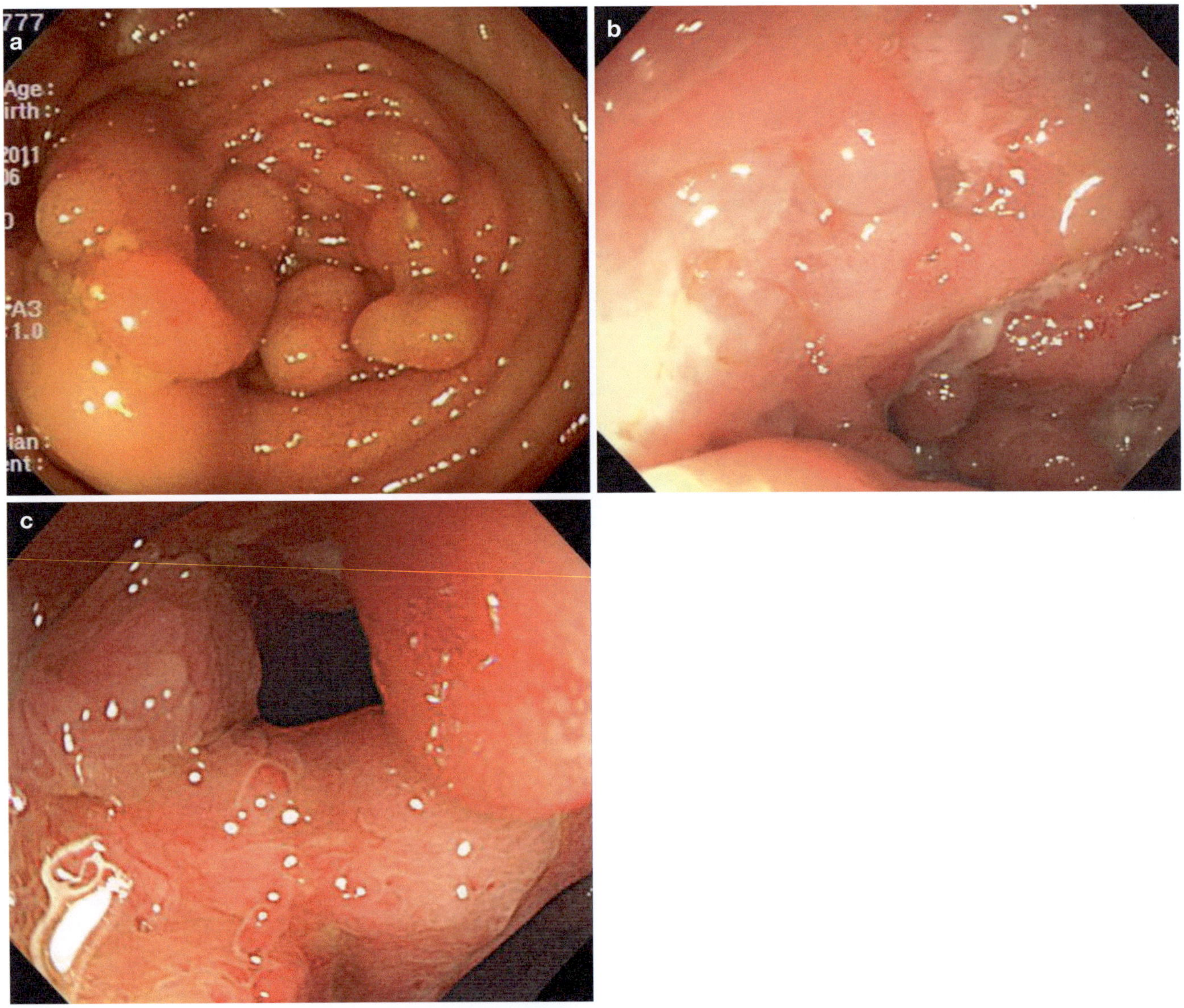

Fig. 2.16 Stricture (**a** ileocecal valve, **b** colon, **c** surgical specimen)

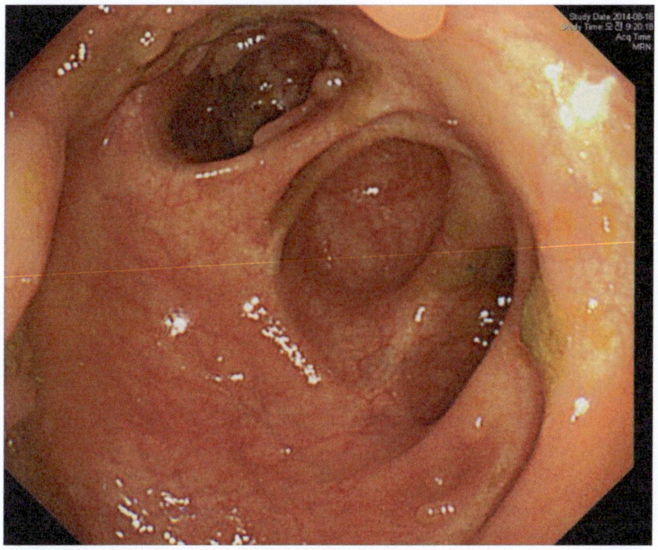

Fig. 2.17 Pseudodiverticulum

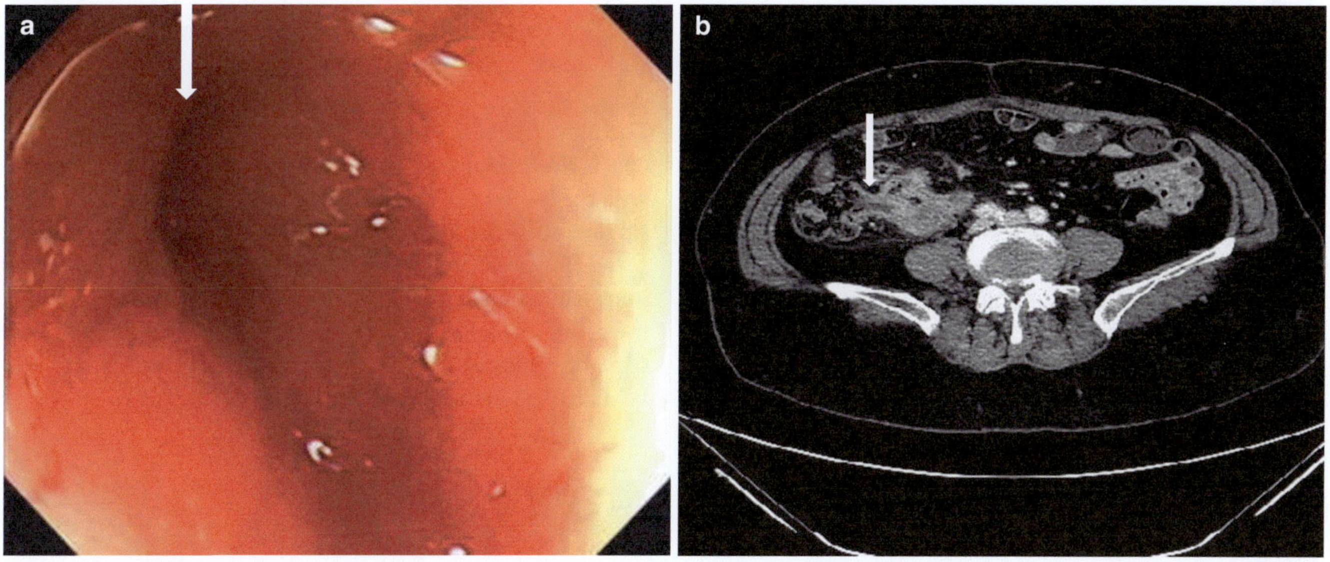

Fig. 2.18 Fistulae (endoscopic features of fistula opening) between cecum and sigmoid colon (**a** suspicious opening (*arrow*) in the sigmoid colon; **b** CT finding (*arrow*))

2.3.2 Histological Findings

Endoscopic biopsy provides diagnostic clues to confirm the diagnosis of CD. Histological findings of CD (Fig. 2.19) can be summarized with transmural inflammation (span the entire depth of the intestinal wall), noncaseating granuloma (cheese-like appearance of granulomas associated with infections), chronicity, and focality. An increased cellularity of lymphocytes and plasma cells in the lamina propria implies chronic inflammations of disease. Crypt irregularity such as distortion, fibrosis extending to the muscularis mucosae, and noncaseating granuloma indicate another possibility of CD [11]. Noncaseating granulomas are observed in only 15–36 % in CD patients, whereas they are regarded as a prominent histopathologic feature of CD [21]. Histological results are just one of various diagnostic tools; therefore clinicians have to remember that biopsies are not meant to tell us everything about the disease.

2.3.3 Diagnostic Criteria for Crohn's Disease [25]

Based on the findings above, the Japanese IBD study group has proposed the diagnostic criteria for Crohn's disease [25] (Table 2.3). These criteria are relatively simple and easy to use in clinical practice. However, all other possible causes of longitudinal or cobblestone-appearing intestinal lesions such as ischemic colitis or ulcerative colitis must be excluded before confirming the diagnosis.

2.3.4 Small Bowel Evaluations

Inflammation is usually presented in the terminal ileum, but in some patients (10–30 %), small bowel proximal to the terminal ileum can be affected. Gastroduodenal and colonic evaluations are relatively easy, while small bowel is not readily accessible by conventional endoscopy. Until recently, the only way to evaluate the small bowel mucosa in a patient with CD was by barium small bowel radiographs and intubation of the distal terminal ileum. However, recent endoscopic modalities such as wireless capsule endoscopy and double-balloon enteroscopy enable direct visualization or biopsy of the deep small bowel mucosa. Typical small bowel lesions of CD (see Chap. 12) show aphthoid, round, or irregular ulcerations with a longitudinal arrangement at the mesenteric border [22]. Both wireless capsule endoscopy and double-balloon enteroscopy allow direct inspection of small bowel and may replace previous radiological methods [2].

2.3.5 Gastroduodenal Involvement of Crohn's Disease

The most frequent finding of gastroduodenal involvement of CD is *Helicobacter pylori*-negative focally active gastritis with the 94 % positive predictive value [15]. Atypical mucosal abnormalities such as erosions and ulcers are able to be seen. However, characteristic appearance such as "bamboo joint-like appearances," which are erosive fissures regularly traversing enlarged folds that longitudinally align the lesser curvature and cardia, can also be observed [26]. Details will be discussed in the following chapter.

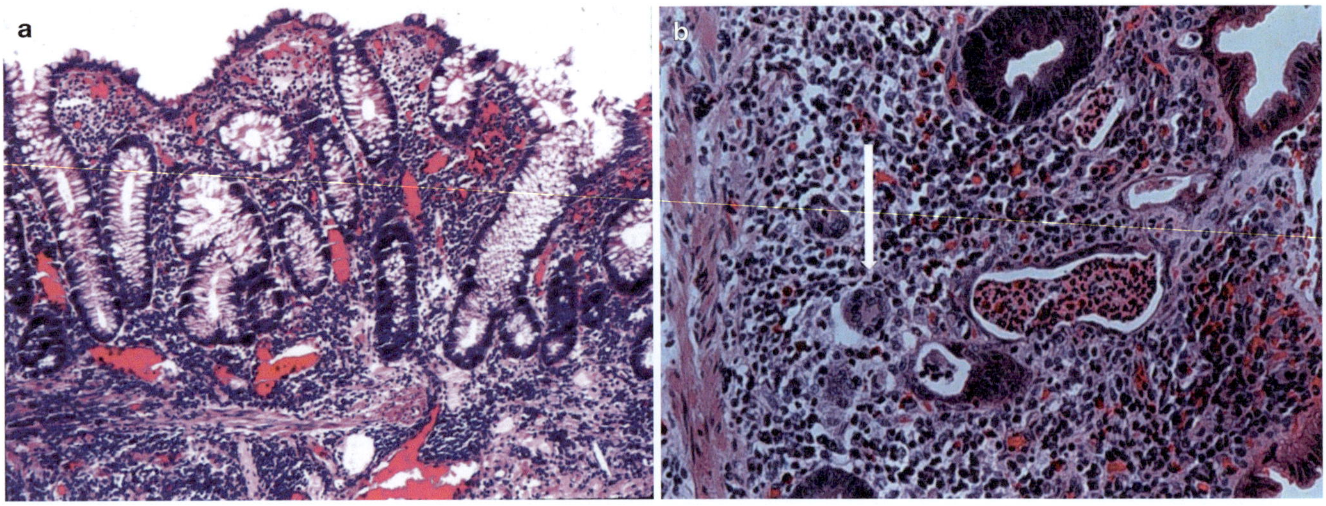

Fig. 2.19 Histologic findings of CD: (**a**) focal crypt distortions (shortening and branching) with increased cellularity of the lamina propria are seen. (**b**) Noncaseating granuloma (*arrow*) has a diagnostic value for CD

Table 2.3 Criteria for definite diagnosis of Crohn's disease

A. One of the following three conditions should be present:
1. Intestinal longitudinal ulcer or deformity induced by a longitudinal ulcer or cobblestone pattern
2. Intestinal small aphthous ulcerations arranged in a longitudinal fashion for at least 3 months, plus noncaseating granulomas
3. Multiple small aphthous ulcerations in both the upper and lower digestive tract, not necessarily with longitudinal arrangement, for at least 3 months, plus noncaseating granulomas
B. The following diseases should be excluded:
1. Ulcerative colitis
2. Ischemic enterocolitis
3. Acute infectious enterocolitis

2.4 Assessment for Disease Extent and Severity

Disease localization helps to determine the prognosis and appropriateness of medical treatment and assists in stratifying the risk of colon cancer. Furthermore, it can help in decision making in patients undergoing surgical therapy. A quantitative endoscopic index of severity (CDEIS) by dividing the bowel into five segments and generating numeric score based on surface involvement by disease and the presence of deep or superficial ulcerations was developed in the 1980s (Table 2.4) [14]. Because of the time-consuming and complicated nature of CDEIS, Daperno and colleagues developed another endoscopic grading system evaluating CD, the Simplified Endoscopic Activity Score for CD (SES-CD) (Table 2.5) [4]. SES-CD was validated to be closely correlated with CDEIS. However, this index has not been used in routine clinical practice.

It is well known that endoscopic severity poorly correlates with clinical symptoms including CD activity index (CDAI, Table 2.6), while endoscopic extent and severity of the disease predict disease course. Therefore, endoscopic appearances in CD might be a better predictor of the future clinical course than CDAI. Moreover, after tumor necrosis factor (TNF)-α blocking agents were launched, endoscopic confirmation of complete mucosal healing is believed to be associated with lower recurrence of the CD. Endoscopic scoring system has been developed and validated for assessing disease activity without interobserver deviation. However, regarding optimal treatment goal of CD (complete recovering of intestinal mucosa), it is still unanswered whether clinicians should rely on clinical, endoscopic, or histological mucosal healing during clinical practice.

Table 2.4 Crohn's disease index of severity (CDEIS)

Parameter	Rectum	Sigmoid and left colon	Transverse colon	Right colon	Ileum	Total
Deep ulcerations (12 if present)						Total 1
Superficial ulcerations (12 if present)						Total 2
Surface involved by disease(cm)						Total 3
Surface involved by ulcerations(cm)						Total 4
Total 1 + Total 2 + Total 3 + Total 4 = Total A						
Number of segments totally or partially explored = *n*						
Total A/*n* = Total B						
If an ulcerated stenosis is present anywhere add 3 = C						
If a nonulcerated stenosis is present anywhere add 3 = D						
Total B + C + D = CDEIS						

Table 2.5 Simple endoscopic score for Crohn's disease (SES-CD score)

	SES-CD score			
Variable	0	1	2	3
Presence of ulcers	None	Aphthous ulcers (Ø 0.1–0.5 cm)	Large ulcers (Ø 0.5–2 cm)	Very large ulcers (Ø >2 cm)
Ulcerated surface	None	<10 %	10–30 %	>30 %
Affected surface	Unaffected segment	<50 %	50–75 %	>75 %
Presence of narrowings	None	Single, can be passed	Multiple, can be passed	Cannot be passed
Number of affected segments	All variables = 0	At least one variable ≥1		

Table 2.6 Crohn's disease activity index (CDAI)

Variable	Description		Multiplier
Number liquid stools	Sum of 7 days		×2
Abdominal pain	Sum of 7 days' ratings	0 = none 1 = mild 2 = moderate 3 = severe	×5
General well being	Sum of 7 days' ratings	0 = generally well 1 = slightly under par 2 = poor 3 = very poor 4 = terrible	×7
Extraintestinal complications	Number of listed complications	Arthritis/arthralgia, iritis/uveitis, erythema nodosum, pyoderma, gangrenosum, aphthous stomatitis, anal fissure/fistula/abscess, fever >37.8 °C	×20
Antidiarrheal drugs	Use in the previous 7 days	0 = no 1 = yes	×30
Abdominal mass		0 = no 2 = questionable 5 = definite	×10
Hematocrit	Expected-observed Hct	Males:47 observed Females:42 observed	×6
Body weight	Ideal/observed ratio	[1–(ideal/observed)] × 100	×1(NOT <–10)

2.5 Follow-Up Colonoscopy During Treatment of Crohn's Disease

There are a lot of guidelines for endoscopic evaluation in managing patients with CD; however, the consensus is that a regular follow-up endoscopy is not generally recommended [20]. Universally recognized indications of endoscopy in patients with CD are gastrointestinal bleeding, severe abdominal pain suggesting intestinal stenosis, and preoperative evaluation (Table 2.7). In one pediatric study, 42 % rate of management change was found after endoscopic evaluation [23]. Follow-up colonoscopy in patients with CD might be deliberate given the invasive nature of endoscopy.

Table 2.7 Guidelines/reviews on the appropriateness of colonoscopy for the clinical management of known Crohn's disease [20]

Endorsement	Main recommendations
American Society for Gastrointestinal Endoscopy (ASGE)	In colonic stricture, a complete examination with biopsy is recommended
European Crohn's and Colitis Organisation (ECCO)	Patients in remission should be clinically assessed on a regular basis. Endoscopy could be of some help but only in specific situations such as surgically induced remission. Endoscopic dilation of a stenosis in Crohn's disease is a preferred technique for the management of short accessible strictures
French Society of Digestive Endoscopy (SFED)	A systematic endoscopic control after a first Crohn's disease treated episode is not justified. Endoscopic procedures should not be systematically performed after each Crohn's disease episode. Colonoscopy/ileoscopy can be used to identify the source of bleeding in Crohn's disease
British Society of Gastroenterology	Colonoscopy should not be repeated in Crohn's disease unless it will alter management or if a surgical decision depends on the result
German Society for Gastroenterological and Metabolic Diseases	Ileoscopy is not necessary in every acute phase or before the introduction of an anti-inflammatory treatment. It can be of some help, although the consequences of this procedure in terms of adaptation of the therapeutic approach often remain unclear. In the elective preoperative phase, an ileoscopy with biopsies is indicated. In the postoperative phase, endoscopy can be necessary if other laboratory and imaging procedures yield unclear results or if complications are suspected
German Society for Gastroenterological Diseases	Endoscopy 3 months after pouch procedure, then once a year. Treatment of strictures in Crohn's disease is the most important indication for endoscopic therapy in inflammatory bowel disease
American College of Gastroenterology (ACG)	Colonoscopic evaluation of surgical anastomoses can be used to predict the likelihood of clinical relapse

2.6 Surveillance for Colitic Cancer

Both CD and ulcerative colitis increase the incidence of colorectal carcinoma (CRC) and need surveillance colonoscopy. It is widely accepted that patients with CD, with a similar extent and duration of colonic involvement, have a similar risk to those with ulcerative colitis [1]. Established risk factors for developing CRC in the setting of colitis include the extent of disease, the duration of disease, and the severity of inflammation. Usually, more than one-third of colonic involvement in CD is a candidate for CRC surveillance. Surveillance programs have evolved with improvement on the understanding of the risk factors associated with CRC and the natural history of dysplasia. Pan-colonic chromoendoscopy with targeted biopsies of abnormal areas in every 1 or 2 years has emerged as the optimal surveillance technique in patients with colitis. In recent years, digital chromoendoscopy such as narrowband imaging has been introduced; however, its role in CRC surveillance in CD is underevaluated. Detailed explanations will follow in the next chapter.

2.7 Assessment for Postoperative Recurrence of Crohn's Disease

Surgical intervention may be considered when treating complications of CD, for example, perforation or strictures that are not amendable to medical or endoscopic therapy. However, CD may recur after surgical therapy, especially at the site of anastomosis and its proximal border (Figs. 2.20, 2.21, and 2.22). It was reported in a meta-analysis that the pooled estimate of patients experiencing severe endoscopic recurrence was as high as 50 % [17]. It was also noted that there is a time lag between the development of endoscopic recurrence and clinical symptoms. Several guidelines have recommended that endoscopic reassessment should be considered at least 6 months after surgery to assess for recurrence, and further medical management may be adjusted according to the endoscopic assessment [24] (Fig. 2.23).

So far, Rutgeerts' score (Table 2.8) is the gold standard scoring system for endoscopic evaluation of postsurgical recurrence in patients with CD [18]. If there is no lesion or mild recurrence less than five aphthoid ulcers on first year after surgery, clinical recurrence rate is 9 % at 7 year, while all patients with severe endoscopic recurrence showed symptomatic relapse within 4 years. However, although endoscopy plays an important role in evaluating postoperative recurrence in CD patients who have undergone prior bowel resections, routine postoperative endoscopic surveillance is still controversial, and it is still imperfect when recurrent lesions occur in the small bowel [2].

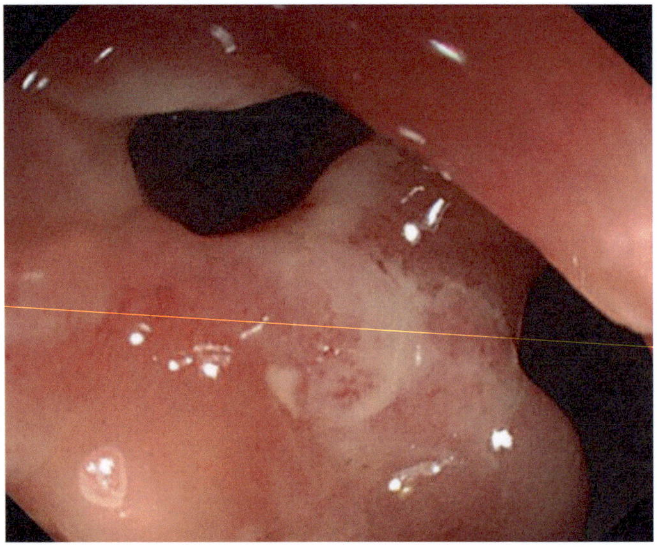

Fig. 2.20 Postoperative recurrence at anastomosis site

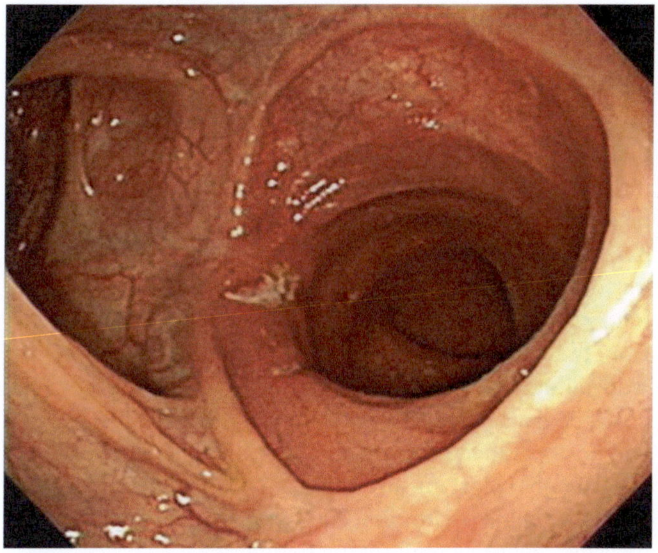

Fig. 2.21 Postoperative recurrence: ulcerations at proximal border of anastomosis site

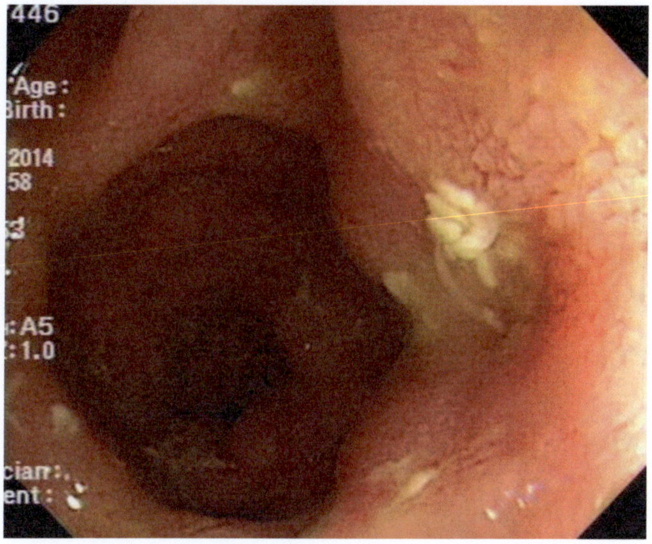

Fig. 2.22 Postoperative recurrence of aphthous and round ulcers in the ileal pouch

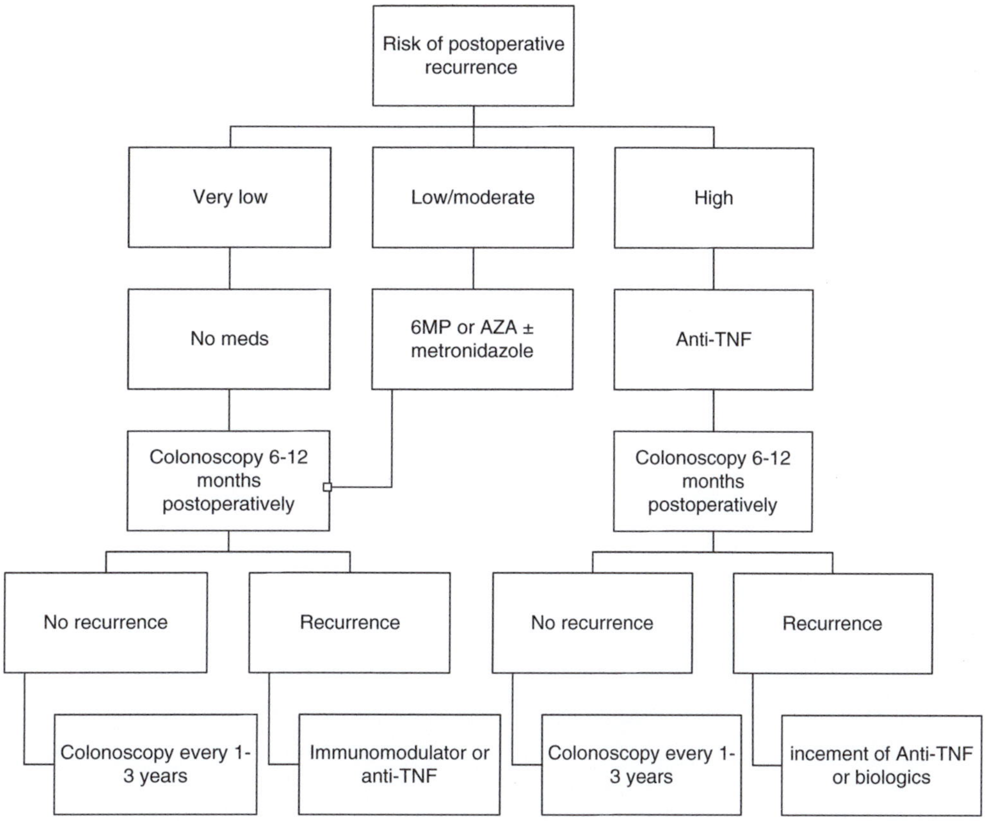

Fig. 2.23 Evaluation and treatment of postoperative Crohn's disease [16]

Table 2.8 Rutgeerts' endoscopic recurrence score after surgery in patients with Crohn's disease

Endoscopic score	Definition
i0	No lesion
i1	≤5 Aphthous lesions
i2	>5 Aphthous lesions with normal mucosa between the lesions or skipped areas of larger lesions or lesions confined to the ileocolonic anastomosis
i3	Diffuse aphthous ileitis with diffusely inflamed mucosa
i4	Diffuse inflammation with already larger ulcers, nodules, and/or narrowing

Remission, endoscopic score of i0 or i1; recurrence, endoscopic score of i2–i4

2.8 Summary

In summary, for any subjects with suspected CD, ileocolonoscopy and biopsies from the terminal ileum to colonic segments are necessary to establish the diagnosis. The introduction of anti-TNFα agents has changed the therapeutic paradigm of patients. Therefore, endoscopic examination has been increasingly used to monitor disease activity and mucosal healing in order to guide therapeutic decision making. Surveillance ileocolonoscopy has also changed recently from multiple random biopsies to pan-colonic dye spraying with targeted biopsies of abnormal areas. Ileocolonoscopy could be considered to assess preoperative risk stratification and postoperative recurrence so that therapy can be tailored accordingly. Most of all, clinicians should require careful judgment about performing endoscopy and making a clinical decision regarding endoscopic findings.

References

1. Cairns SR, Scholefield JH, Steele RJ, Dunlop MG, Thomas HJ, Evans GD, Eaden JA, Rutter MD, Atkin WP, Saunders BP, Lucassen A, Jenkins P, Fairclough PD, Woodhouse CR; British Society of Gastroenterology; Association of Coloproctology for Great Britain and Ireland. Guidelines for colorectal cancer screening and surveillance in moderate and high risk groups (update from 2002). Gut. 2010;59(5):666–89. doi:10.1136/gut.2009.179804.
2. Cheon JH, Kim WH. Recent advances of endoscopy in inflammatory bowel diseases. Gut Liver. 2007;1(2):118–25. doi:10.5009/gnl.2007.1.2.118.
3. Crohn BB, Ginzburg L, Oppenheimer GD. Regional ileitis: a pathologic and clinical entity. 1932. Mt Sinai J Med. 2000;67(3):263–8.
4. Daperno M, D'Haens G, Van Assche G, Baert F, Bulois P, Maunoury V, Rutgeerts P. Development and validation of a new, simplified endoscopic activity score for Crohn's disease: the SES-CD. Gastrointest Endosc. 2004;60(4):505–12.
5. Freeman HJ. Application of the Montreal classification for Crohn's disease to a single clinician database of 1015 patients. Can J Gastroenterol. 2007;21(6):363–6.
6. Gasche C, Scholmerich J, Brynskov J, D'Haens G, Hanauer SB, Irvine EJ, Sutherland LR. A simple classification of Crohn's disease: report of the working party for the world congresses of gastroenterology, Vienna 1998. Inflamm Bowel Dis. 2000;6(1):8–15.
7. Geboes K, Ectors N, D'Haens G, Rutgeerts P. Is ileoscopy with biopsy worthwhile in patients presenting with symptoms of inflammatory bowel disease? Am J Gastroenterol. 1998;93(2):201–6. doi:10.1111/j.1572-0241.1998.00201.x.
8. Hanauer SB, Sandborn W. Management of Crohn's disease in adults. Am J Gastroenterol. 2001;96(3):635–43. doi:10.1111/j.1572-0241.2001.3671_c.x.
9. Hassan C, Zullo A, De Francesco V, Ierardi E, Giustini M, Pitidis A, Morini S. Systematic review: endoscopic dilatation in Crohn's disease. Aliment Pharmacol Ther. 2007;26(11–12):1457–64. doi:10.1111/j.1365-2036.2007.03532.x.
10. Lind E, Fausa O, Elgjo K, Gjone E. Crohn's disease. Clinical manifestations. Scand J Gastroenterol. 1985;20(6):665–70.
11. Magro F, Langner C, Driessen A, Ensari A, Geboes K, Mantzaris GJ, Villanacci V, Becheanu G, Borralho Nunes P, Cathomas G, Fries W, Jouret-Mourin A, Mescoli C, de Petris G, Rubio CA, Shepherd NA, Vieth M, Eliakim R; European Society of Pathology (ESP); European Crohn's and Colitis Organisation (ECCO). European consensus on the histopathology of inflammatory bowel disease. J Crohns Colitis. 2013;7(10):827–51. doi:10.1016/j.crohns.2013.06.001.
12. Marshall JK, Cawdron R, Zealley I, Riddell RH, Somers S, Irvine EJ. Prospective comparison of small bowel meal with pneumocolon versus ileo-colonoscopy for the diagnosis of ileal Crohn's disease. Am J Gastroenterol. 2004;99(7):1321–9. doi:10.1111/j.1572-0241.2004.30499.x.
13. Mills S, Stamos MJ. Colonic Crohn's disease. Clin Colon Rectal Surg. 2007;20(4):309–13. doi:10.1055/s-2007-991030.
14. Modigliani R, Mary JY, Simon JF, Cortot A, Soule JC, Gendre JP, Rene E. Clinical, biological, and endoscopic picture of attacks of Crohn's disease. Evolution on prednisolone. Groupe d'Etude Therapeutique des Affections Inflammatoires Digestives. Gastroenterology. 1990;98(4):811–8.
15. Oberhuber G, Puspok A, Oesterreicher C, Novacek G, Zauner C, Burghuber M, Wrba F. Focally enhanced gastritis: a frequent type of gastritis in patients with Crohn's disease. Gastroenterology. 1997;112(3):698–706.
16. Regueiro M. Management and prevention of postoperative Crohn's disease. Inflamm Bowel Dis. 2009;15(10):1583–90. doi:10.1002/ibd.20909.
17. Renna S, Camma C, Modesto I, Cabibbo G, Scimeca D, Civitavecchia G, Cottone M. Meta-analysis of the placebo rates of clinical relapse and severe endoscopic recurrence in postoperative Crohn's disease. Gastroenterology. 2008;135(5):1500–9. doi:10.1053/j.gastro.2008.07.066.
18. Rutgeerts P, Geboes K, Vantrappen G, Kerremans R, Coenegrachts JL, Coremans G. Natural history of recurrent Crohn's disease at the ileocolonic anastomosis after curative surgery. Gut. 1984;25(6):665–72.
19. Satsangi J, Silverberg MS, Vermeire S, Colombel JF. The Montreal classification of inflammatory bowel disease: controversies, consensus, and implications. Gut. 2006;55(6):749–53. doi:10.1136/gut.2005.082909.
20. Schusselé Filliettaz S, Juillerat P, Burnand B, Arditi C, Windsor A, Beglinger C, Dubois RW, Peytremann-Bridevaux I, Pittet V, Gonvers JJ, Froehlich F, Vader JP; EPAGE II Study Group. Appropriateness of colonoscopy in Europe (EPAGE II). Chronic diarrhea and known inflammatory bowel disease. Endoscopy. 2009;41(3):218–26. doi:10.1055/s-0028-1119627.
21. Shen B. Endoscopic, imaging, and histologic evaluation of Crohn's disease and ulcerative colitis. Am J Gastroenterol. 2007;102:S41–5.
22. Sunada K, Yamamoto H, Hayashi Y, Sugano K. Clinical importance of the location of lesions with regard to mesenteric or antimesenteric side of the small intestine. Gastrointest Endosc. 2007;66(3 Suppl):S34–8. doi:10.1016/j.gie.2007.02.036.
23. Thakkar K, Lucia CJ, Ferry GD, McDuffie A, Watson K, Tsou M, Gilger MA. Repeat endoscopy affects patient management in pediatric inflammatory bowel disease. Am J Gastroenterol. 2009;104(3):722–7. doi:10.1038/ajg.2008.111.
24. Van Assche G, Dignass A, Reinisch W, van der Woude CJ, Sturm A, De Vos M, Lindsay J. The second European evidence-based consensus on the diagnosis and management of Crohn's disease: special situations. J Crohns Colitis. 2010;4(1):63–101. doi:10.1016/j.crohns.2009.09.009.
25. Yao T, Matsui T, Hiwatashi N. Crohn's disease in Japan: diagnostic criteria and epidemiology. Dis Colon Rectum. 2000;43(10 Suppl):S85–93.
26. Yokota K, Saito Y, Einami K, Ayabe T, Shibata Y, Tanabe H, Kohgo Y. A bamboo joint-like appearance of the gastric body and cardia: possible association with Crohn's disease. Gastrointest Endosc. 1997;46(3):268–72.

Differential Diagnosis: Intestinal Behçet's Disease

3

Jae Jun Park, Jae Hee Cheon, and Won Ho Kim

3.1 Clinical Features

Behçet's disease (BD) is a chronic relapsing multisystemic vasculitic disorder characterized by recurrent oral and genital ulcers, ocular lesions, skin manifestations, arthritis, as well as vascular, neurologic, and intestinal involvement. The prevalence of BD is higher in the Middle and East Asia than in Western countries. Intestinal BD is a specific subtype of BD, characterized by intestinal ulcers and associated gastrointestinal symptoms. The frequency of GI involvement varies depending on geographic location, ranging from 3 to 50 % [3]. Symptomatic or documented intestinal involvement is rare in Mediterranean patients with BD, whereas it is common in East Asian countries including Korea and Japan. The most frequently affected site is the ileocecal region, and common clinical symptoms include abdominal pain, diarrhea, and bleeding. Although the diagnosis of systemic BD is usually made according to the criteria suggested by the Behçet's Disease Research Committee of Japan or the International Study Group for Behçet's Disease, adequate diagnosis of intestinal BD using these criteria is limited due to various extraintestinal manifestations that emerge at different time points throughout the disease course. Therefore, novel diagnostic criteria for intestinal BD were recently proposed, which may be particularly useful in patients with ileocolonic ulcers that do not fully satisfy the diagnostic criteria for systemic BD (Fig. 3.1) [4]. Histologic findings of intestinal BD are generally nonspecific, showing lymphocytic or neutrophilic infiltration rather than vasculitis (Fig. 3.2).

Similar to inflammatory bowel disease (IBD), including Crohn's disease and ulcerative colitis, intestinal BD exhibits a fluctuating disease course with repeated episodes of relapse and remission. As a result, the primary goals of intestinal BD management are induction and maintenance of symptom remission to minimize recurrences, surgical procedures, and irreversible bowel damage. Medical treatment of intestinal BD is largely empirical since well-controlled studies have been difficult to perform due to the heterogeneity and rarity of the disease [2]. To date, 5-aminosalicylic acids, systemic corticosteroids, and immunomodulators have been used anecdotally to treat intestinal BD. Regarding prognostic factors of intestinal BD, several clinical variables including younger age, higher disease activity at the time of diagnosis, volcano-type ulcers, absence of mucosal healing, higher C-reactive protein level, history of surgery, and lack of initial response to medical therapy have been repeatedly shown as poor prognosticators in patients with intestinal BD [6].

J.J. Park, MD, PhD (✉) • J.H. Cheon, MD, PhD (✉)
W.H. Kim, MD, PhD
Department of Internal Medicine, Institute of Gastroenterology,
Yonsei University College of Medicine,
50-1 Yonsei-ro, Seodaemun-gu, Seoul 120-752, South Korea
e-mail: jaejpark@yuhs.ac; geniushee@yuhs.ac

W.H. Kim, J.H. Cheon (eds.), *Atlas of Inflammatory Bowel Diseases*,
DOI 10.1007/978-3-642-39423-2_3, © Springer-Verlag Berlin Heidelberg 2015

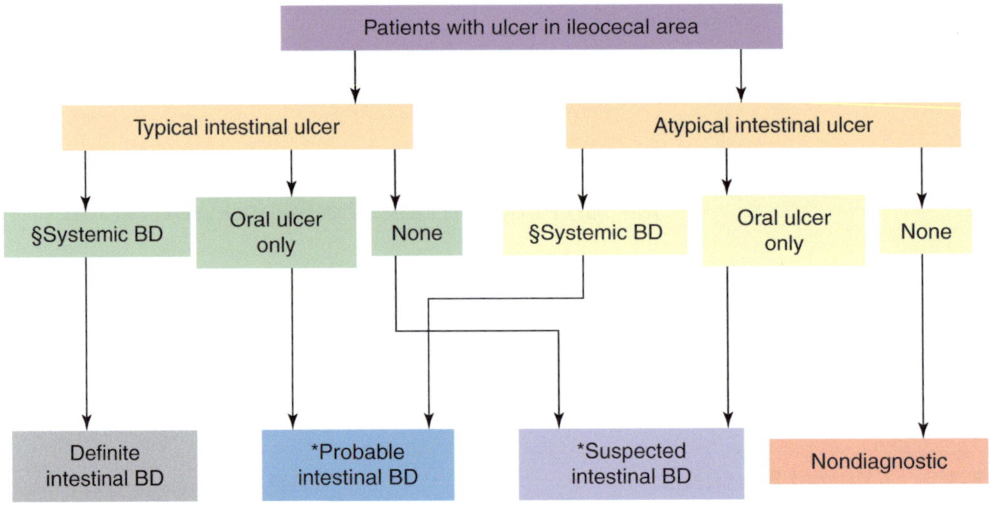

Fig. 3.1 Algorithm for the diagnosis of intestinal Behçet's disease (BD) based on the type of ileocolonic ulcerations and clinical manifestations (Adapted from Cheon et al. [4]). §Complete, incomplete, and suspected subtypes of systemic BD were classified according to the diagnostic criteria of the Research Committee of Japan. *Close follow-up is necessary

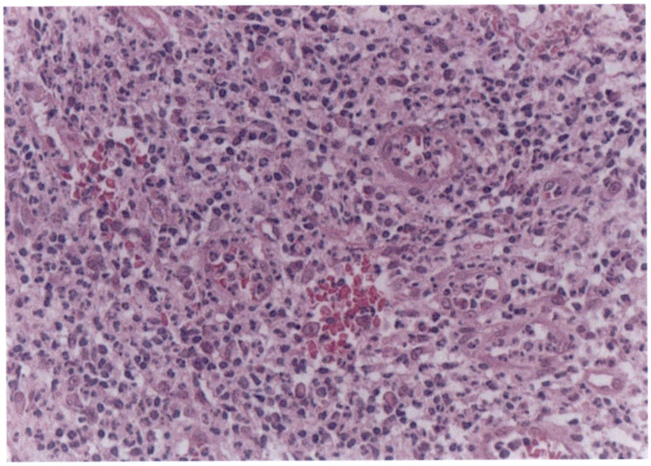

Fig. 3.2 Microscopic examination from ulcers of the colon showed inflammatory infiltration consisting of lymphocytic or neutrophilic infiltration accompanying vasculitis (H&E stain, ×200)

3.2 Endoscopic Findings

Although the ileocecal area is the most common site (80–95 %) of intestinal BD involvement, it can affect any site of gastrointestinal tract, from oral cavity to anus [3, 5]. The locations of ulcers in intestinal BD are depicted in Fig. 3.3. Esophageal involvement is quite uncommon (less than 5 %), and it usually involves the middle part of the esophagus (Fig. 3.4) [3]. Moreover, the stomach is the least frequently involved part of the gastrointestinal tract (Fig. 3.5). Usually, the number of ulcers is one (60–65 %) or several (Fig. 3.5); however, diffuse involvement can occasionally be present. Although the size of ulcer can vary from small to large size, patients with intestinal BD usually have relatively large ulcers (70–80 % of patient have more than 1 cm-sized ulcers). When the ulcer was small, it appears like an aphthous lesion or small well-demarcated circular or oval-shaped ulcer with normal adjacent mucosa (Fig. 3.6). As the size of ulcer increase, deeply penetrating ulcer which is "typical" to intestinal BD is formed; however, the ulcer shape is maintained with circular or oval shape with discrete, elevated margin, and the ulcer base is covered with whitish, thick exudate (Fig. 3.7). These intestinal BD ulcers can cause clinical complications such as bleeding (Fig. 3.8) or perforation. Meanwhile, irregular-shaped ulcers can present in patients with intestinal BD (Fig. 3.9). As mentioned above, ulcer type has a prognostic implication for patients with intestinal BD, and intestinal BD ulcers showing large, well-demarcated nodular margins, deeply penetrating feature, are known as a "volcano-type" ulcer (Fig. 3.10), and patients having these type ulcers show less favorable response to medical treatment, a more frequent requirement for surgery, and more frequent relapse [6, 7]. Ileocecal valve deformity can be seen due to shrinkage of adjacent mucosa by inflammatory or scaring change (Fig. 3.11). In addition, luminal stricture can be seen in active stage (Fig. 3.12). Various findings of healing of ulcerative lesions after medical therapy are presented in Fig. 3.13. During the disease course of intestinal BD, a substantial number of patients eventually undergo bowel resective surgery due to complications or medically refractory diseases. After surgery, intriguingly, most recurrences occur at the anastomotic site or within the vicinity of the site (Fig. 3.14).

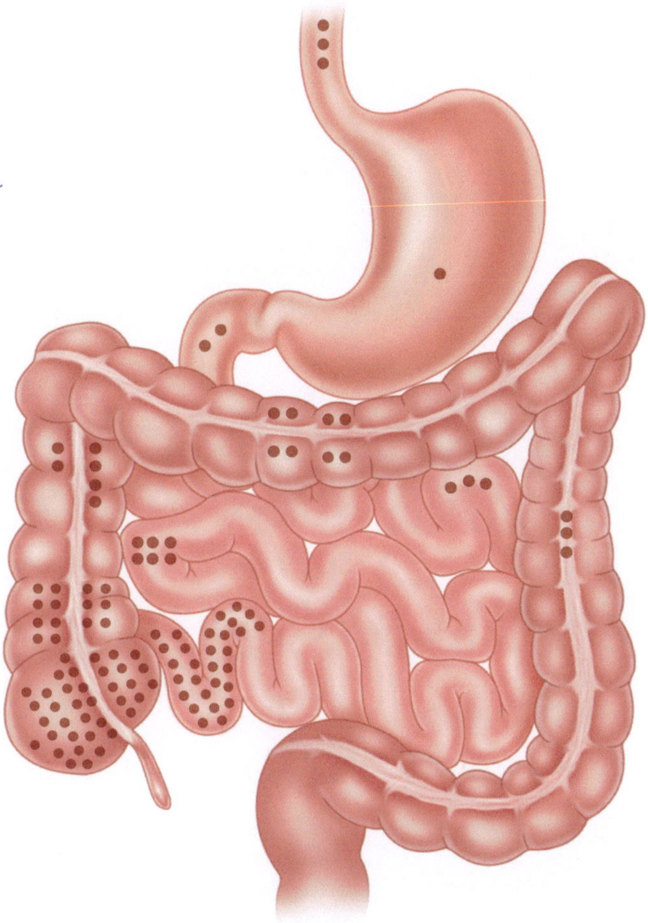

Fig. 3.3 Location of ulcers in intestinal BD (Adapted from Kasahara et al. [1])

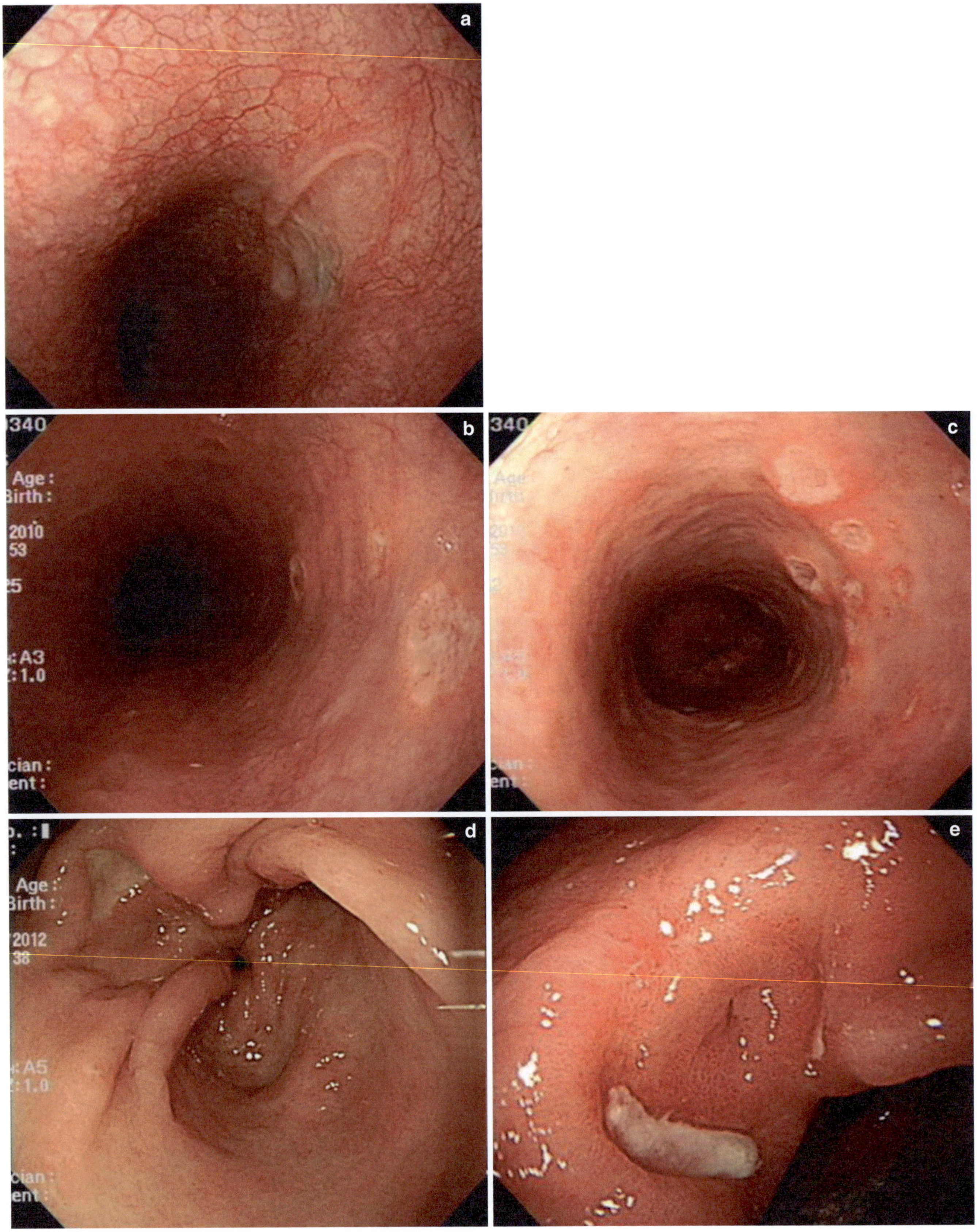

Fig. 3.4 Upper gastrointestinal involvement in intestinal BD. (**a**) An oval-shaped mid-esophageal ulcer with discrete margin. (**b**) Several shallow ulcers in the mid-esophagus. (**c**) The number of esophageal ulcers (figure **b**) is increased on follow-up endoscopy after 2 years. (**d**). A well-defined active ulcer in the gastric antrum. The lesion was suspected for gastric involvement of intestinal BD. (**e**) Although the previous ulcer (figure **d**) is healed, another active ulcer is noted after 1 year

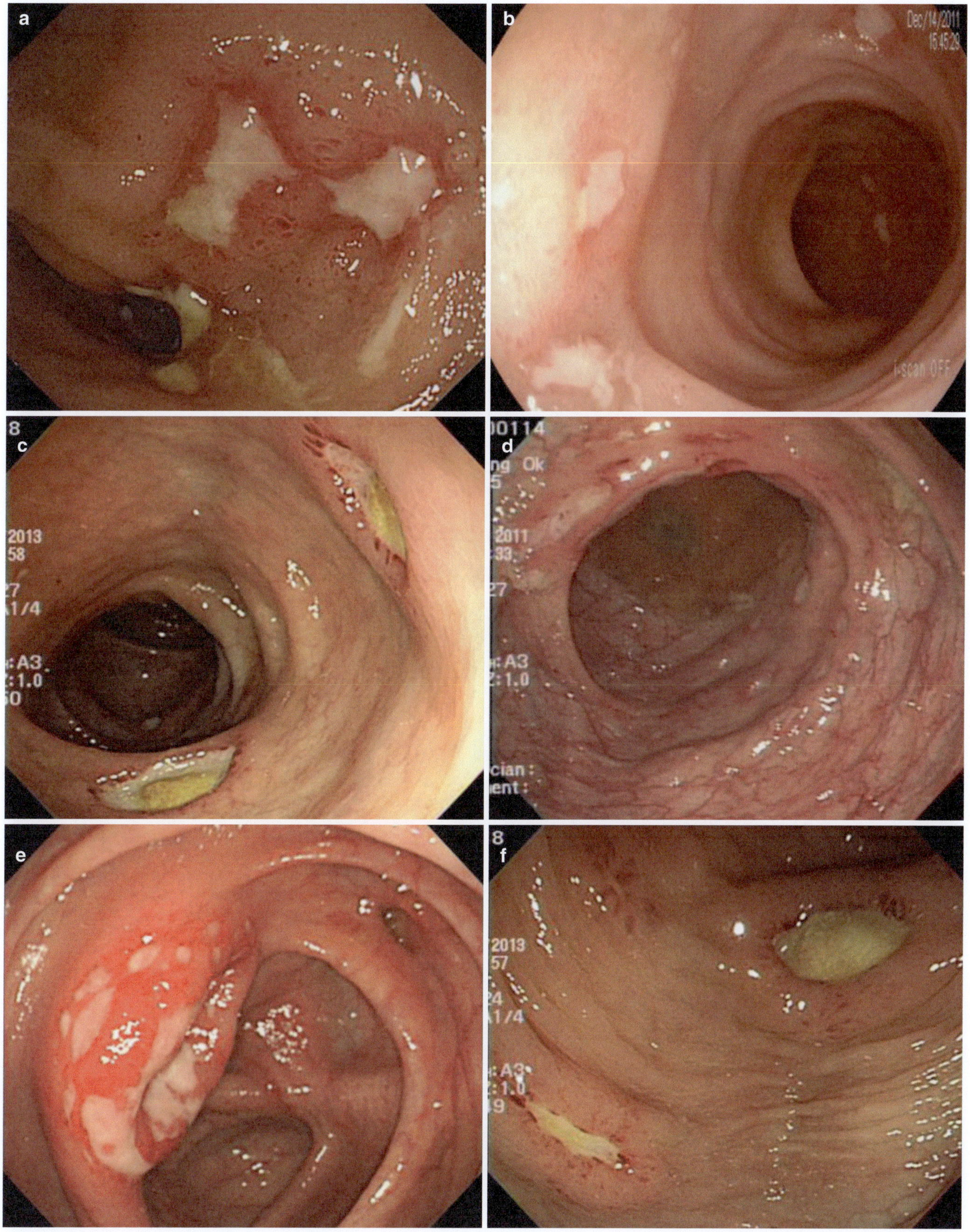

Fig. 3.5 Multiple ulcers in intestinal BD. (**a**) Multiple active ulcers with irregular margin in the terminal ileum. (**b**) Multiple irregular-shaped small ulcers in the terminal ileum. (**c**) Multiple circular-shaped ulcers with yellowish exudate in the transverse colon. (**d**) Multiple small ulcers and aphthous lesions in the ileocecal area. (**e**) Multiple active ulcers accompanying erythematous mucosa in the ileocecal valve. (**f**) Oval-shaped ulcers in the descending colon

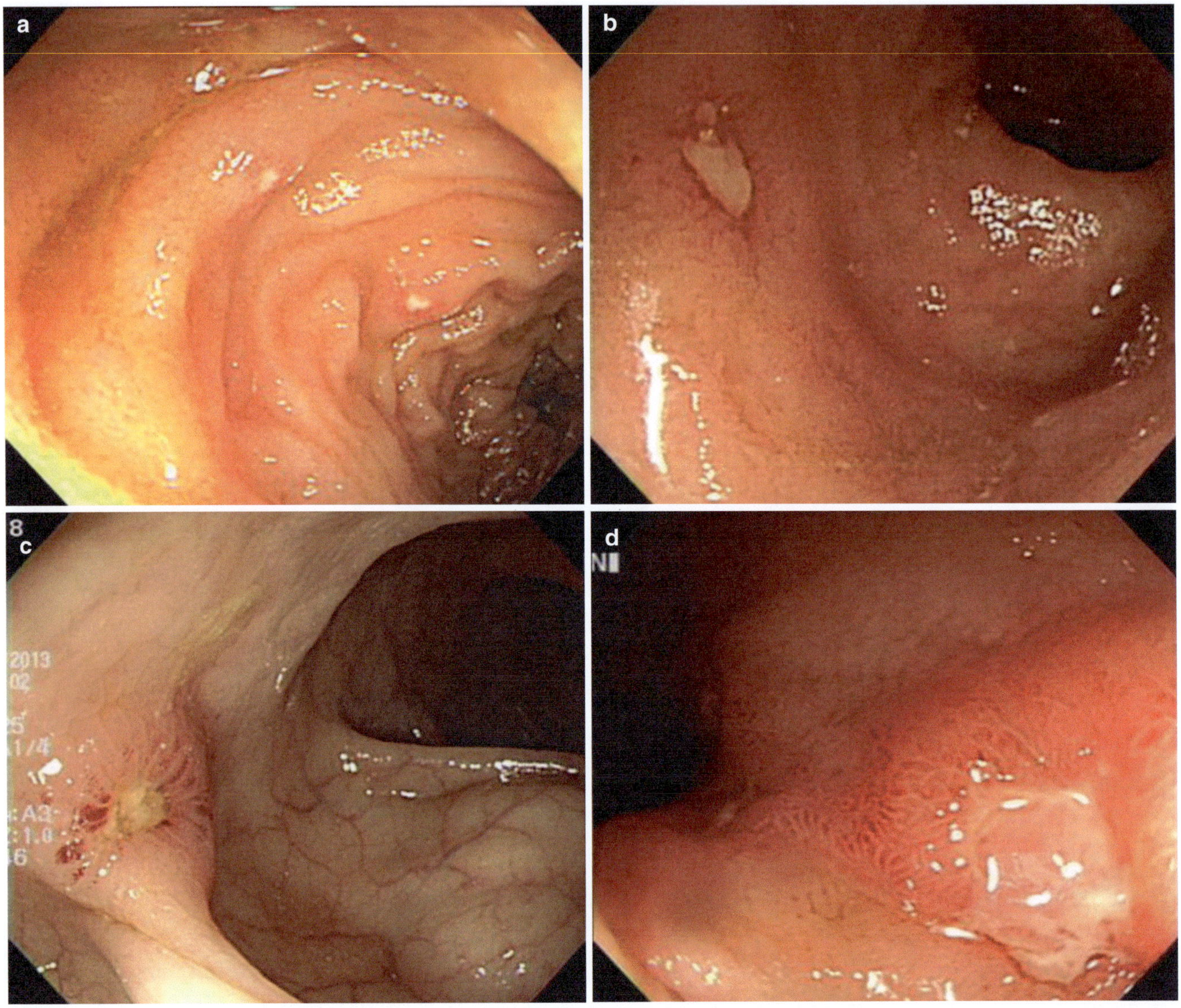

Fig. 3.6 Small ulcers in intestinal BD. (**a**) Two aphthous lesions in the terminal ileum. (**b**) A small oval-shaped ulcer in the terminal ileum. (**c**) A small circular-shaped ulcer in the sigmoid colon. (**d**) A small ulcer in the terminal ileum. (**e**) A small irregular-shaped ulcer in the ileocecal valve. (**f**) A circular-shaped small ulcer in the ileocecal valve. (**g**) A small oval-shaped ulcer in the terminal ileum. (**h**) Several circular-shaped ulcers covered with whitish exudate in the transverse colon

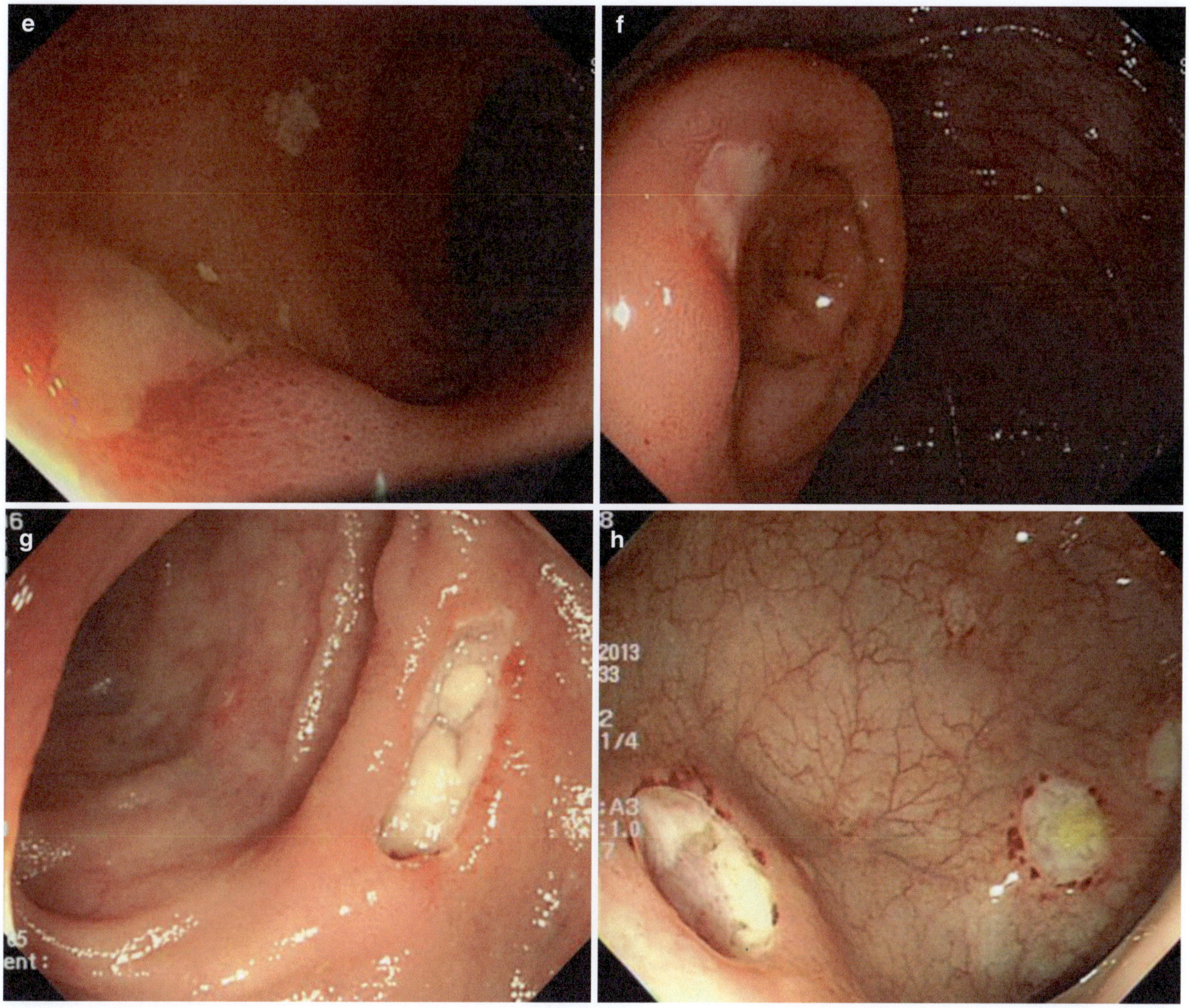

Fig. 3.6 (continued)

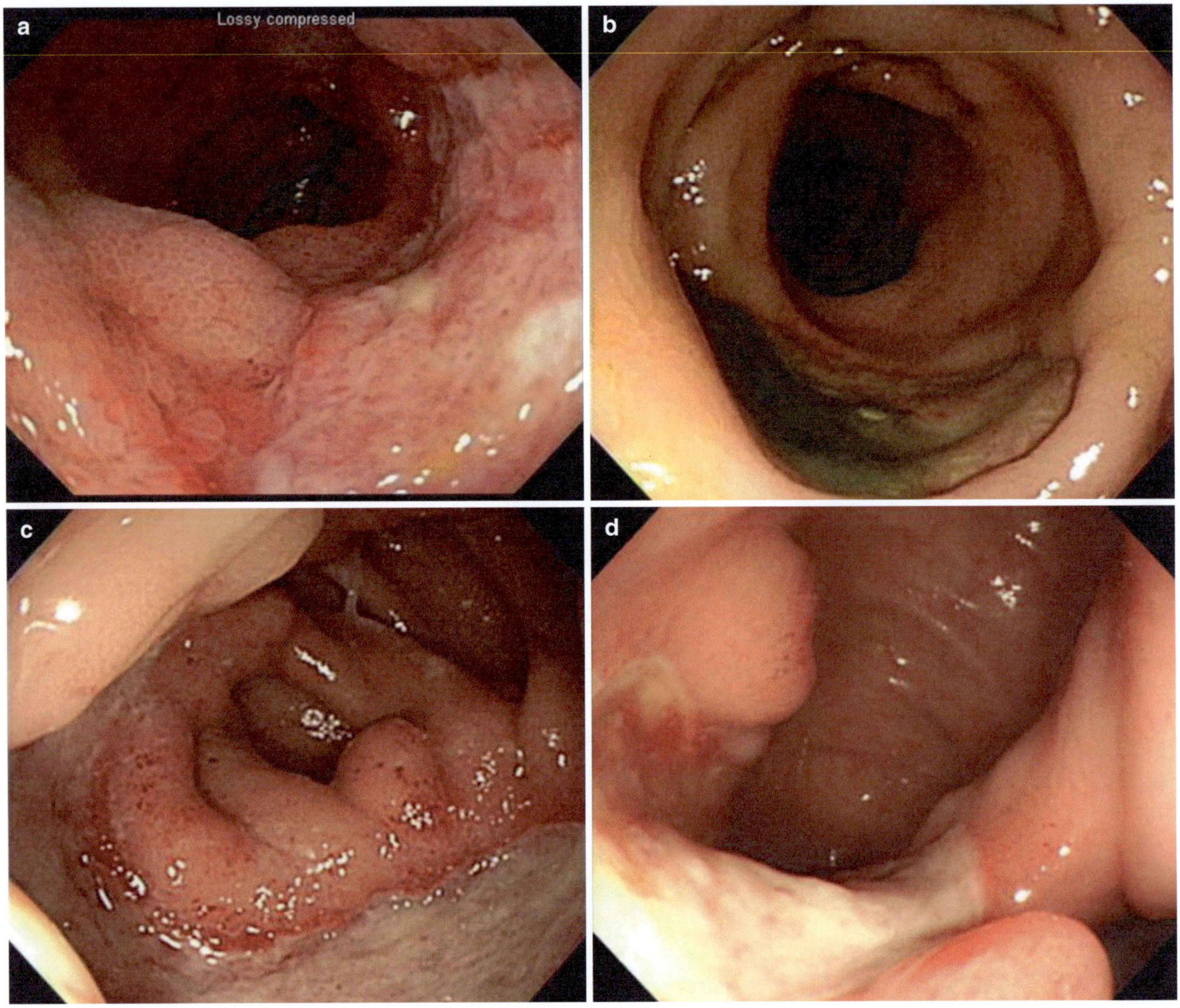

Fig. 3.7 Typical intestinal ulcers in intestinal BD. (**a**) A large deep ulcer in the terminal ileum. (**b**) A round-shaped ulcer with discrete border in the transverse colon. (**c**) A large deep round-shaped cecal ulcer accompanying sharply demarcated, elevated border and whitish thick exudate. (**d**) A large round-shaped cecal ulcer with discrete margin. (**e**) A huge active ulcer with elevated margin is located over the ileocecal valve and proximal ascending colon. (**f**) A deep round shaped ulcer covered with thick exudate in the terminal ileum. The lesion accompanied by the ileocecal valve stricture preventing colonoscope passage

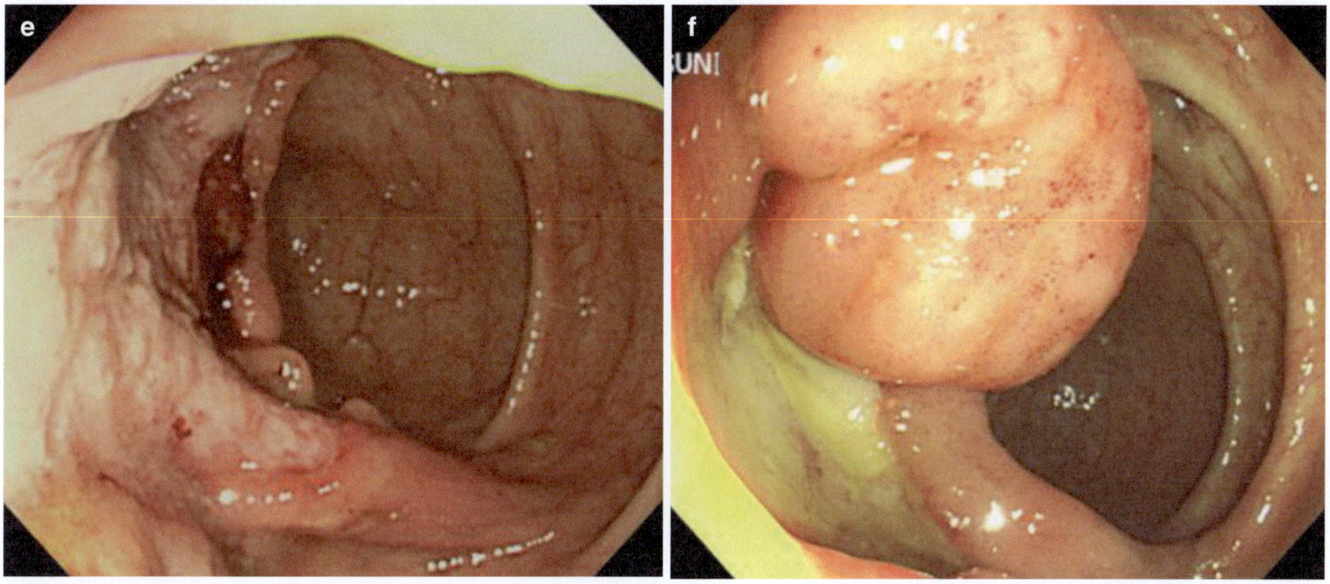

Fig. 3.7 (continued)

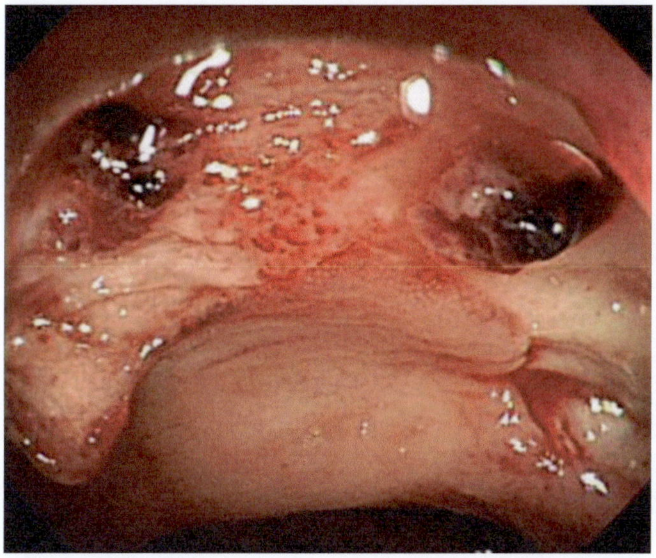

Fig. 3.8 Active ulcers in a patient with intestinal BD presented with hematochezia. An active cecal ulcer with two visible vessels

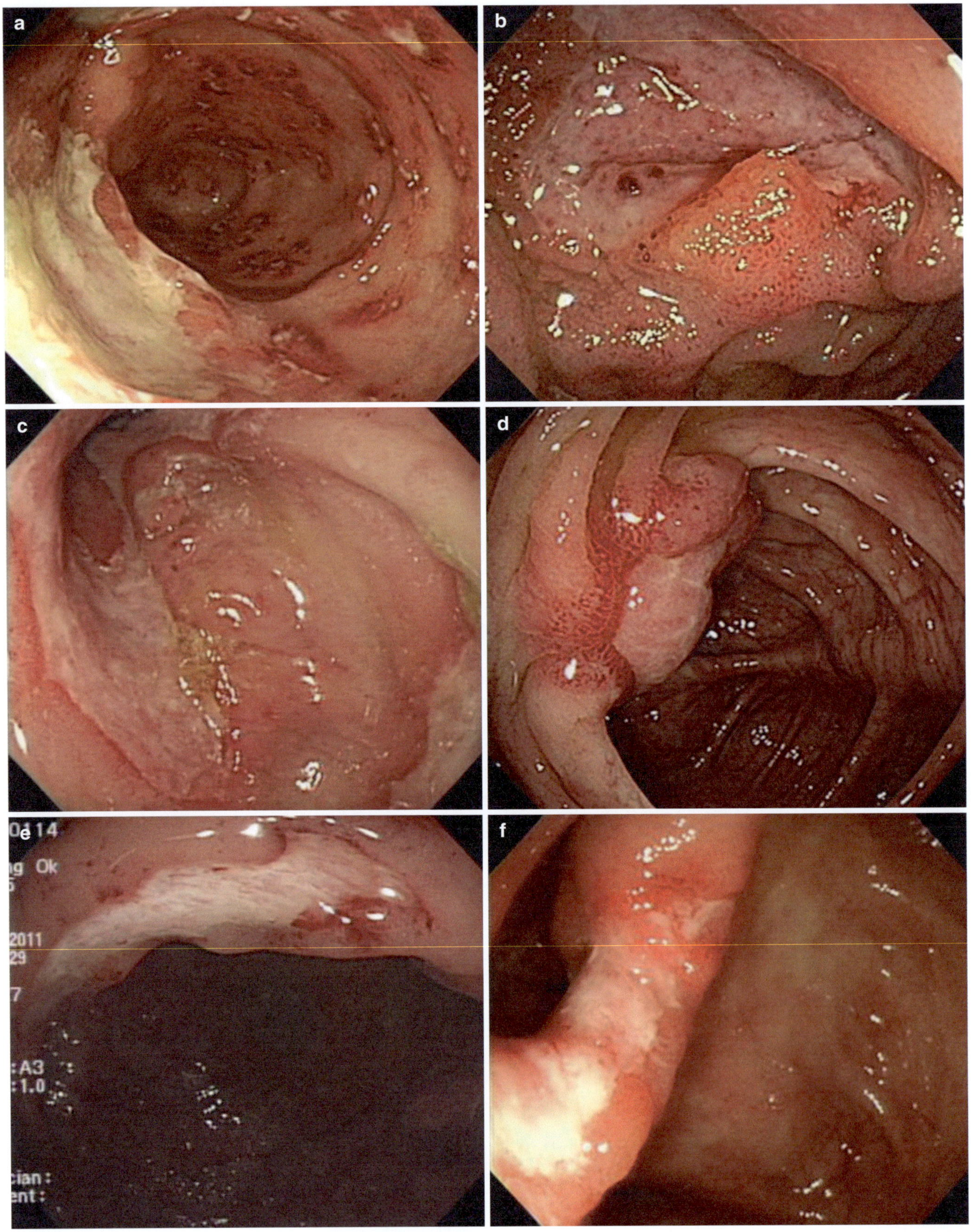

Fig. 3.9 Irregular-shaped ulcers in intestinal BD. (**a**) A large active ulcer covered with thick whitish exudate accompanying geographic margin in the proximal ascending colon. Multiple aphthous lesions are also shown in the ileocecal area. (**b**) An irregular-shaped ulcer in the terminal ileum. (**c**) A geographic-shaped ulcer in the transverse colon. (**d**) An ileocecal ulcer with irregular erythematous border. (**e**) A circumferential-shaped active ulcer. (**f**) An ulcer in the ileocecal valve with ill-defined margin

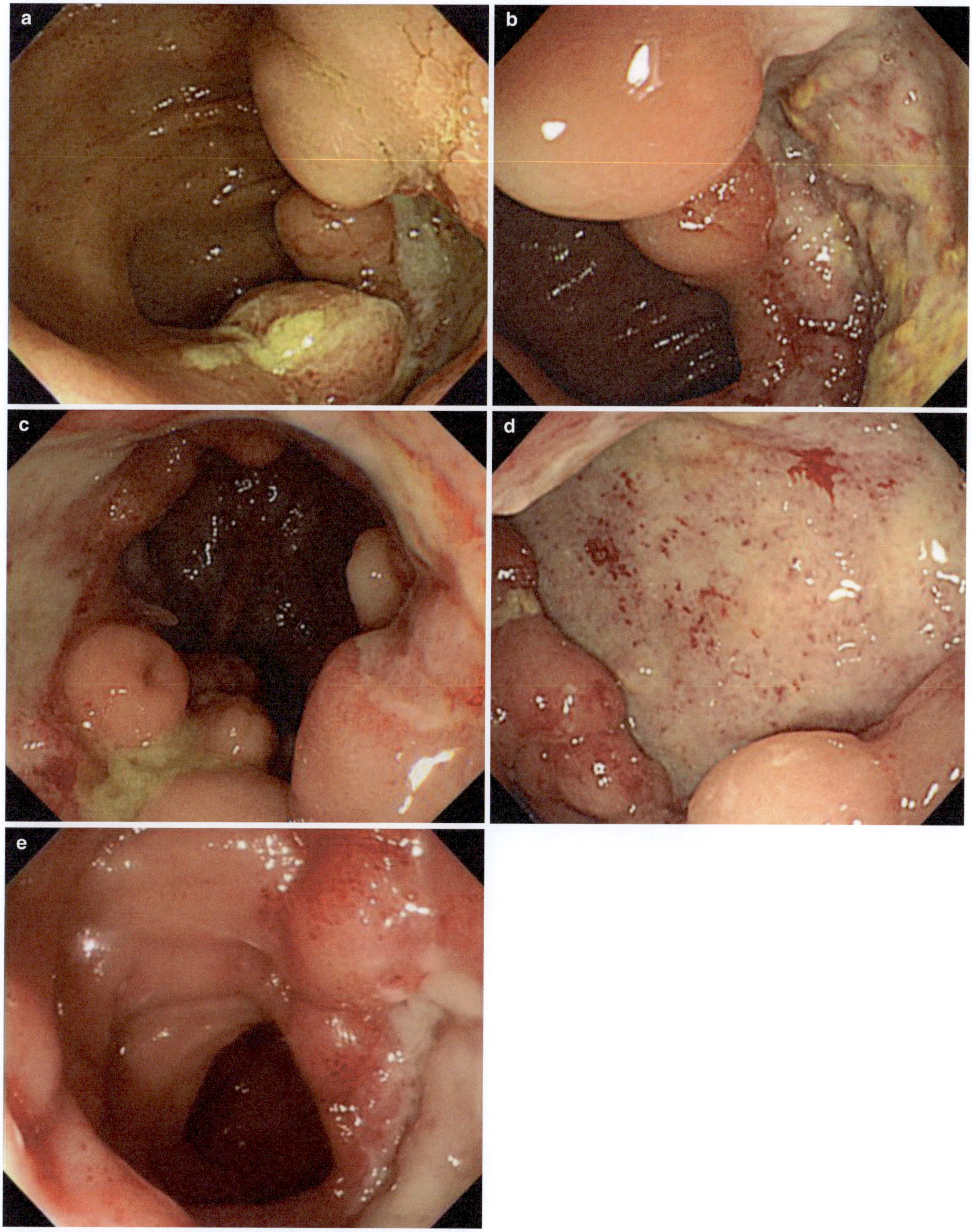

Fig. 3.10 Volcano-type ulcers in intestinal BD. (**a**) A deep penetrating ulcer with nodular margins in the terminal ileum. (**b**) A deep penetrating circular-shaped ulcer in the terminal ileum. (**c**) A huge cecal ulcer accompanying nodular margins and whitish surface exudate. (**d**) A large cecal ulcer with nodular border and whitish exudate. (**e**) A deep terminal ileal ulcer with nodular erythematous margin

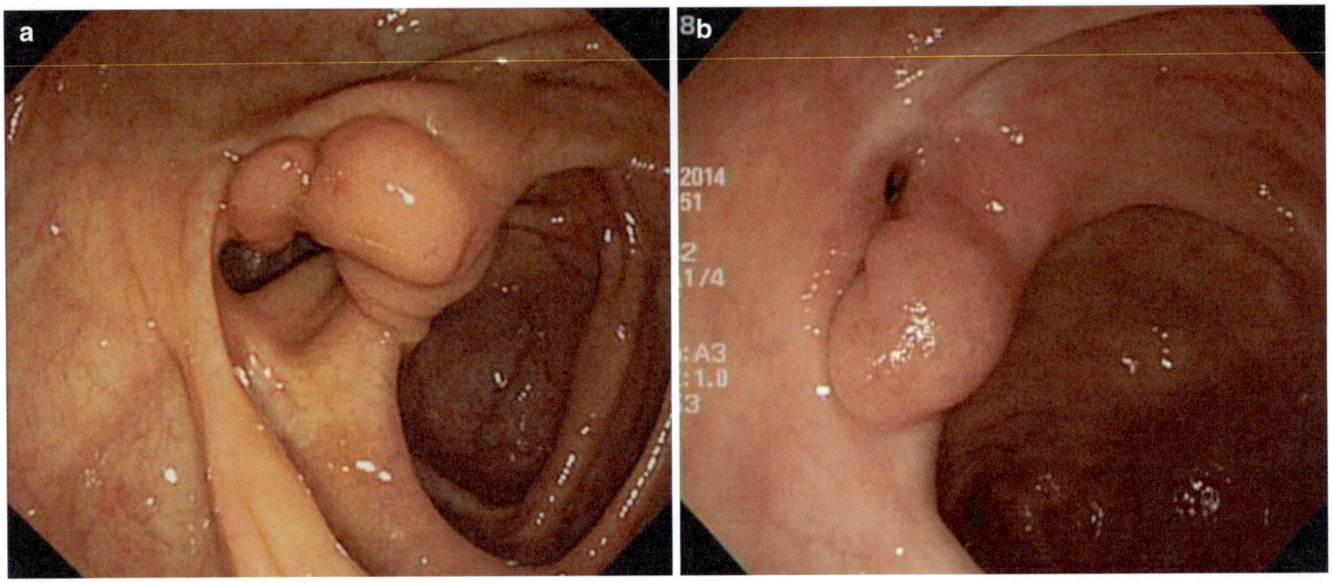

Fig. 3.11 Ileocecal valve deformities in intestinal BD. (**a**) Fixed opening of ileocecal valve with scaring change is noted. (**b**) Scaring change with ileocecal valve stricture

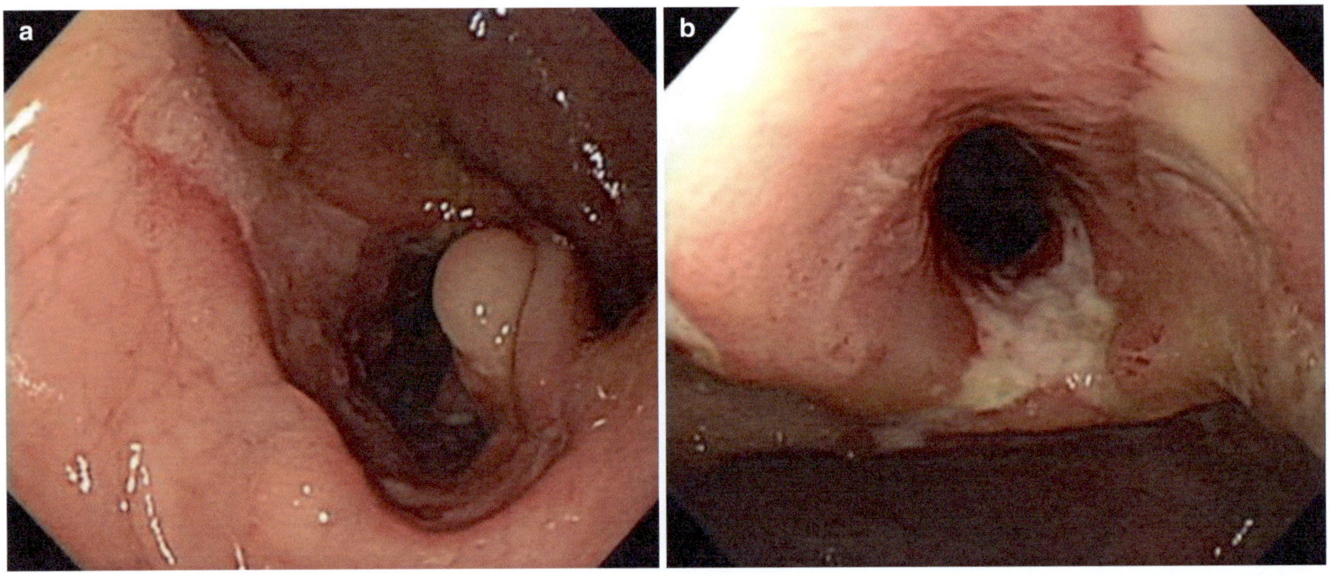

Fig. 3.12 Stricture in intestinal BD. (**a**) Irregular-shaped ulcer with luminal stricture in the transverse colon. (**b**) Luminal stricture with active ulcer in the splenic flexure

Fig. 3.13 Various findings of healing of active ulcers after medical treatment. (**a**) Several active ulcers are noted in the ileocecal area. (**b**) Active ulcers (Figure **a**) are healed into scar after 1 year of medical treatment. (**c**) A huge deep penetrating ulcer showing nodular ulcer base in the cecum. Multiple circular-shaped ulcers are also seen in the vicinity. (**d**) After 6 months of immunomodulator therapy, a huge ulcer (figure **c**) is substantially improved into shallow ulcers. (**e**) A deep active ulcer in the ileocecal valve. (**f**) After 10 months of medical therapy, the active ulcer (figure **e**) is completely healed into scar. (**g**) A small active ulcer is observed in the ileocecal valve. (**h**) The active ulcer (figure **g**) is completely healed after 6 months of medical therapy. (**i**) An irregularly bordered active ulcer in the terminal ileum. (**j**) After 1 year of medical treatment, the active ulcer (figure **i**) is completely healed into scar. (**k**) A small circular-shaped ulcer in the terminal ileum. (**l**) After 3 year, the small ulcer (figure **k**) is aggravated into a large deep ulcer with nodular margin

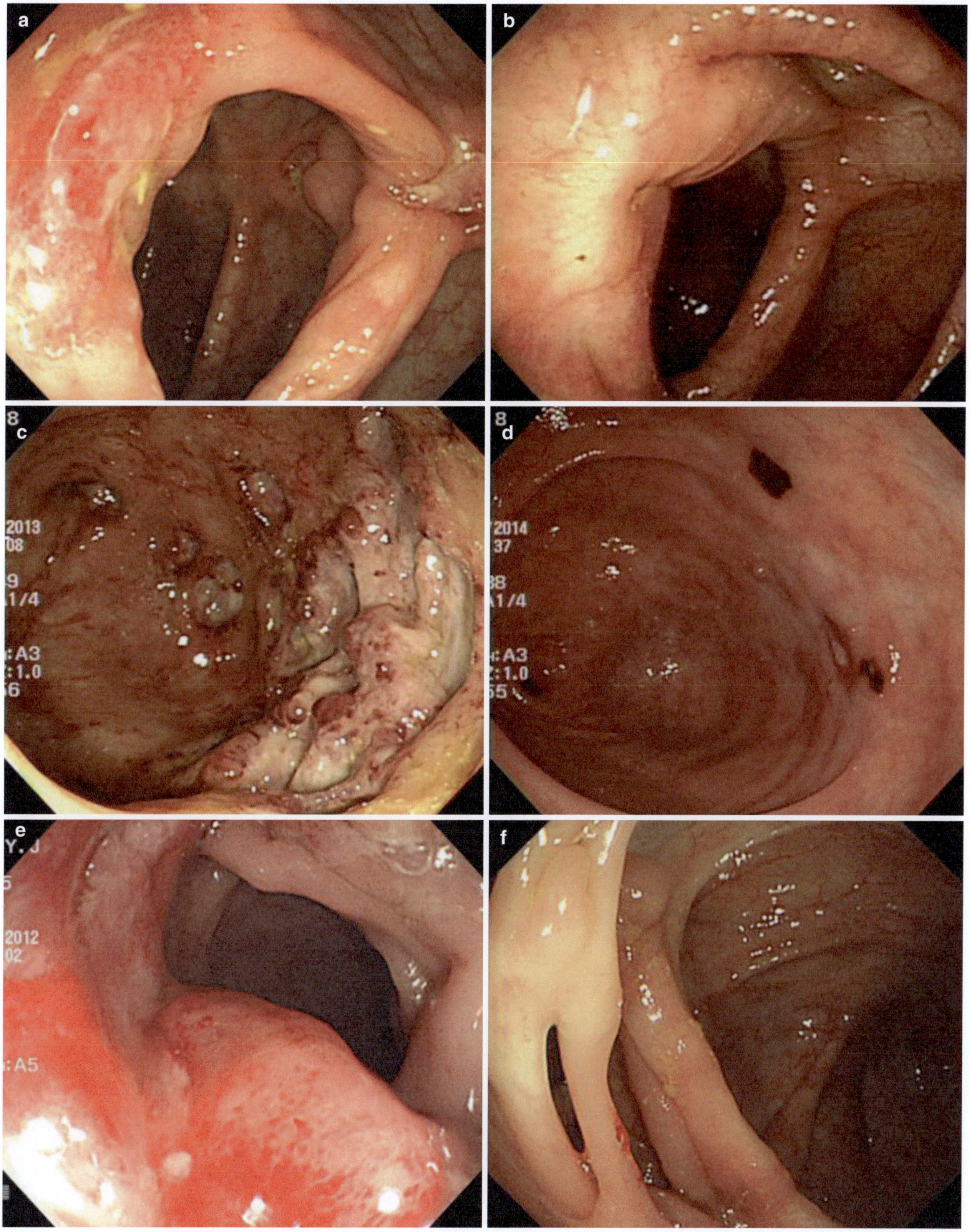
a
b
c
d
e
f

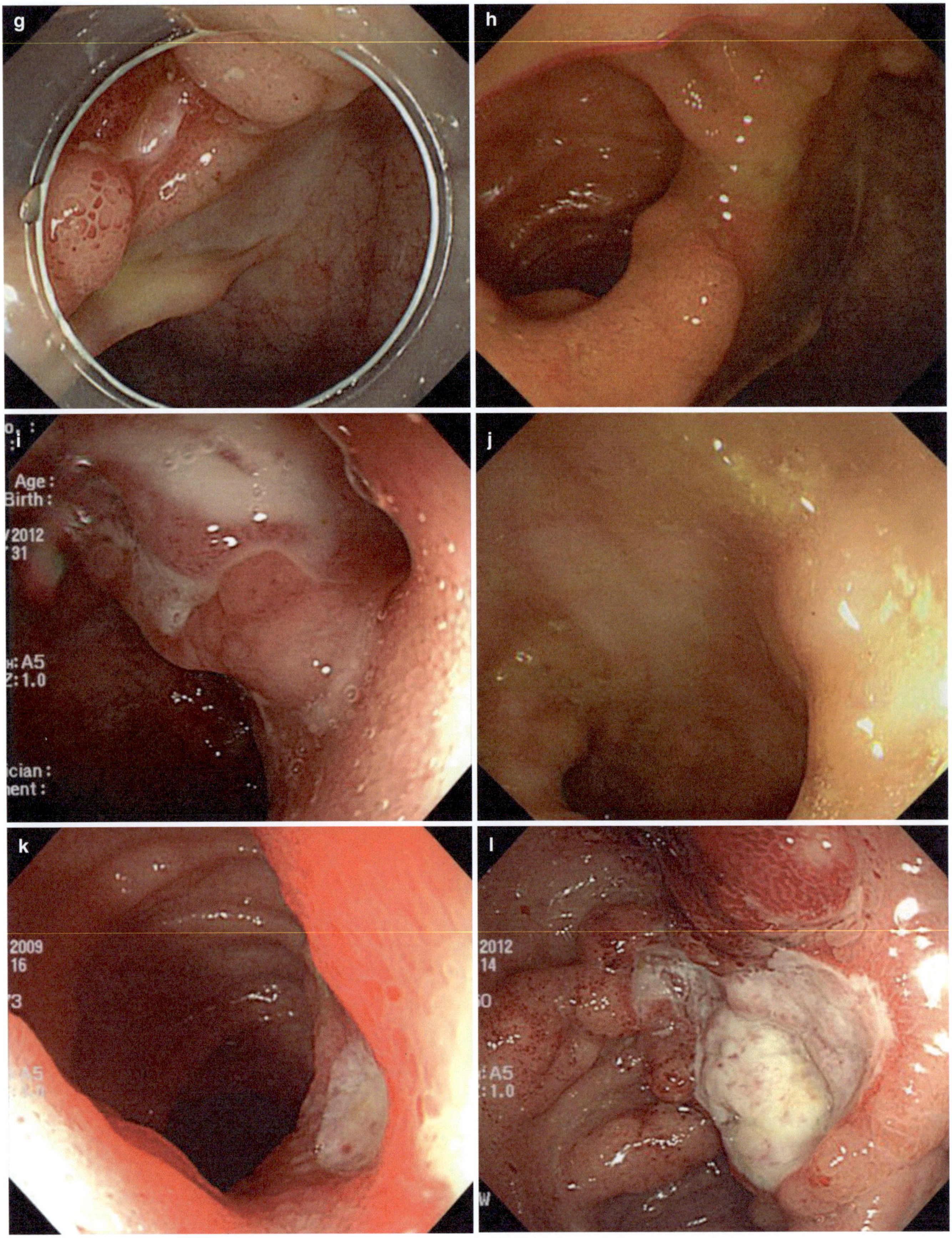

Fig. 3.13 (continued)

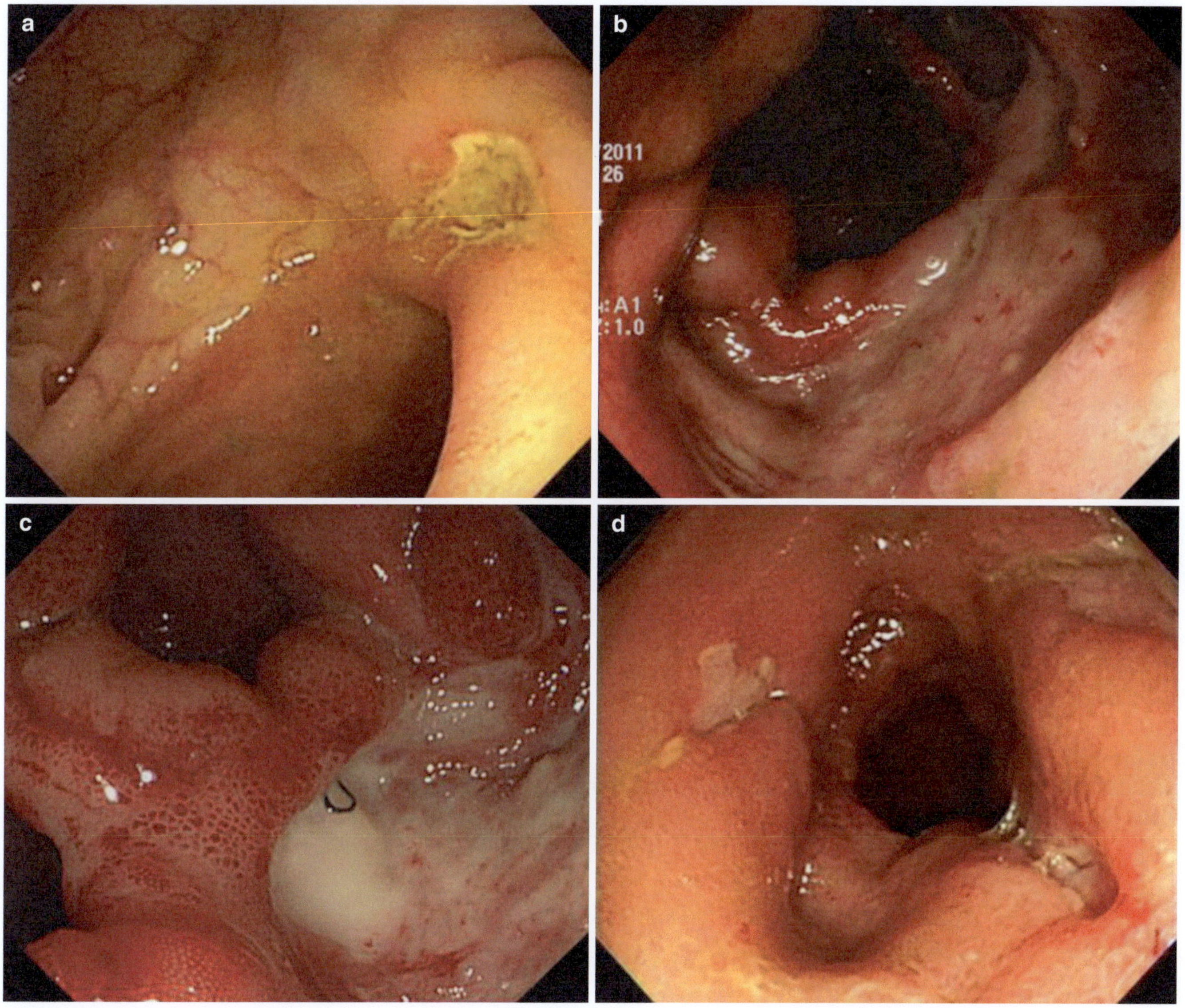

Fig. 3.14 Postoperative endoscopic recurrence in intestinal BD. (**a**) A small active ulcer is noted at the anastomotic site in an intestinal BD patient after right hemicolectomy. (**b**) A huge active ulcer is observed at the anastomotic site in an intestinal BD patient who underwent right hemicolectomy. (**c**) A deeply penetrating discrete ulcer at the anastomotic site after ileocecectomy. (**d**) Variable-shaped multiple active ulcers are noted in the neo-terminal ileum in a patient with intestinal BD who underwent right hemicolectomy

3.3 Endoscopic Differential Diagnosis

Despite the typical findings of intestinal BD, the appropriate differential diagnosis of intestinal BD and other intestinal diseases especially those with Crohn's disease (CD) can be problematic in some cases. Therefore, clinicians should make diagnosis after full consideration of clinical, endoscopic, and pathologic findings and long-term follow-up can occasionally be needed for definite differentiation. For proper differentiations between intestinal BD and CD, endoscopic features of ulcers and its distribution can be informative (Table 3.1) [8]. Regarding distribution pattern, diffuse or segmental involvement is more frequent in CD than in intestinal BD. Meanwhile, localized focal involvement is more frequent in intestinal BD than in CD. Moreover, unlike in CD, anorectal involvement is rare in intestinal BD. With respect to the number of ulcers, intestinal BD usually has single or several number of ulcers; on the other hand, CD commonly presents with multiple ulcers. Ulcers of intestinal BD are usually larger, deeper, and more obviously demarcated than those of CD. In addition, longitudinal ulcers and cobblestonings which are occasionally shown in CD are rare in intestinal BD. A simple distinguishing strategy including two endoscopic characteristics including ulcer shape (round, irregular/geographical, longitudinal) and distribution of lesion (focal single/focal multiple, segmental/diffuse) has been proposed, yielding 92 % of correct diagnosis either intestinal BD or CD on internal validation cohort (Fig. 3.15) [8].

Table 3.1 Differential features between intestinal BD and Crohn's disease

Endoscopic findings	Intestinal Behçet's disease	Crohn's disease
Anorectal involvement	Rare	Common
Ulcer		
Distribution	Mainly ileocecal area	More wide distribution other than ileocecal area
Number	1 ~ several	Several ~ multiple
Size	Usually large	Various
Shape	Round, oval	Longitudinal, various shape
Border	Discrete, elevated	Relatively irregular

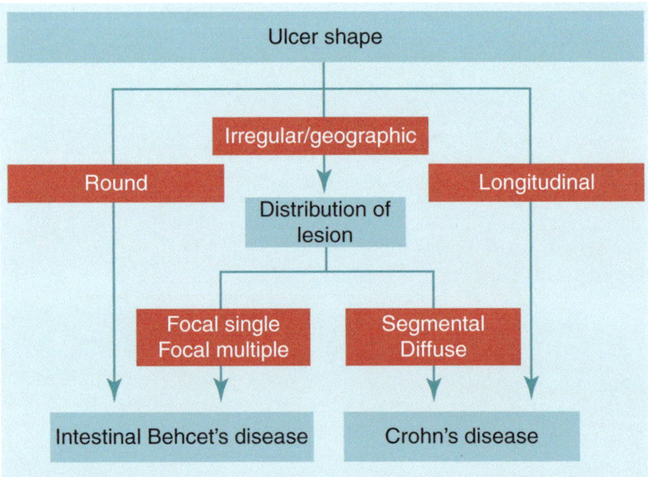

Fig. 3.15 The simple decision tree model for endoscopic differentiations between intestinal BD and Crohn's disease (Adapted from Lee et al. [8])

References

1. Kasahara Y, Tanaka S, Nishino M, Umemura H, Shiraha S, Kuyama T. Intestinal involvement in Behçet's disease: review of 136 surgical cases in the Japanese literature. Dis Colon Rectum. 1981;24:103–6.
2. Kobayashi K, Ueno F, Bito S, Iwao Y, Fukushima T, Hiwatashi N, et al. Development of consensus statements for the diagnosis and management of intestinal Behçet's disease using a modified Delphi approach. J Gastroenterol. 2007;42:737–45.
3. Ebert EC. Gastrointestinal manifestations of Behçet's disease. Dig Dis Sci. 2009;54:201–7.
4. Cheon JH, Kim ES, Shin SJ, Kim TI, Lee KM, Kim SW, Kim JS, Kim YS, Choi CH, Ye BD, Yang SK, Choi EH, Kim WH. Development and validation of novel diagnostic criteria for intestinal Behçet's disease in Korean patients with ileocolonic ulcers. Am J Gastroenterol. 2009;104:2492–9.
5. Lee CR, Kim WH, Cho YS, Kim MH, Kim JH, Park IS, et al. Colonoscopic findings in intestinal Behçet's disease. Inflamm Bowel Dis. 2001;7:243–9.
6. Park JJ, Kim WH, Cheon JH. Outcome predictors for intestinal Behçet's disease. Yonsei Med J. 2013;54:1084–90.
7. Choi IJ, Kim JS, Cha SD, Jung HC, Park JG, Song IS, et al. Long-term clinical course and prognostic factors in intestinal Behçet's disease. Dis Colon Rectum. 2000;43:692–700.
8. Lee SK, Kim BK, Kim TI, Kim WH. Differential diagnosis of intestinal Behçet's disease and Crohn's disease by colonoscopic findings. Endoscopy. 2009;41:9–16.

4 Differential Diagnosis: Intestinal Tuberculosis

Jae Jun Park and Jae Hee Cheon

4.1 Clinical Features

Tuberculosis (TB) is a chronic granulomatous infectious disease caused by *Mycobacterium tuberculosis* (*M. tuberculosis*). The gastrointestinal tract is the sixth most frequent form of extrapulmonary TB (after lymphatic, genitourinary, bone and joint, miliary, and meningeal tuberculosis) [1]. Intestinal TB (ITB) can develop via swallowing infected sputum, hematogenous spread, ingestion of contaminated milk or food, and/or contiguous spread from adjacent organs [3]. The ileocecal region is the most common site of intestinal involvement, likely due to the relative stasis and abundant lymphoid tissue in this region.

The symptoms and signs of ITB are relatively vague and nonspecific. Nonspecific chronic abdominal pain is the most common symptom, occurring in 80–90 % of patients. Anorexia, fatigue, fever, night sweat, weight loss, diarrhea, constipation, or blood in the stool may be present. Moreover, palpable right lower quadrant abdominal mass or ascites also may be observed [1, 2, 3].

A presumptive diagnosis of ITB can be made in the setting of known active pulmonary TB, together with clinical, endoscopic, and/or radiographic findings suggestive of ITB. The definite diagnosis of ITB can be confirmed when caseating granulomas (Fig. 4.13) or acid-fast bacilli (Fig. 4.14) are identified during the histologic examination of colonoscopic biopsy specimens or when *M. tuberculosis* is isolated from the culture of biopsy specimens; however, in real clinical practice, these findings are positive in less than 50 % of patients with ITB. Recently, detection of tubercle bacilli DNA by polymerase chain reaction (PCR) has been reported as a rapid and accurate diagnostic tool for ITB, but application of PCR in clinical settings still requires validation and false-positive results of PCR limit its active use [1]. Because initial definite diagnosis of intestinal TB is not made in a substantial number of patients, an empiric initiation of antituberculous therapy is frequently used for situations in which there is a high index of suspicion for ITB based on clinical, radiographic, and endoscopic findings (in the absence of histological and/or microbiologic confirmation) [8]. Patients with ITB generally demonstrate clinical improvement within 2 weeks on empiric therapy and complete healing of active ulcers and erosions in colonoscopic follow-up after 2–3 months of anti-TB therapy. For nonresponding cases, drug-resistant TB or enteritides other than TB should be considered.

In general, treatment of ITB is similar to that of pulmonary TB, with the combinations of conventional antituberculous chemotherapies (rifampicin, isoniazid, pyrazinamide, and ethambutol) for 2 months, followed by rifampicin, ethambutol, and isoniazid for an additional 4 months. The cure rate after medical treatment exceeds 95 %. Surgery is warranted for patients with complications such as perforation, massive bleeding, and/or high-grade obstruction.

J.J. Park, MD, PhD (✉) • J.H. Cheon, MD, PhD (✉)
Department of Internal Medicine, Institute of Gastroenterology, Yonsei University College of Medicine,
50-1 Yonsei-ro, Seodaemun-gu, Seoul 120-752, South Korea
e-mail: jaejpark@yuhs.ac; geniushee@yuhs.ac

W.H. Kim, J.H. Cheon (eds.), *Atlas of Inflammatory Bowel Diseases*,
DOI 10.1007/978-3-642-39423-2_4, © Springer-Verlag Berlin Heidelberg 2015

4.2 Endoscopic Findings

The ileocecal involvement is observed in the majority (80–90 %) of patients with ITB [5]. In approximately 20 % of cases, segmental colonic involvement occurs in the absence of ileocecal lesions. ITB less commonly involves as head toward left-side colon and rectum or small intestine.

The gross endoscopic findings of intestinal ITB are mainly divided into three groups: ulcerative (60 %) type, characterized by multiple superficial ulcers; hypertrophic type (10 %), characterized by scarring, fibrosis, and pseudotumor lesions; and ulcerohypertrophic type (30 %), characterized by an inflammatory mass around the ileocecal valve with thickened and ulcerated intestinal walls [3]. The ulcers of ITB typically show in a transverse/circumferential orientation relative to the long axis of the gut lumen (Fig. 4.1), and these types of ulcers are identified in 40–60 % of patients with ITB, which is the single most important endoscopic clue for differentiation from Crohn's disease (CD). Additionally, the multiple ulcers occasionally show circumferential arrangement (Fig. 4.2). Besides circumferential ulcers, other types of ulcers including geographic, round, longitudinal, and irregular shape can also be observed (Fig. 4.3). The surrounding mucosa of ulcers is usually inflamed and shows nodular feature. Although small ulcers can be seen in ITB, aphthous lesions are not common (<20 %) (Fig. 4.4). Among the three endoscopic types of ITB, ulcerohypertrophic-type ITB particularly necessitates differential diagnosis with colon cancer (Fig. 4.5). Ileocecal valve deformity can be seen, and ileocecal valve occasionally shows fixed-open or patulous feature due to shrinkage of adjacent mucosa by inflammatory or scarring change (Fig. 4.6). In addition, luminal stricture can be seen in active stage, and this can grow worse or emerge during healing process (Fig. 4.7). Small ulcers can disappear without scar, but most ulcers of ITB remain scarring change after healing (Fig. 4.8). Some scars make diverticulum-like lesion (pseudodiverticulum) (Fig. 4.9). Variable-sized inflammatory polyps are occasionally seen (Fig. 4.10). Diverse findings of healing of ulcerative lesions after antituberculous chemotherapy are shown in Fig. 4.11.

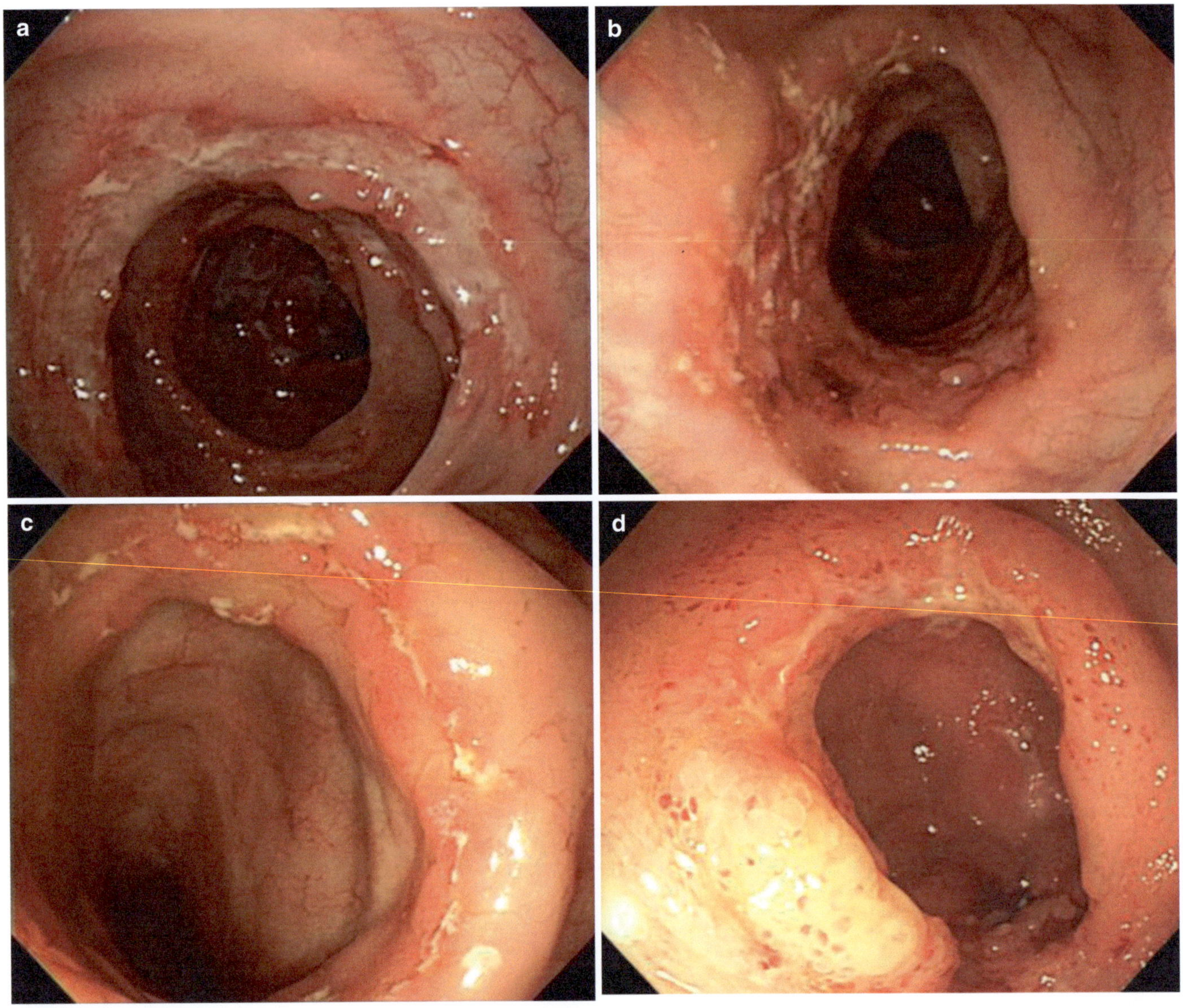

Fig. 4.1 Circumferential-shaped ulcers in ITB. (**a**) Deep transverse ulcer travels colonic lumen about half. (**b**) Wide transverse ulcer encircling colonic lumen. (**c**) Shallow circumferential ulcer encircling colonic lumen is noted. (**d**) Circumferential-shaped ulcer is noted in the terminal ileum

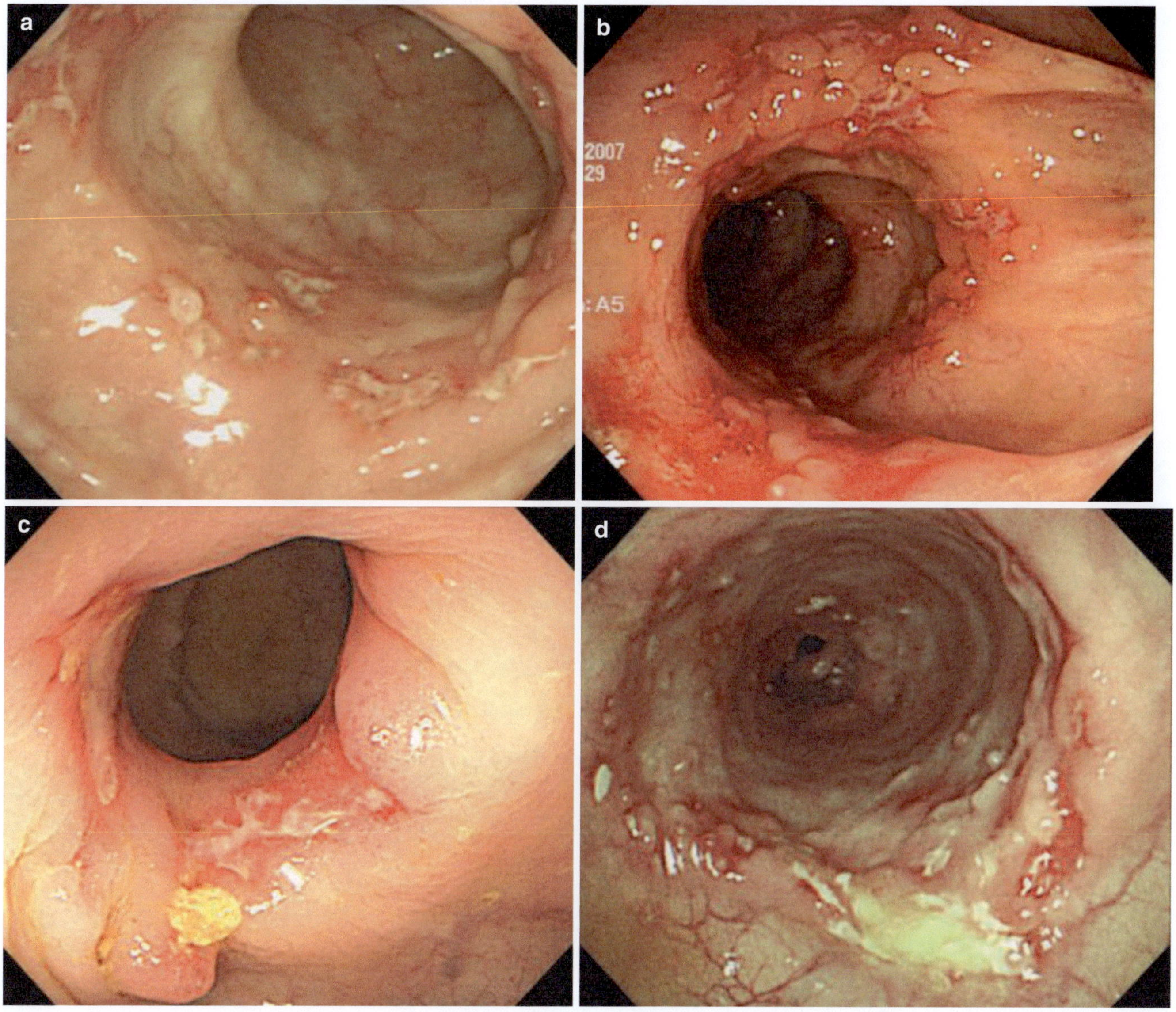

Fig. 4.2 Multiple ulcers with circumferential arrangement. (**a**) Multiple ulcers are arranged in a transverse direction. (**b**) Several active ulcers are arranged in a circular direction accompanying nodular change and hyperemia. (**c**) Two active ulcers are arrayed in a circumferential direction accompanying luminal narrowing. (**d**) Multiple active ulcers are circumferentially positioned encircling colonic lumen

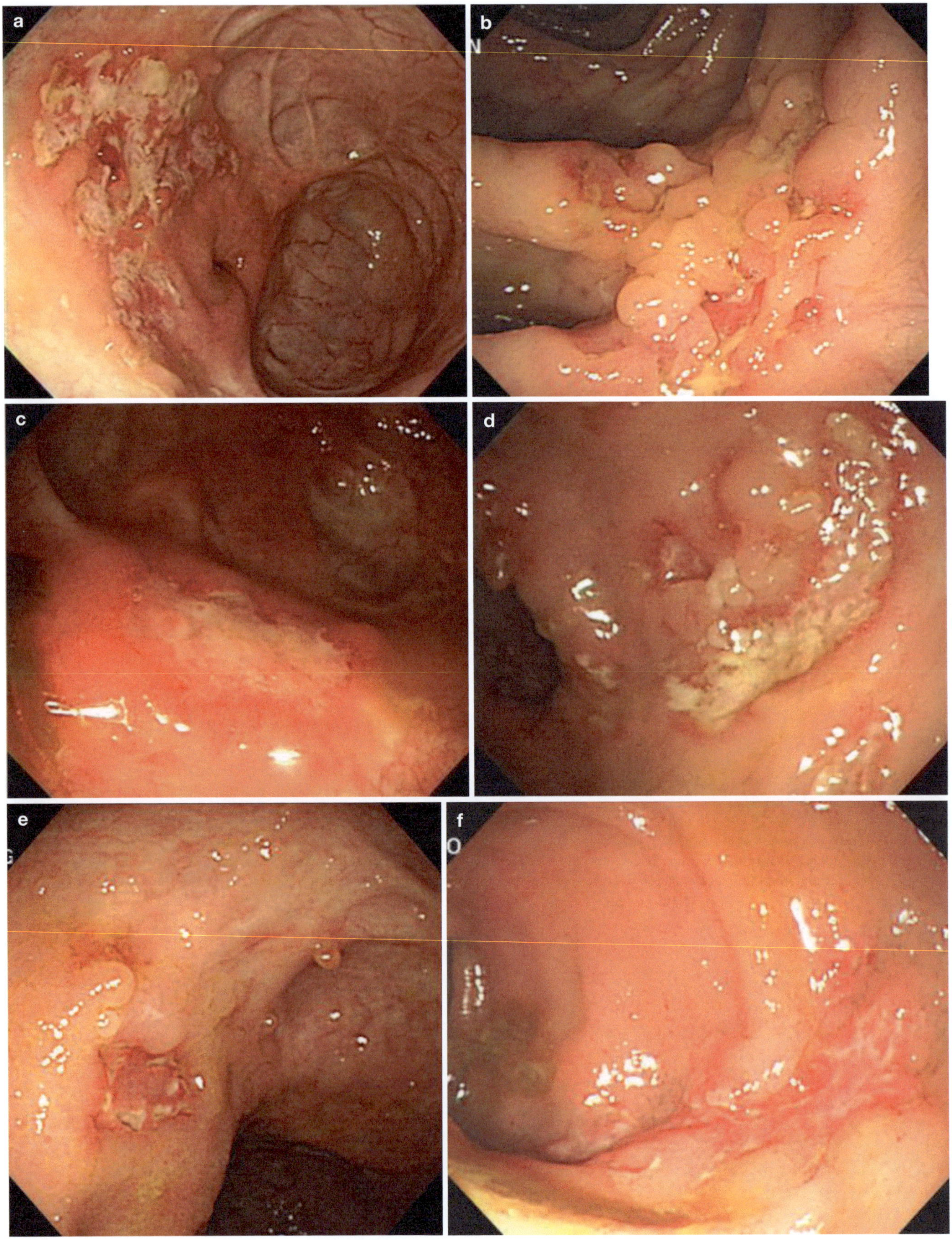

Fig. 4.3 Various shapes of ulcers in ITB. (**a**) Geographic-shaped ulcer contiguous to the ileocecal valve. Scarring change of cecum is also observed. (**b**) Starlike-shaped ulcer in the colon accompanying nodular change. (**c**) Round-shaped ulcer in the cecum base. (**d**) Irregular-shaped ulcers with exudate. (**e**) Square-shaped ulcer. Pseudopolyps and scarring change also are noted. (**f**) Longitudinal-shaped ulcer in the terminal ileum

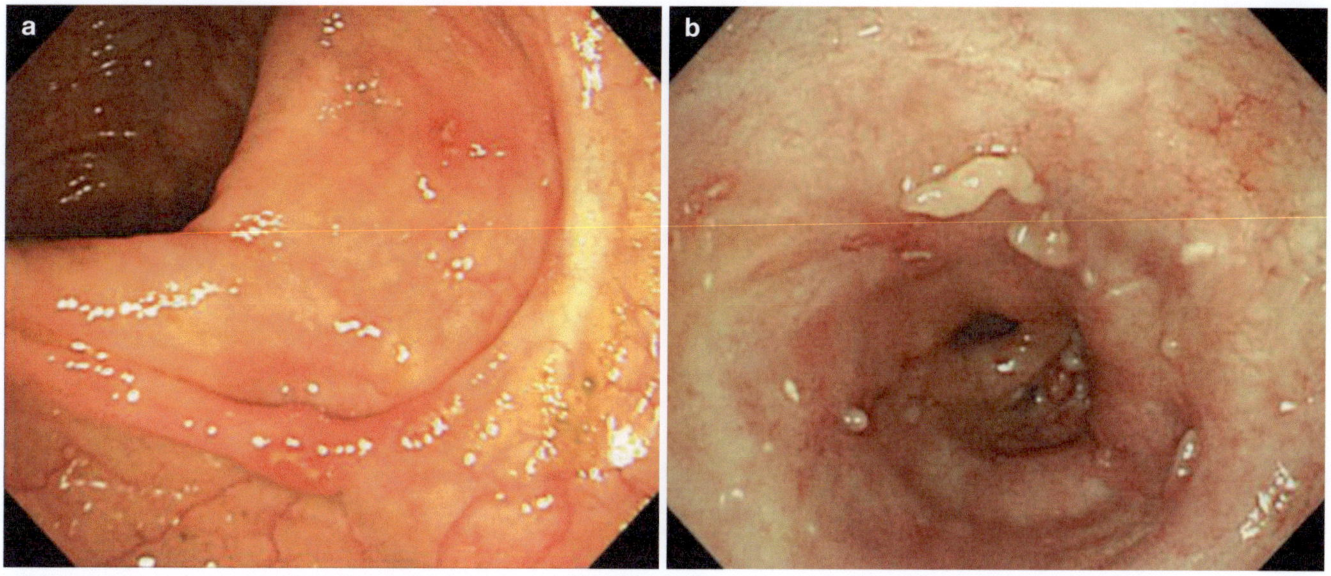

Fig. 4.4 Small ulcers in ITB. (**a**) Small ulcers in the colon. (**b**) Aphthous lesions with scarring change and inflammatory polyps. Irregular vascularity is also observed on scar

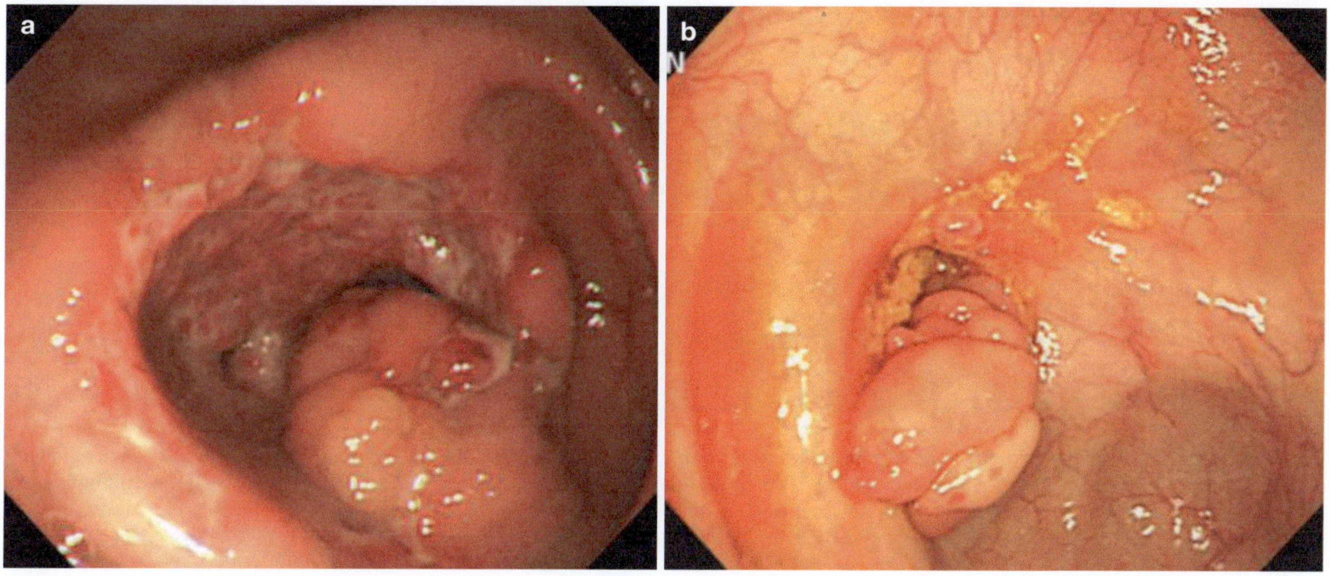

Fig. 4.5 Ulcerohypertrophic type of ITB. (**a**) A protruding polypoid mass with surface nodularity is noted at the ileocecal area. On adjacent mucosa, discrete and deep ulcerations are accompanied. (**b**) Colonoscopic findings after 2 months of antituberculous treatment. The size of the polypoid mass (**a**) is reduced, and active ulcer is healed into scar

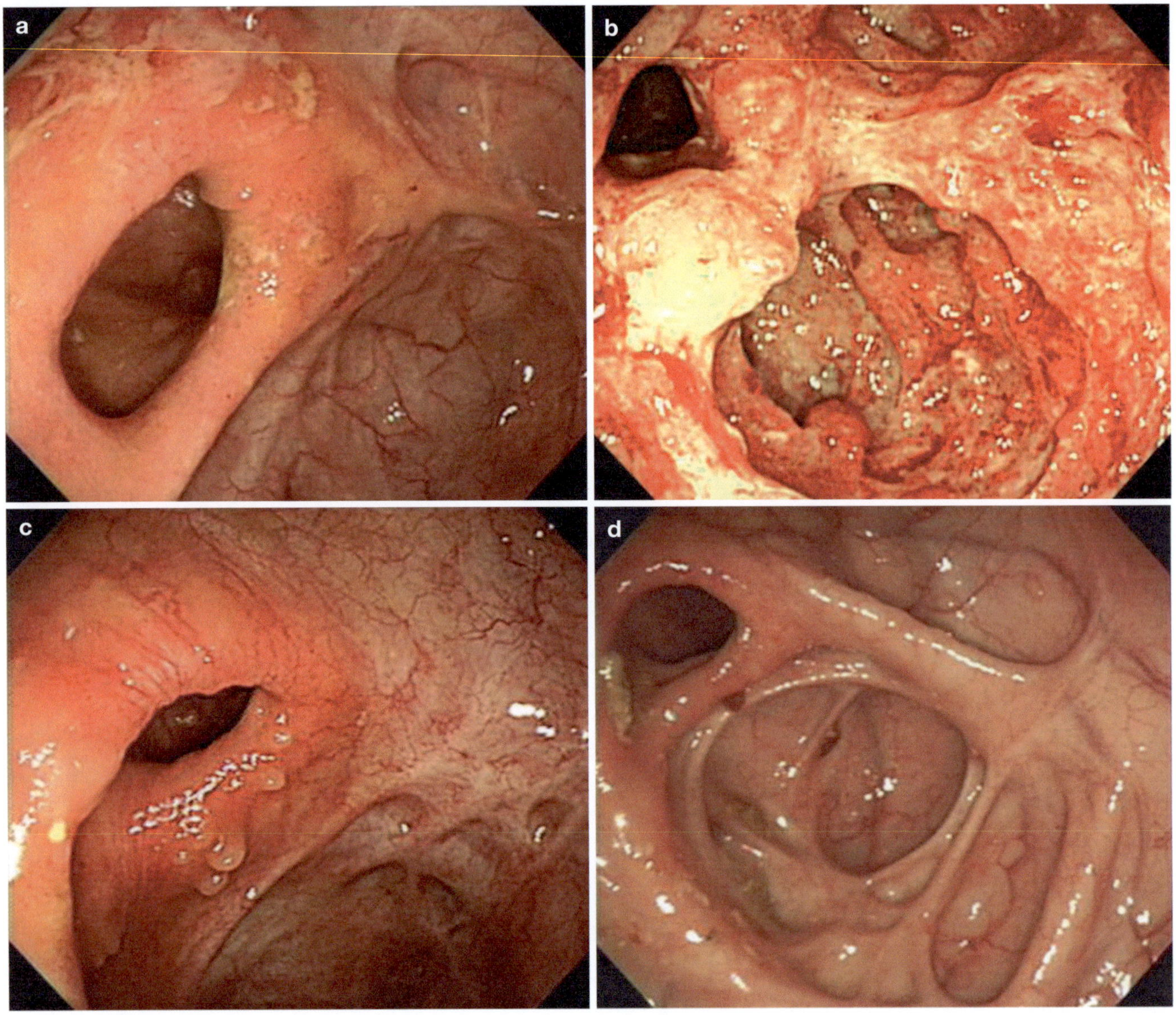

Fig. 4.6 Patulous ileocecal valve. (**a**) Widely opened ileocecal valve with adjacent active ulcer and cecal scarring change. (**b**) Fixed opening of ileocecal valve was observed accompanying adjacent deep ulcers with friability and nodular change. (**c**) Fixed opening of ileocecal valve with inflammatory polyps. Scarring change with pseudodiverticula is also noted in the cecum. (**d**) Patulous ileocecal valve and multiple pseudodiverticula are noted after completion of antituberculous chemotherapy

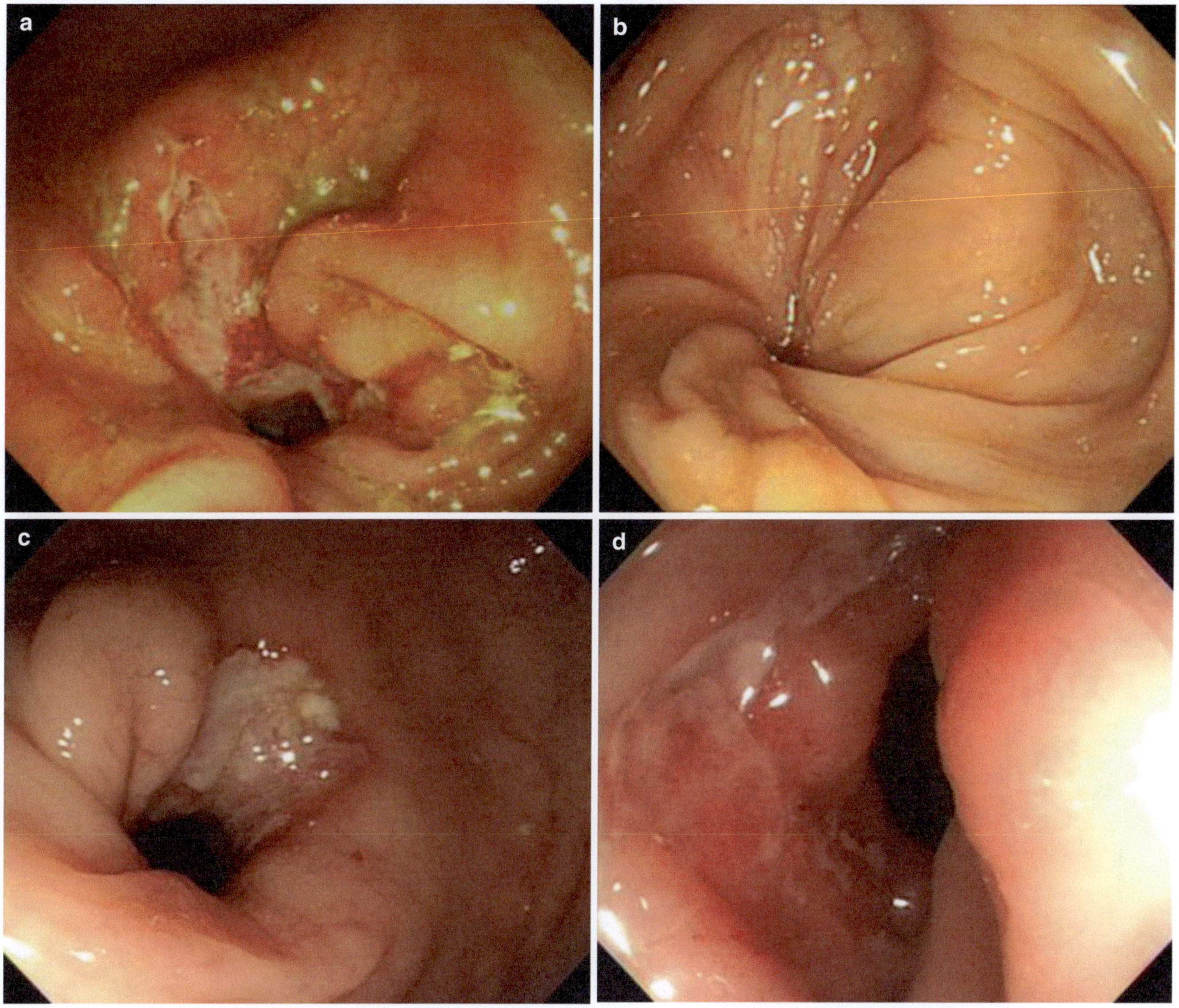

Fig. 4.7 Strictures in ITB. (**a**) Ileocecal valve stenosis with active ulcer was noted. Colonoscope could not pass ileocecal valve. (**b**) Active ulcer in the ileocecal valve (figure **a**) was healed into scar after 6 months of antituberculous therapy. Ileocecal stricture was more worsened. (**c**) Luminal stricture with active ulcer in the hepatic flexure. (**d**) Luminal stricture with circumferential ulcer in the ascending colon. (**e**) Active transverse ulcer with stricture preventing colonoscope passage in the descending colon. (**f**) After completion of 6 months of antituberculous therapy, although active ulcer (figure **e**) was completely healed, luminal stricture is still sustained. (**g**) A wide circumferential ulcer in the proximal transverse colon. (**h**) After 2 months of antituberculous therapy, active ulcer (figure **g**) was substantially healed into scar; however, newly developed luminal narrowing was observed

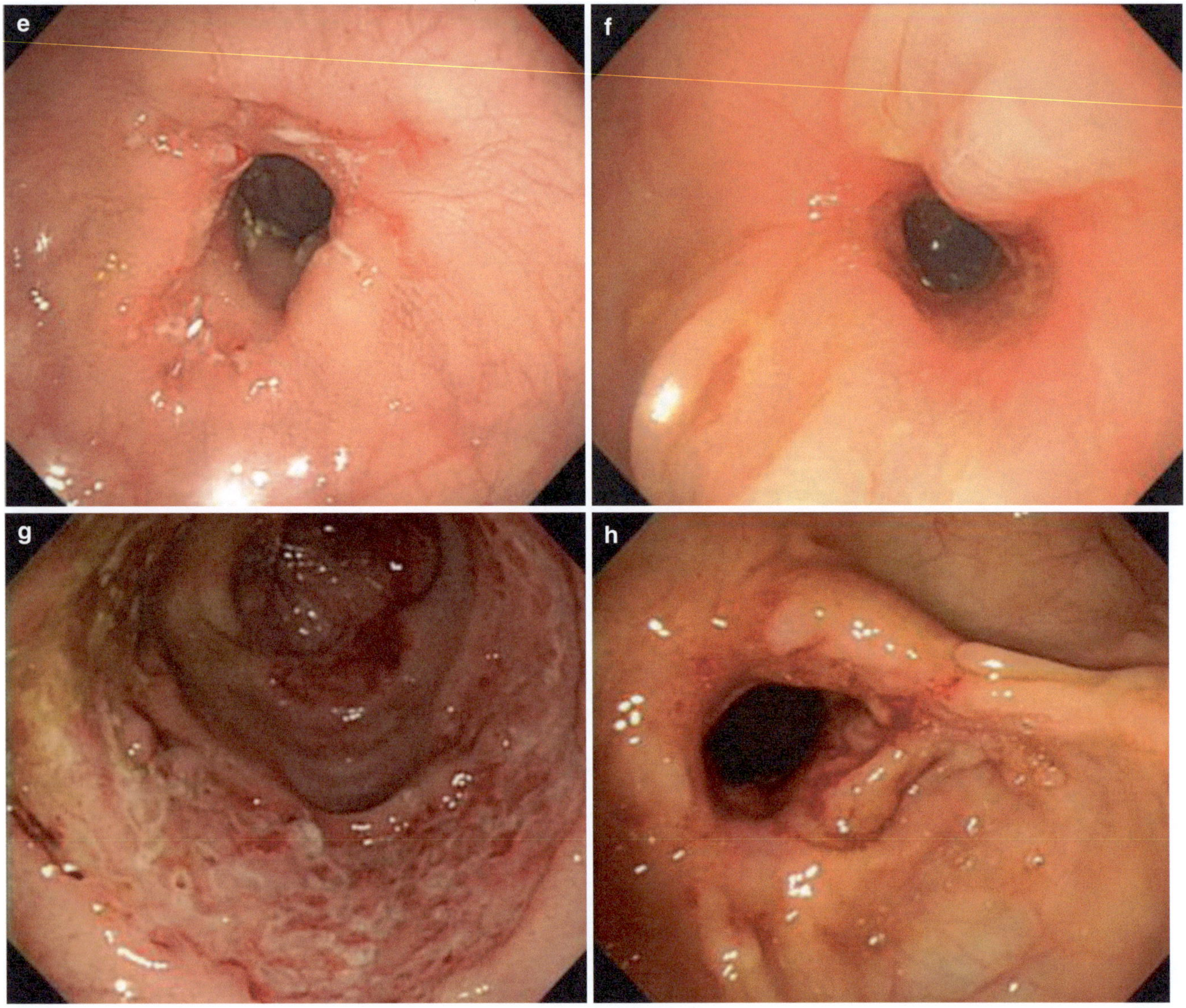

Fig. 4.7 (continued)

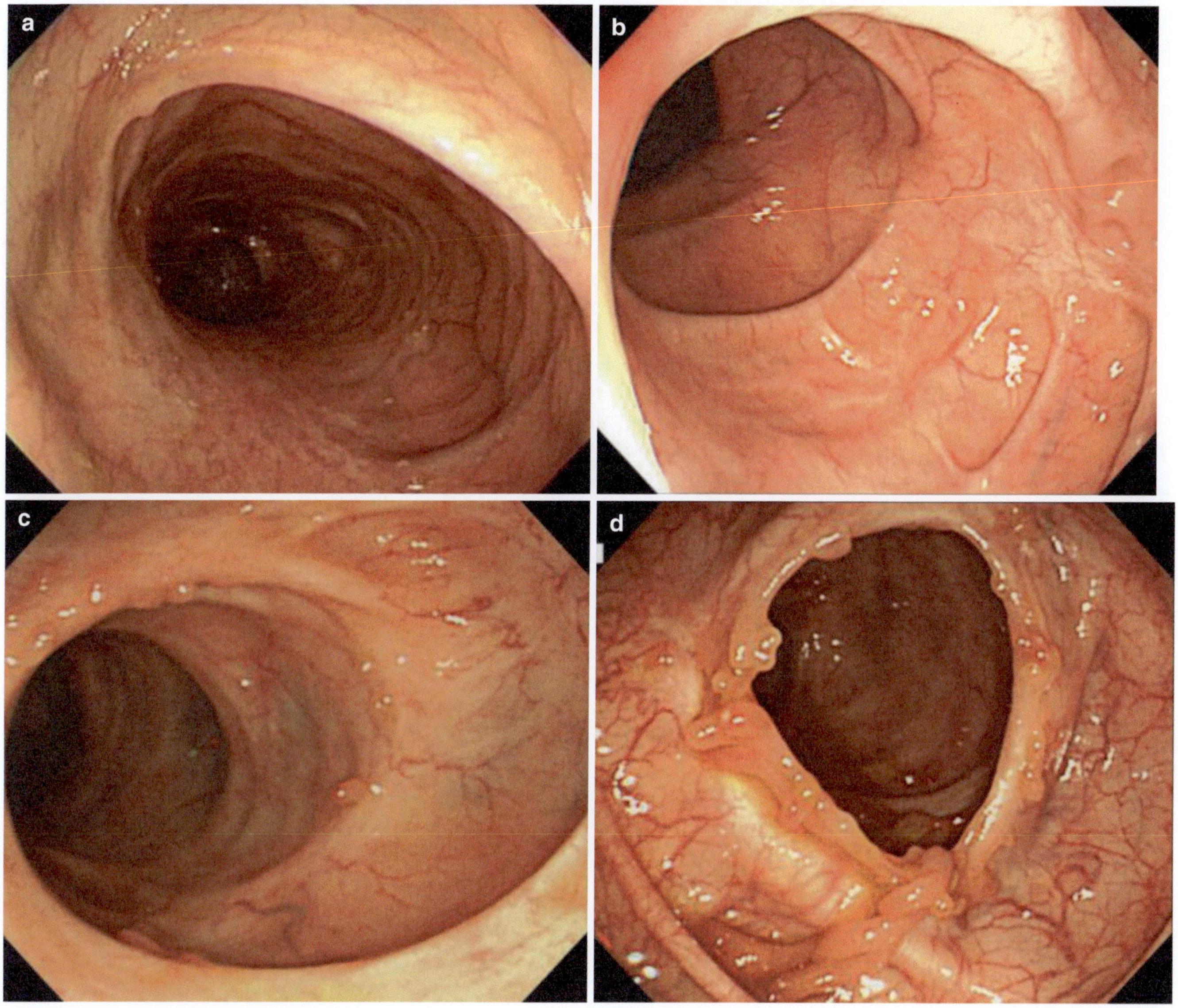

Fig. 4.8 Scars in ITB. (**a**) Diffuse scarring change in the ascending colon. (**b**) Scar in the colon. (**c**) Circumferential scar with inflammatory polyps. (**d**) Circular scar with multiple inflammatory polyps

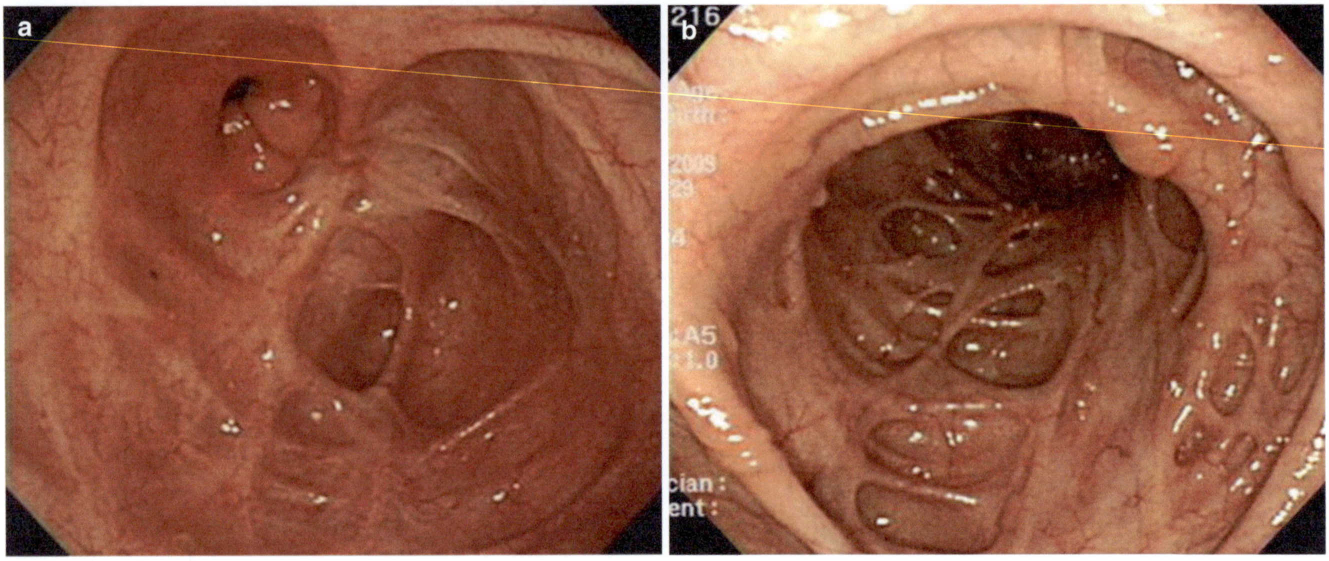

Fig. 4.9 Pseudodiverticula in ITB. (**a**) Several pseudodiverticula in the cecum. (**b**) After completion of antituberculous therapy, multiple pseudodiverticula and mucosal bridges are observed in the ascending colon

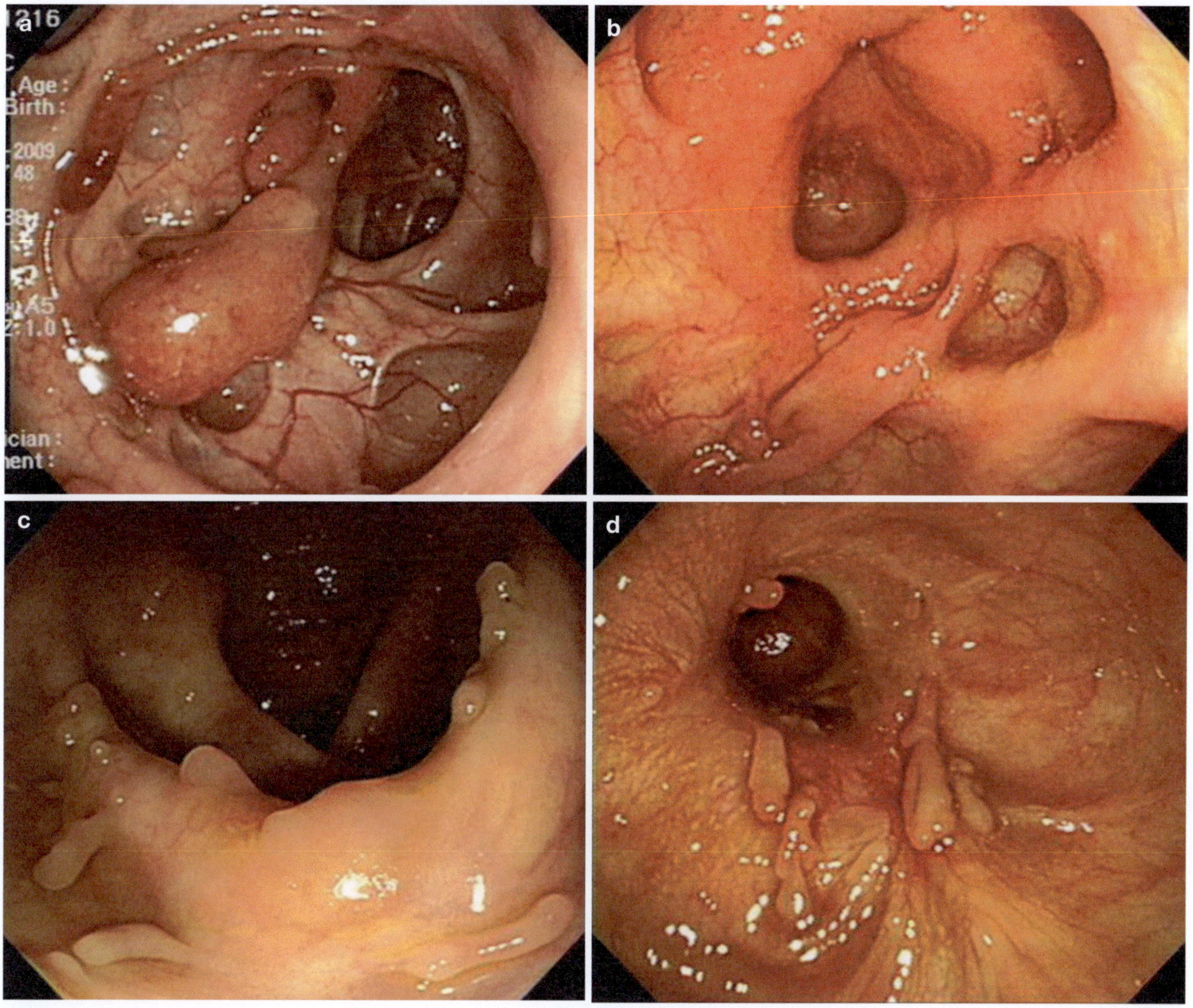

Fig. 4.10 Inflammatory polyps in ITB. (**a**) Several large inflammatory polyps are clinging to the cecal wall, and multiple pseudodiverticula also are noted. (**b**) An inflammatory polyp is attached in the cecum. (**c**) Multiple inflammatory polyps are seen along the semilunar folds in the ascending colon. (**d**) Multiple inflammatory polyps are attached in the cecum. Ileocecal valve shows patulous feature

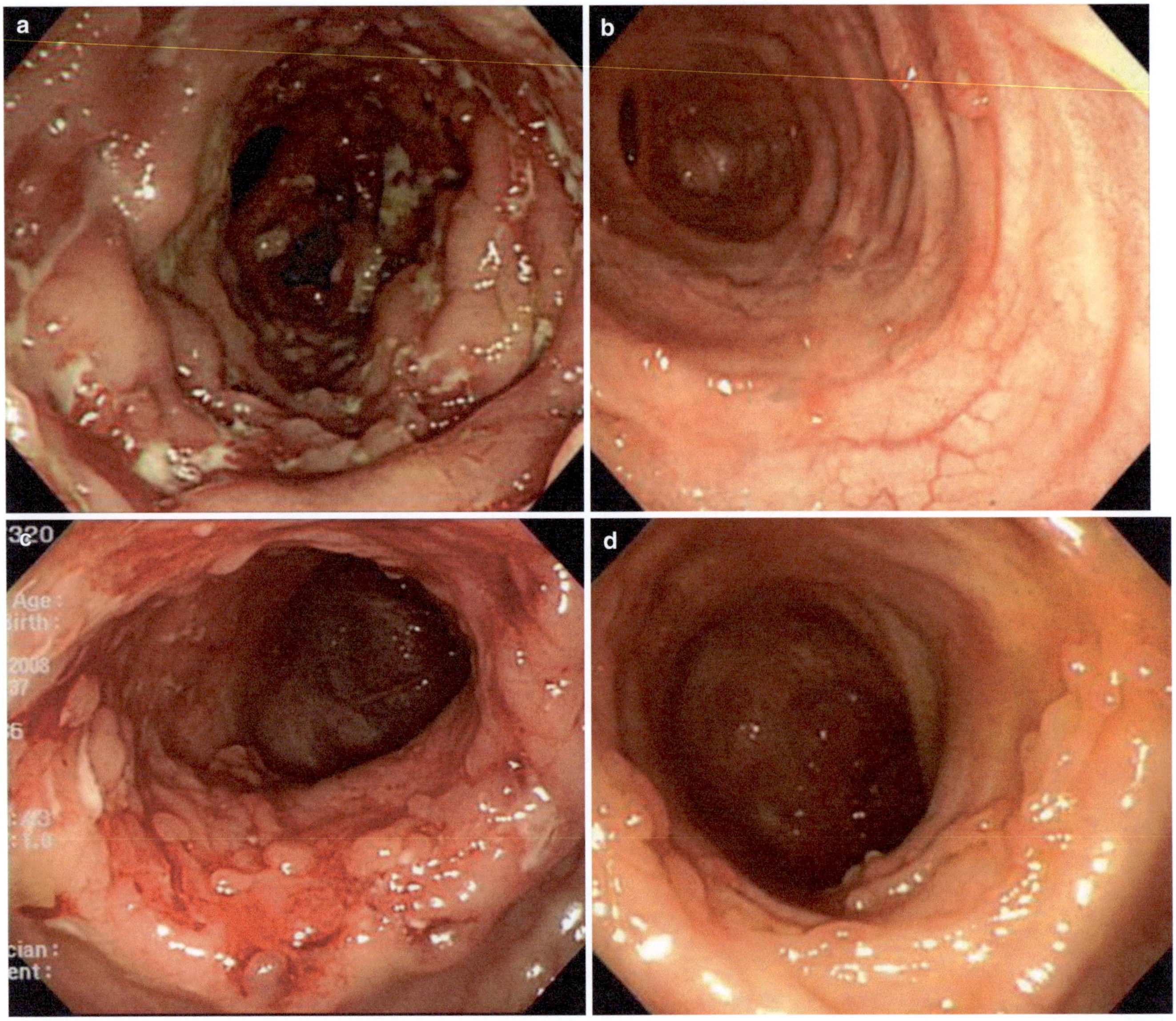

Fig. 4.11 Diverse findings of healing of active ulcers after antituberculous chemotherapy. (**a**) Multiple active ulcers are connected with each other; the intervening protruded mucosa appears like cobblestone. (**b**) After completion of antituberculous therapy, active ulcers (figure **a**) completely healed into scar. (**c**) A wide circumferential ulcer completely encircling colonic lumen. (**d**) After 3 months of antituberculous therapy, active ulcer (figure **c**) healed with the remaining several inflammatory polyps. (**e**) Variable-shaped ulcers with exudate are scattered in the colonic segment. (**f**) After 3 months of antituberculous therapy, active ulcers (figure **e**) completely healed into scar and multiple inflammatory polyps. (**g**) Two transverse ulcers are arranged side by side in the ascending colon. (**h**) After 2 months of antituberculous therapy, two active circumferential ulcers (figure **g**) substantially healed into scar

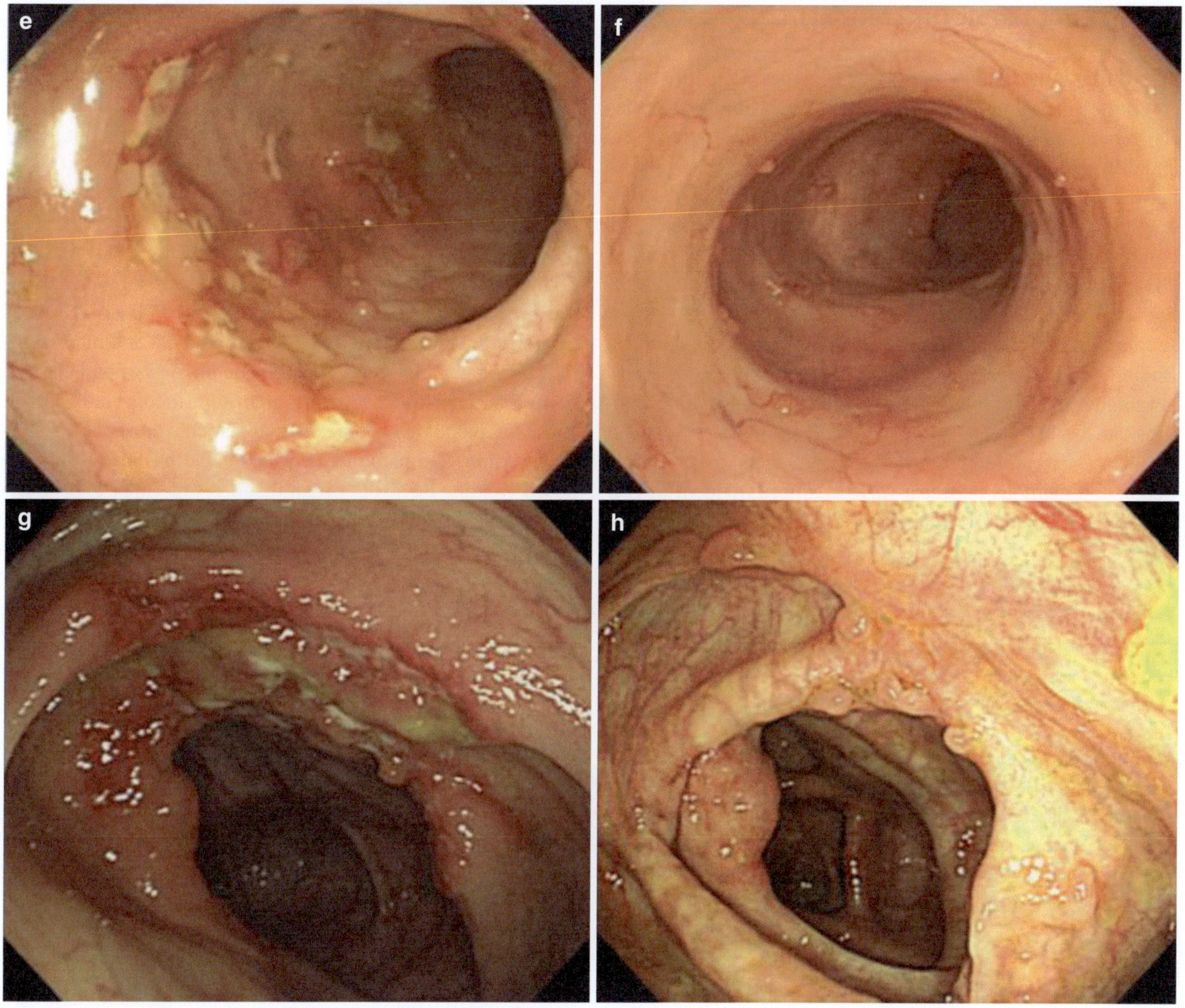

Fig. 4.11 (continued)

4.3 Endoscopic Differential Diagnosis

The differential diagnosis of ITB includes CD, infectious enteritides including actinomycosis, histoplasmosis, amebiasis, yersiniosis, typhlitis, lymphoma, colon cancer, mucoceles, and drug-induced lesions. Among them, differential diagnosis between ITB and CD is the most frequently encountered challenging problem for clinicians especially in Asia where ITB continues to be highly prevalent, and where the incidence of CD is increasing, since these two diseases overlap in clinical, endoscopic, and histological features [4]. Regarding endoscopic differentiation, although there is no single diagnostic finding for definite differentiation between the two diseases, comprehensive assessment of characteristic endoscopic findings can be helpful in initial differentiation. To be specific, transverse-/circumferential-shaped ulcers, scars, pseudodiverticula, and patulous ileocecal valve are more frequent in ITB than in CD, whereas longitudinal-shaped ulcers, presence of skipped lesions and aphthous lesions, cobblestone appearance, pseudopolyps, and multi-segment and anorectal involvement are more common in CD than ITB. With respect to distribution, focal distribution is more common in ITB than CD; on the other hand, segmental or diffuse distributions are more frequent in CD than ITB. Based on difference of these findings between the two diseases, ileocolonoscopy-based scoring system including eight endoscopic parameters has been proposed for the differential diagnosis of ITB and CD (Table 4.1) [5]. According to the external validation data using this scoring system, the diagnosis of either ITB or CD could have been made correctly in 78 % of patients and incorrectly in 8 % and would not have been made in 14 % of patients [6]. Even a simpler differentiating algorithm incorporating three variables including anorectal involvement, presence of aphthous lesion, and patulous ileocecal valve has also been proposed yielding 82 % of correct diagnosis of either ITB or CD on internal validation cohort (Fig. 4.12) [7].

Table 4.1 Ileocolonoscopic differential diagnosis between ITB and CD

(A) Findings suggestive of intestinal tuberculosis	(B) Findings suggestive of Crohn's disease
Less than 4-segment involvement[a]	Anorectal lesions
A patulous ileocecal valve	Longitudinal ulcer
Transverse ulcer	Aphthous ulcer
Scar or pseudopolyp	Cobblestone appearance
Putative diagnosis	
1. Intestinal tuberculosis: number of (A) findings > number of (B) findings	
2. Crohn's disease: number of (A) findings < number of (B) findings	
3. Undetermined diagnosis: number of (A) findings = number of (B) findings	

[a]Segment classification: ileocecal area, ascending colon, transverse colon, descending colon, sigmoid colon, anorectum

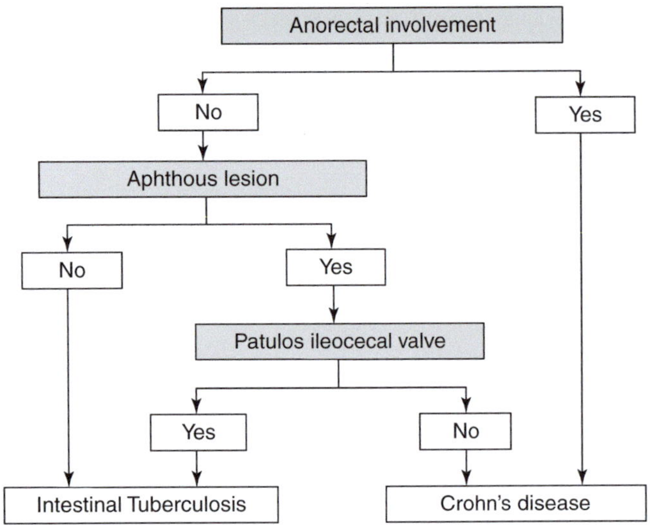

Fig. 4.12 Ileocolonoscopy-based simple decision tree model for differential diagnosis between intestinal tuberculosis (ITB) and Crohn's disease (CD)

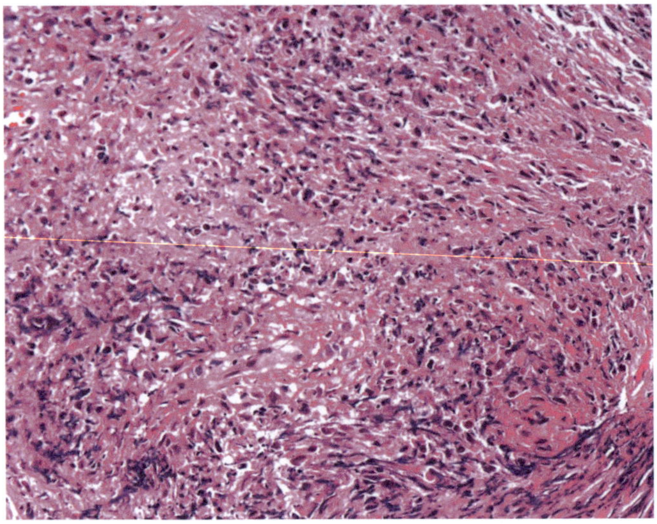

Fig. 4.13 Caseating granuloma in endoscopic mucosal biopsy specimen of intestinal tuberculosis. Epithelioid cells surround a central area of necrosis that appears irregular, amorphous, and pink (H&E stain, x200)

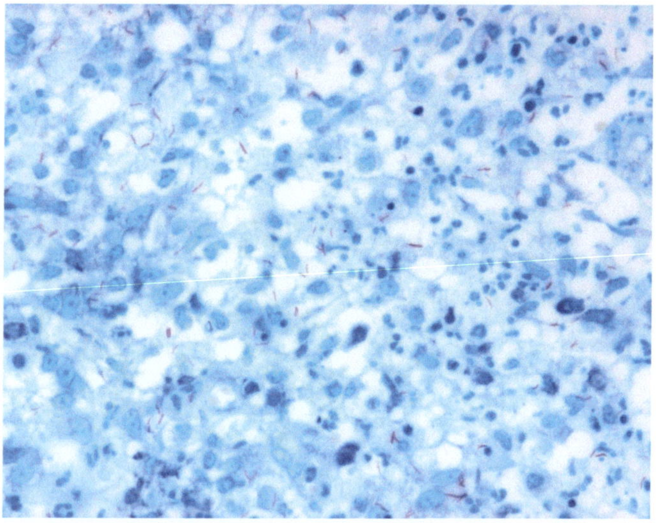

Fig. 4.14 Mycobacterium tuberculosis visualized using special stain. Zielen-Nielson stain reveals many acid-fast bacilli in endoscopic biopsy specimen of patients with intestinal tuberculosis (Zielen-Nielson stain, x400)

References

1. Donoghue HD, Holton J. Intestinal tuberculosis. Curr Opin Infect Dis. 2009;22:490.
2. Haddad FS, Ghossain A, Sawaya E, Nelson AR. Abdominal tuberculosis. Dis Colon Rectum. 1987;30:724–35.
3. Marshall JB. Tuberculosis of the gastrointestinal tract and peritoneum. Am J Gastroenterol. 1993;88:989–99.
4. Kirsch R, Pentecost M, Hall Pde M, Epstein DP, Watermeyer G, Friederich PW. Role of colonoscopic biopsy in distinguishing between Crohn's disease and intestinal tuberculosis. J Clin Pathol. 2006;59:840–4.
5. Lee YJ, Yang SK, Byeon JS, Myung SJ, Chang HS, Hong SS, Kim KJ, Lee GH, Jung HY, Hong WS, Kim JH, Min YI, Chang SJ, Yu CS. Analysis of colonoscopic findings in the differential diagnosis between intestinal tuberculosis and Crohn's disease. Endoscopy. 2006;38:592–7.
6. Park YM, Park JJ, Park SJ, Hong SP, Kim TI, Kim WH, Cheon JH. External validation of ileocolonoscopy based scoring system for differential diagnosis between intestinal tuberculosis and Crohn's disease. U Eur Gastroenterol J. 2013;1 Suppl 1:1432.
7. Park JJ, Park SJ, Hong SP, Kim TI, Cheon JH. Differential diagnosis between intestinal tuberculosis and Crohn's disease by ileocolonoscopic findings. U Eur Gastroenterol J. 2013;1 Suppl 1:1415.
8. Horvath KD, Whelan RL. Intestinal tuberculosis: return of an old disease. Am J Gastroenterol. 1998 May;93(5):692–6.

5 Differential Diagnosis Between Inflammatory Bowel Diseases and Other Intestinal Disorders

Sung Pil Hong

Inflammatory bowel disease shares similar several clinical or endoscopic features with many other enterocolitides. Because of the absence of definite confirmative diagnostic tests, misdiagnosis is frequently made. Careful history taking and physical examinations are the first step to differentiate those diseases. In this chapter, we show differential points of endoscopic features in other enterocolitides from IBD (Table 5.1).

Table 5.1 Differential diagnosis between inflammatory bowel diseases and other intestinal disorders

Disease	Differential diagnosis
Ischemic colitis	Clinical symptoms, abrupt transition to normal mucosa with sparing rectum
Radiation proctitis	A history of exposure to radiation
Lymphoma	Clinical symptoms
Vasculitis	Clinical symptoms and signs of systemic disease
Infectious colitis	Clinical symptoms and signs
Drug-induced colitis	A history of NSAID use

S.P. Hong
Department of Internal Medicine and Institute of Gastroenterology, Yonsei University College of Medicine, Seoul, South Korea
e-mail: sphong@yuhs.ac

W.H. Kim, J.H. Cheon (eds.), *Atlas of Inflammatory Bowel Diseases*,
DOI 10.1007/978-3-642-39423-2_5, © Springer-Verlag Berlin Heidelberg 2015

5.1 Ischemic Colitis

5.1.1 Clinical Manifestations

Ischemic colitis is caused by reduction in blood flow into the colon, which often affects the elderly [1, 2]. Patients with age older than 60; patients who are on hemodialysis; those with hypertension, hypoalbuminemia, or diabetes mellitus; and those who are taking constipation-inducing or constipation-relieving medications have been known as risk factors. The typical presentations are a sudden and cramping abdominal pain with an urgent desire to defecate and passage of bright red or bloody diarrhea. Other manifestations include systemic symptoms such as fever, hypotension, or shock due to bowel necrosis, perforation, peritonitis, and sepsis.

5.1.2 Endoscopic Features

The splenic flexure, descending colon, and sigmoid colon, which are called as the "watershed" area, are most commonly involved, whereas the rectum is usually spared [3, 4]. Endoscopic appearances include edematous and friable mucosa, erythema, scattered erosions, ulcerations, petechial hemorrhages, and purple hemorrhagic nodules. These endoscopic findings are typically limited to the affected mucosa with abrupt transit to normal mucosa (Fig. 5.1).

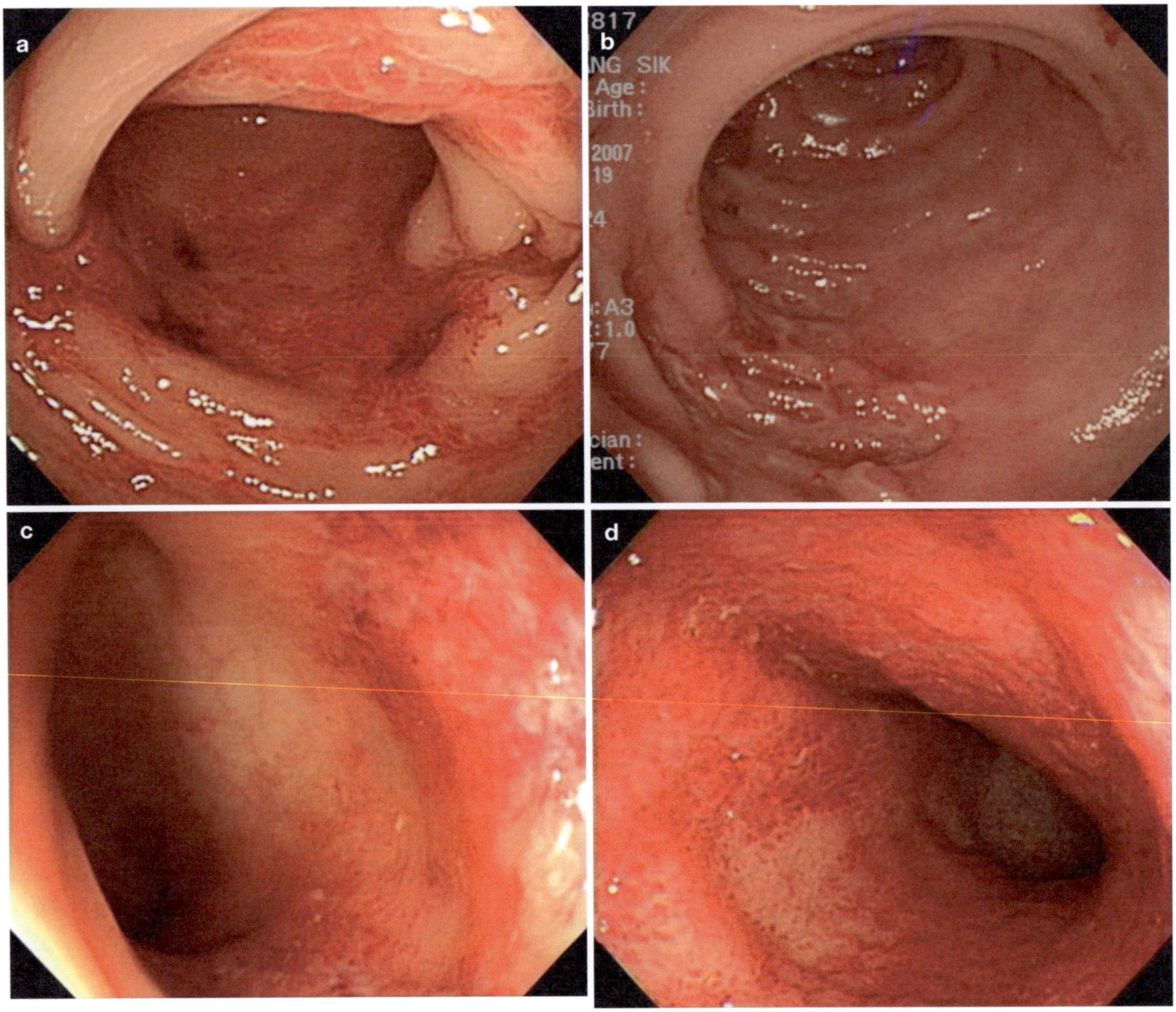

Fig. 5.1 Ischemic colitis. (**a**) Erythematous and edematous mucosa is noted in the sigmoid colon with petechial hemorrhages. (**b**) Discrete ulceration is noted with demarcated normal mucosa. (**c**) Friable and edematous mucosa with erosion is noted in the sigmoid colon. The affected mucosa was abruptly transit to normal mucosa. (**d**) Edematous and erythematous mucosa with ease touch bleeding is noted in the sigmoid colon, mimicking ulcerative colitis

5.2 Radiation Proctitis

5.2.1 Clinical Manifestations

Radiation injury to the colorectum results from epithelial damage following radiation treatment of cancers located in the rectum, anus, cervix, uterus, prostate, urinary bladder, or testis [1, 2]. The rectum and sigmoid colon are most frequently affected. Acute radiation injury occurs during or within 6 weeks of radiation treatment. Chronic injury usually occurs 9–14 months after radiation treatment but can occur any time postirradiation up to 30 years after exposure. Clinical symptoms of radiation proctitis include diarrhea, mucus discharge, urgency, tenesmus, and bleeding.

5.2.2 Endoscopic Features

Endoscopic findings include mucosal friability, pallor, and telangiectasias [3, 4]. These lesions tend to be continuous but can vary in intensity. Chronic radiation proctitis shows various manifestations from pallor mucosa with telangiectasia to ulceration, fistula, stricture, and mucosal bleeding (Fig. 5.2).

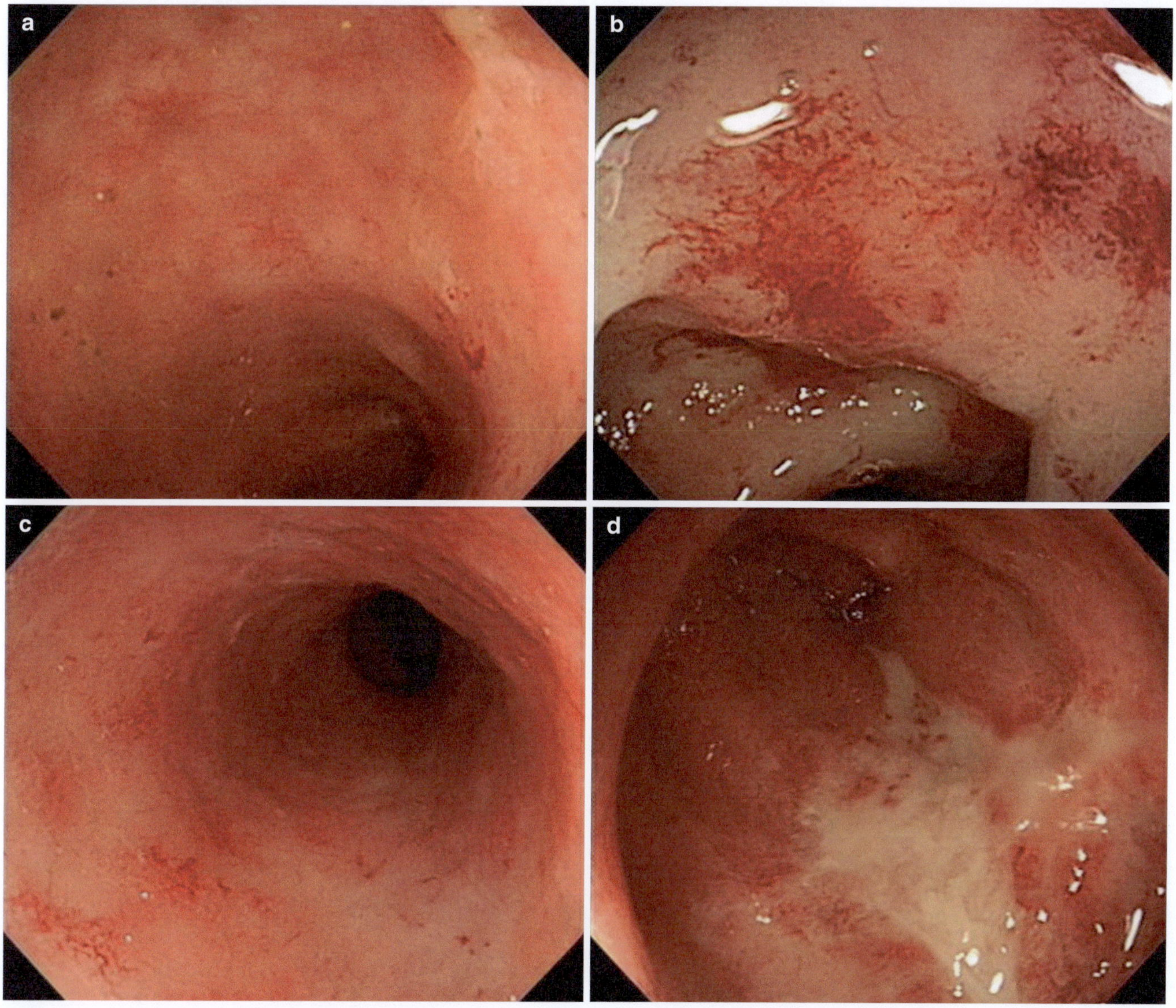

Fig. 5.2 Radiation proctitis. (**a**) Pale mucosa with telangiectasia is observed in the rectum. (**b**) Telangiectasia with oozing blood is noted in the rectum. (**c**) Pale mucosa with telangiectasia is noted in the sigmoid colon. The sigmoid colon looks like a pipe without mucosal folds, mimicking long-standing ulcerative colitis. (**d**) A geographic ulcer with surrounding mucosal edema and erythema is noted in the rectum. (**e**) Ulcer scarring with deformity is noted at rectum. Surrounding mucosa shows typical pale and telangiectatic change. (**f**) Chronic radiation injury evokes circumferential ulceration with stricture in the rectosigmoid junction. The scope could not be passed through the stricture

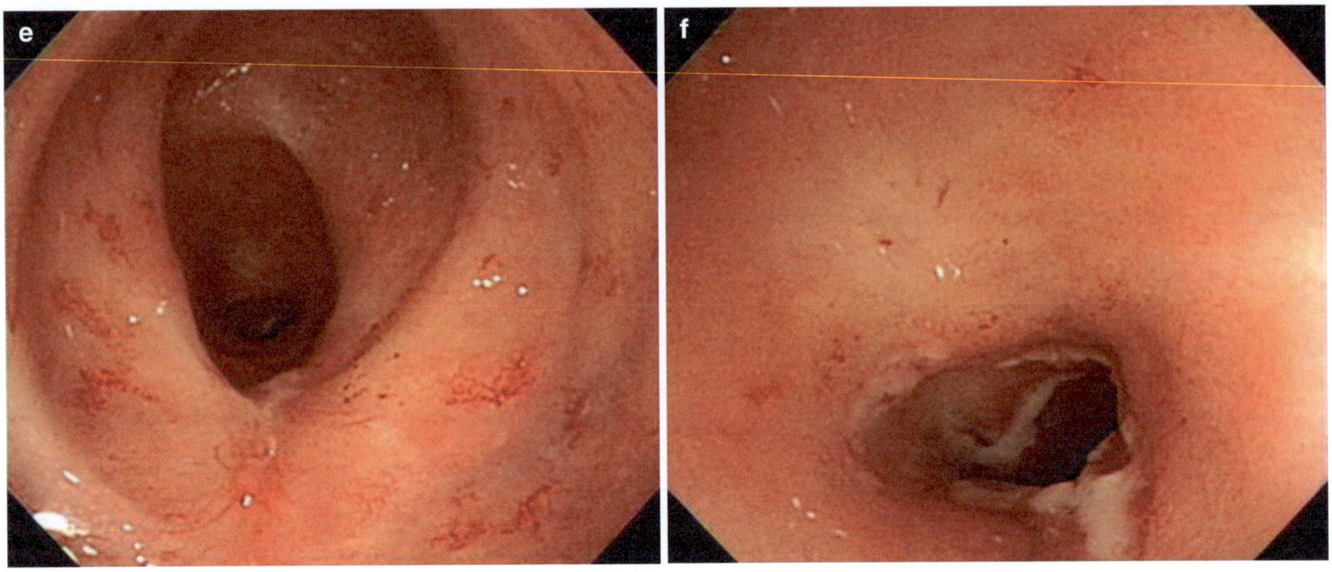

Fig. 5.2 (continued)

5.3 Lymphoma

5.3.1 Clinical Manifestations

Primary gastrointestinal tract lymphoma is rare, while secondary gastrointestinal involvement is relatively common [1, 2]. Colorectal lymphoma accounts for 3 % of the gastrointestinal lymphomas and 0.3 % of colorectal malignancies. There is a male predominance. The common histologies include mantle cell lymphoma, Burkitt lymphoma, follicular lymphoma, and diffuse large B-cell lymphoma. The cecum is the most common site for primary colorectal lymphoma, followed by the rectum.

5.3.2 Endoscopic Features

Colonoscopy findings of primary colorectal lymphoma commonly show large and polypoid lesions, but mucosal irregularity or ulceration can also be found [3, 4]. Mantle cell lymphoma shows typical small nodular or polypoid (2 mm to more than 2 cm in size) lesions with or without normal intervening mucosa. Sometimes, mantle cell lymphoma presents stricture with ulceration, mimicking Crohn's disease. Some authors claim that B-cell lymphoma often forms mass-like lesions, while T-cell lymphoma is more likely to have ulcerative lesions (Fig. 5.3).

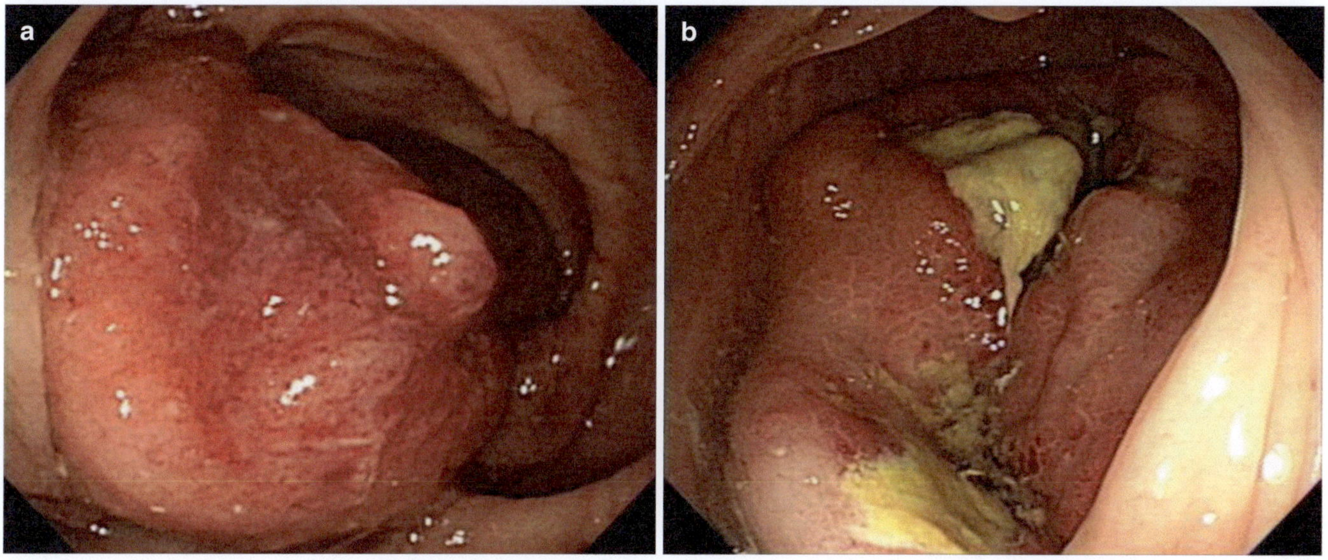

Fig. 5.3 Colon lymphoma. (**a**) A 4-cm-sized mass-like lesion with mucosal friability is noted in the ascending colon. The histology showed diffuse large B-cell lymphoma. (**b**) A huge deep ulceration with surrounding mucosal edema and covering mucus is noted in the ascending colon. The histology showed Burkitt lymphoma. (**c**) Thickened mucosa with induration and mucus is noted at the ileocecal valve. Ulceration was not definite, and the scope could not be passed into the terminal ileum. The histology showed Burkitt lymphoma. (**d**) Mucosal thickening and edema with small-sized multiple nodules and prominent capillaries are noted in the rectum. The histology showed MALT lymphoma. (**e**) Longitudinal ulceration with mucosal edema and erythema is noted in the descending colon. The lesion is segmental, mimicking inflammatory bowel disease. The histology showed MALT lymphoma. (**f**) Short segmental stricture with ulceration covering exudate is noted at the ileocecal valve. The ulcer is longitudinal and surrounding mucosa is edematous, mimicking Crohn's disease. The histology showed mantle cell lymphoma

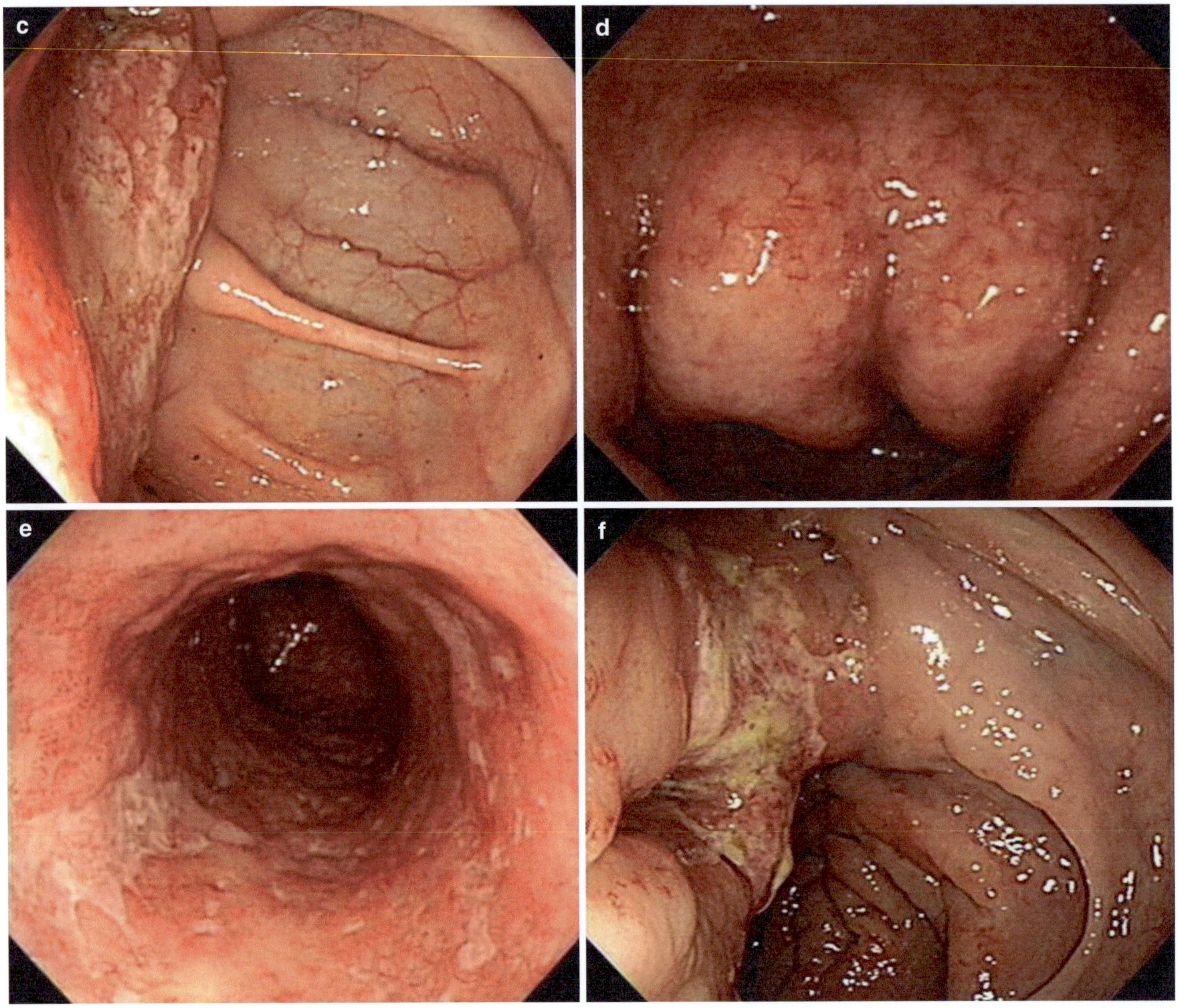

Fig. 5.3 (continued)

5.4 Vasculitis

5.4.1 Clinical Manifestations

Vasculitis involving the gastrointestinal tract is usually the progress of systemic disease, such as polyarteritis nodosa, Henoch-Schonlein purpura, or systemic lupus erythematosus. The signs and symptoms result from mesenteric ischemia secondary to vasculitis [1, 2].

5.4.2 Endoscopic Features

Endoscopic appearances show various features, including hyperemia, edema, erosions, ulcerations, and necrosis [3, 4] (Fig. 5.4).

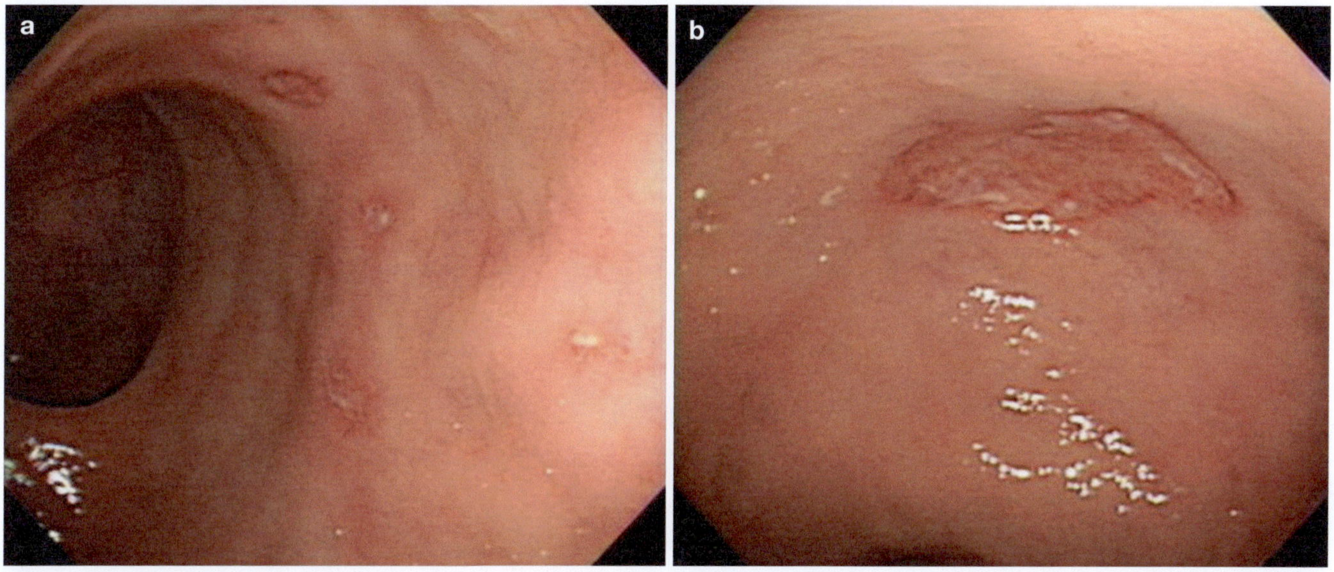

Fig. 5.4 Vasculitis. (**a**) Multiple shallow and small ulcerations are noted in the sigmoid colon in patients with microscopic polyangiitis. (**b**) Discrete shallow ulceration with exudates and clear margin is noted in the sigmoid colon in patients with microscopic polyangiitis. The surrounding mucosa looks normal

5.5 Drug-Induced Colitis

5.5.1 Clinical Manifestations

Nonsteroidal anti-inflammatory drugs (NSAIDs) are the most common agents to evoke inflammation in the gastrointestinal tract [1, 2]. The distal small bowel and colon are vulnerable to NSAIDs. It has been reported that approximately 10–12 % of newly diagnosed colitis may be related to NSAID administration. The elderly and long-term NSAID users are at high risk. Clinical symptoms and signs include occult blood loss, iron-deficiency anemia, abdominal pain, bowel obstruction, massive bleeding, and perforation.

5.5.2 Endoscopic Features

Endoscopic appearances are quite nonspecific, including hyperemia, erosions, different-sized shallow or deep ulcerations, and strictures [3, 4] (Fig. 5.5).

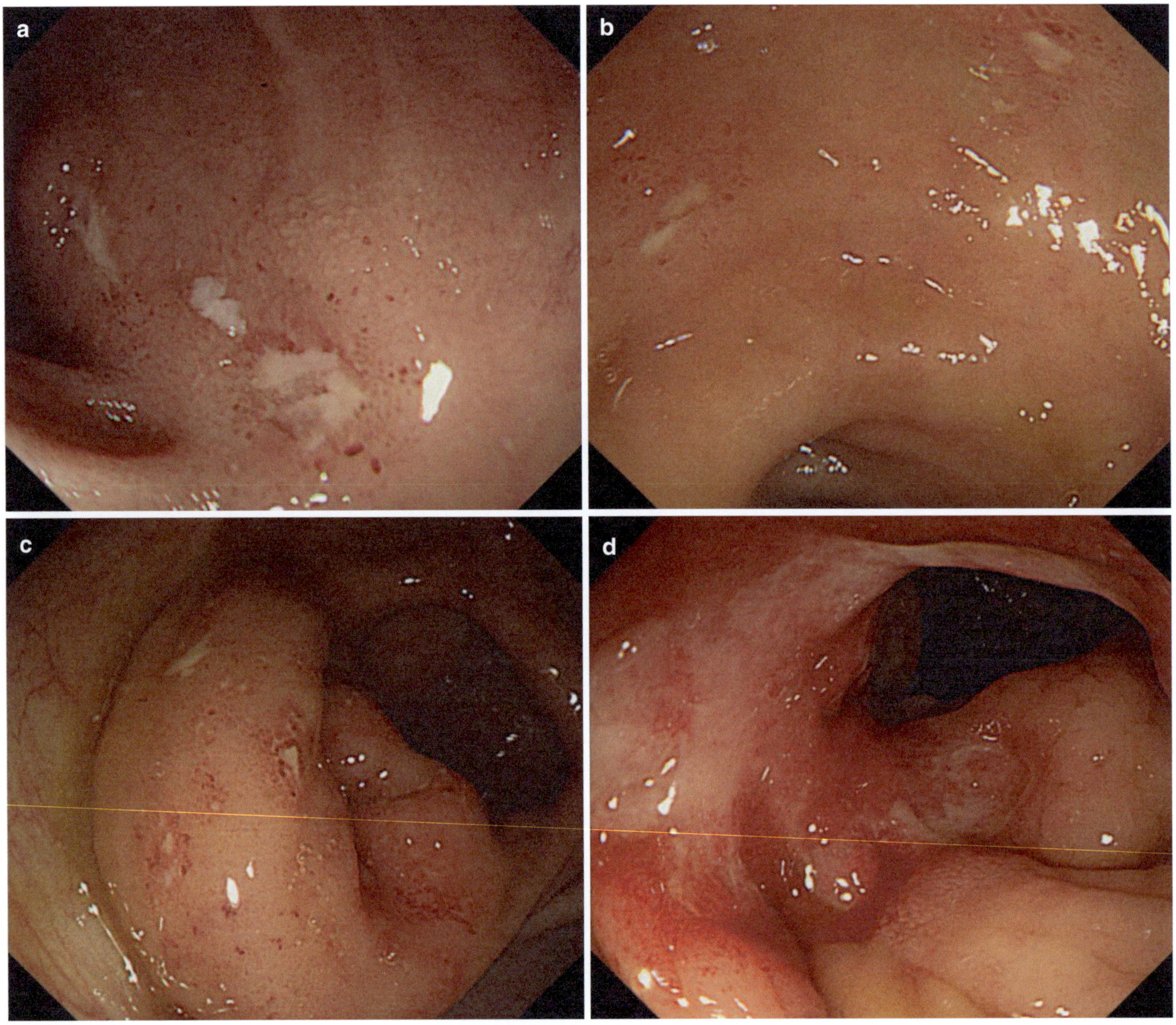

Fig. 5.5 Drug-induced colitis. (**a**) Several 5-mm-sized aphthous ulcers are noted in the terminal ileum. (**b**) Several aphthous ulcers with less than 5 mm in size are noted in the cecum. (**c**) Multiple shallow ulcers with erythema are noted in the ileocecal valve. (**d**) A huge geographic ulcer with hyperemia and easy touch bleeding is noted in the ileocecal area. (**e**) Geographic ulceration with exudates and nodular mucosal change is noted in the ascending colon. (**f**) Circumferential ulcer with stricture is noted in the descending colon

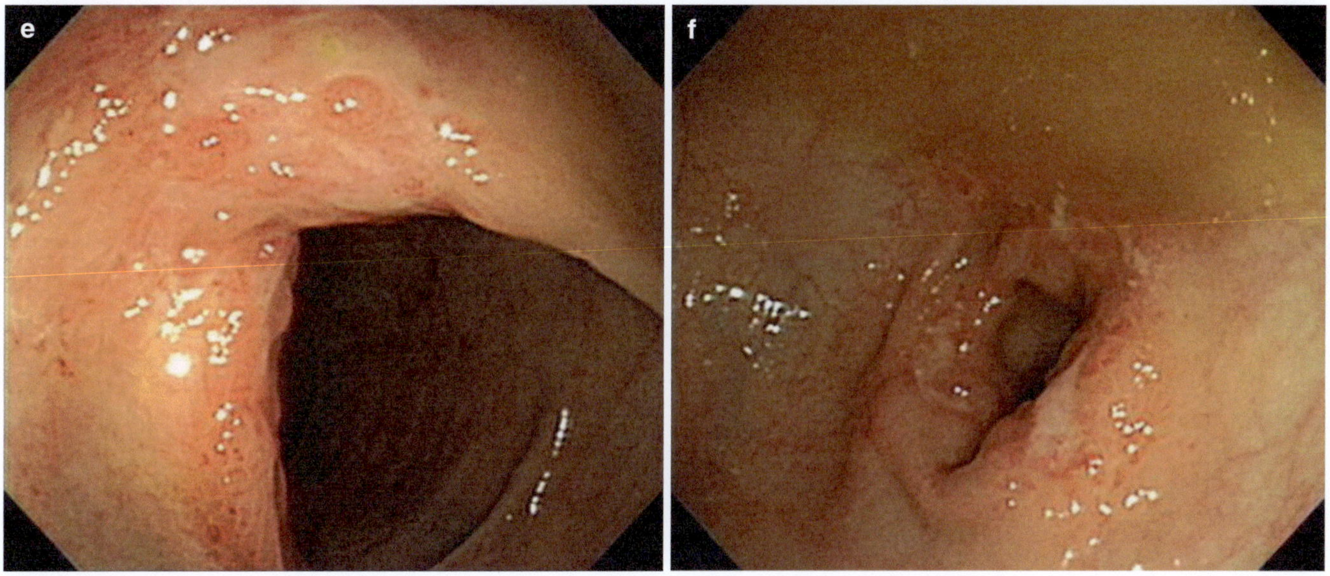

Fig. 5.5 (continued)

5.6 Infectious Colitis

5.6.1 Clinical Manifestations

Various infections can occur in the small bowel and colon. Most infections resolve within 1–2 weeks. The differential points from IBD here are clinical manifestations (see Chap. 1 and Table 1.6). When the disease course is unusually long or atypical or an urgent decision is necessary, a sigmoidoscopy or colonoscopy could be performed.

5.6.2 Endoscopic Features

Endoscopic features may vary. In acute stage, nonspecific inflammatory changes including mucosal exudate, erythema, and edema can occur. Mucosal friability, shallow ulcers, or hemorrhage develops in severe cases. In recovering stage, small aphthae, hemorrhagic spots, or focal erythema may be seen (Fig. 5.6).

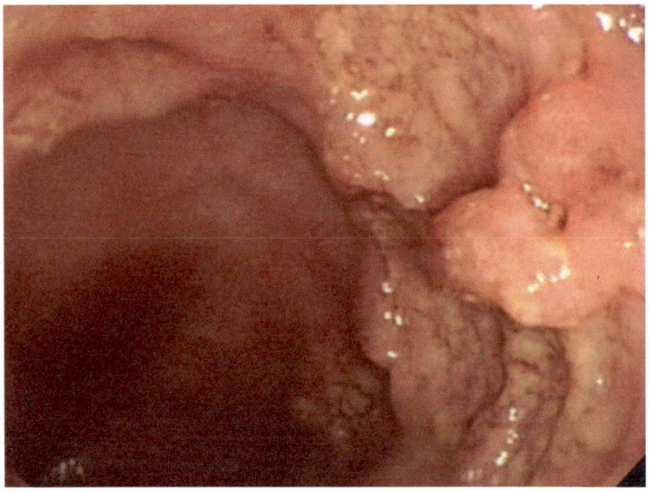

Fig. 5.6 Salmonella enteritis. Several shallow ulcerations with exudate are observed in the terminal ileum. No scar or surrounding fibrosis is found. Salmonella infection usually occurs in the right colon or terminal ileum. Blood and tissue cultures revealed it was salmonellosis

References

1. Feldman M, et al. Sleisenger and Fordtran's gastrointestinal and liver disease. 9th ed. Atlanta: Saunders; 2010.
2. Waye SP, et al. Colonoscopy: principles and practice. 2nd ed. Hoboken: Wiley-Blackwell; 2009.
3. Yang SK. Colonoscopy: diagnosis and treatment. Seoul: Koonja; 2009.
4. Kim CD, et al. Atlas of gastrointestinal endoscopy. Seoul: Medbook; 2011.

6 Small Bowel Endoscopy

Fumihito Hirai and Toshiyuki Matsui

6.1 Small Bowel Endoscopy: Introduction

Currently, we have two balloon-assisted enteroscopy (BAE) systems to observe the entire small bowel. One is double balloon enteroscopy (Fujifilm Medical Co., Tokyo, Japan) that Dr. Yamamoto developed [1], and the other one is single balloon enteroscopy (Olympus Co., Tokyo, Japan). Both of them enable the endoscopist not only to observe the small bowel directly but also to perform the endoscopic treatments in the small bowel. This new modality led us to obtain much knowledge about small bowel diseases. BAE has some advantages, including the ability of directly observing the small bowel and performing biopsy, compared with other small bowel modalities. CT or MRI are the least invasive methods; however, these methods are not able to evaluate the small bowel mucosal lesions directly or in detail. Capsule endoscopy (CE) is also a noninvasive method and it can directly observe the small bowel mucosa. Therefore, this modality has been frequently used for evaluating small bowel disorders in the world. However, it has several limitations including the possibility of retention in case of intestinal strictures [2] and impossibility of the biopsy [3]. On the other hand, the biopsy can be done easily by using the BAE. BAE is quite useful for the correct diagnosis of small bowel diseases, particularly small bowel tumors and inflammatory diseases. However, BAE also has some disadvantages in terms of its invasiveness and technical difficulty of insertion. We should select the best one among these modalities for small bowel observation according to the status, indication, purpose, and suspicious diagnosis of each case [4–12].

In the diagnosis of Crohn's disease, gastroenterologists should be aware of the morphological characteristics of the disease (Table 6.1). Moreover, it is very important that infectious and other enteritides, such as drug-induced enterocolitis [13, 14], intestinal tuberculosis [15–17], intestinal Behçet's disease [18], chronic nonspecific multiple ulcers of the small intestine [19, 20], ischemic enteritis, etc., should be excluded before confirming the diagnosis of Crohn's disease (Table 6.2). In this section, endoscopic findings of various small bowel disorders using BAE and CE will be demonstrated, which are useful for the differential diagnosis of inflammatory small bowel diseases.

F. Hirai (✉) • T. Matsui
Department of Gastroenterology,
Fukuoka University Chikushi Hospital, 1-1-1 Zokumyoin,
Chikushino, Fukuoka 818-8502, Japan
e-mail: fuhirai@cis.fukuoka-u.ac.jp

W.H. Kim, J.H. Cheon (eds.), *Atlas of Inflammatory Bowel Diseases*,
DOI 10.1007/978-3-642-39423-2_6,

Table 6.1 Endoscopic features of small bowel lesions in Crohn's disease

Feature
Distribution
Discontinuous pattern of inflammation
Skip lesions
Ulcerous lesion
Longitudinal ulcer (mesenteric side)
Fissuring ulcer
Round ulcer (longitudinal arrangement)
Aphthous ulcer (longitudinal arrangement)
Elevated lesion
Cobblestone appearance
Inflammatory polyp
Deformity
Asymmetrical deformity
Pseudodiverticular formation
Others
Stricture
Fistula

Table 6.2 Major differential diagnosis (small bowel disorders) of Crohn's disease

Category	Cause	Disease
Acute infectious enteritis	Bacterial	Vibrio enteritis
		Salmonella enteritis
		Campylobacter enteritis
		Yersinia enteritis
	Viral	Cytomegalovirus enteritis
	Parasitic	Anisakiasis
Chronic infectious enteritis	Bacterial	Intestinal tuberculosis
	Parasitic	Giardiasis
		Strongyloidiasis
		Isosporiasis
Acute noninfectious enteritis	Inflammatory	Eosinophilic gastroenteritis
		Henoch-Schönlein purpura
	Vascular	Ischemic enteritis
Chronic noninfectious enteritis	Inflammatory	Behçet's disease
		Radiation enteritis
		Chronic nonspecific multiple ulcers of the small intestine
	Toxic	NSAID-induced enteritis
	Others	Amyloidosis
		Benign lymphoid hyperplasia

6.2 Small Bowel Enteroscopy

6.2.1 Normal Findings

Figure 6.1.

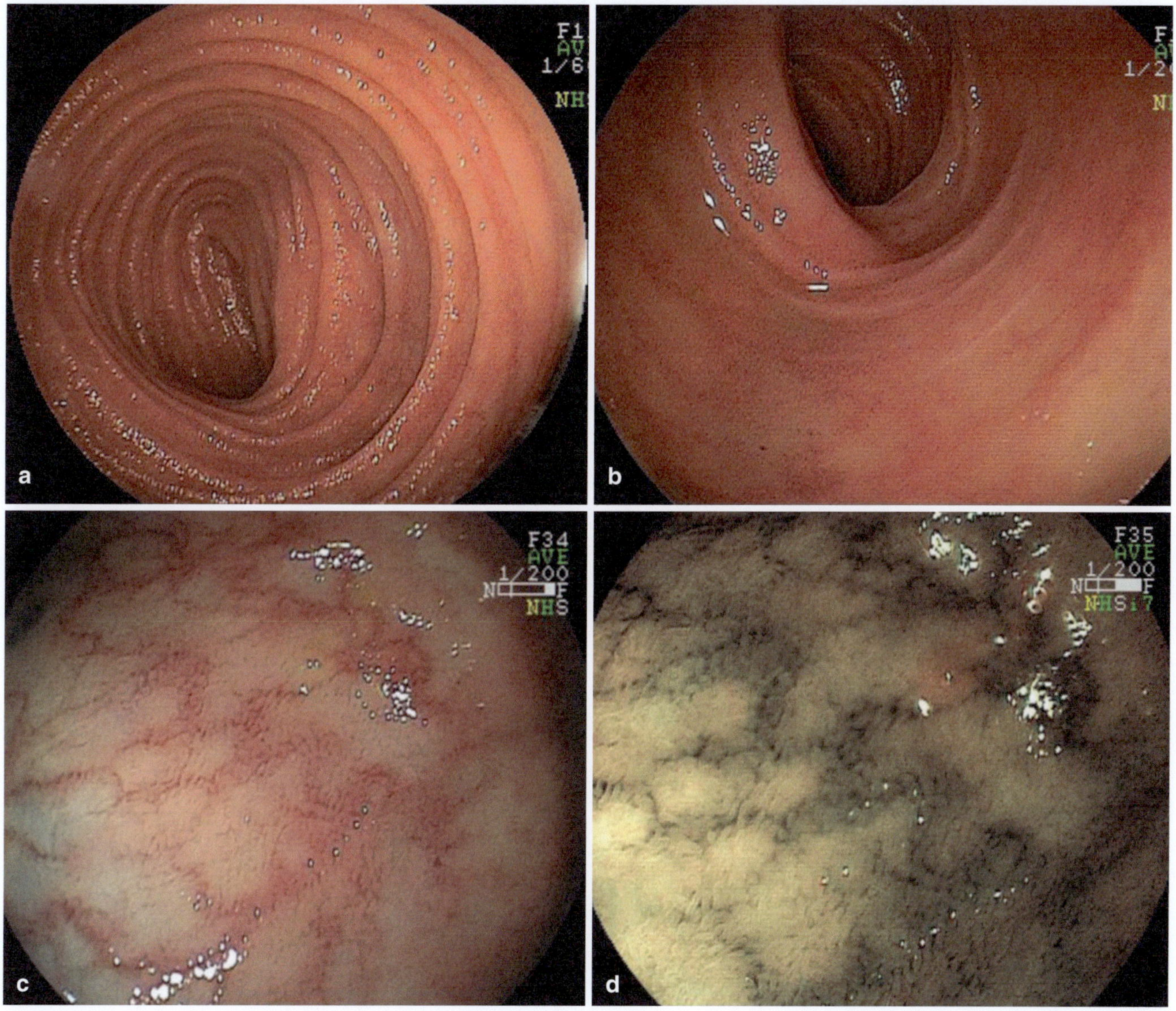

Fig. 6.1 Normal findings of the small intestine (**a**) Normal jejunal mucosa. The Kerckring's folds are prominent. (**b**) Normal ileal mucosa. The folds in the ileum are less prominent and villi are rather flattened compared to the jejunum. (**c**) Normal ileal vessels (white light). (**d**) Normal ileal vessels are observed by FUJI Intelligent Color Enhancement (FICE). (**e**, **f**) Normal ileal villi are observed by magnifying view (**e** white light, **f** after dye spraying)

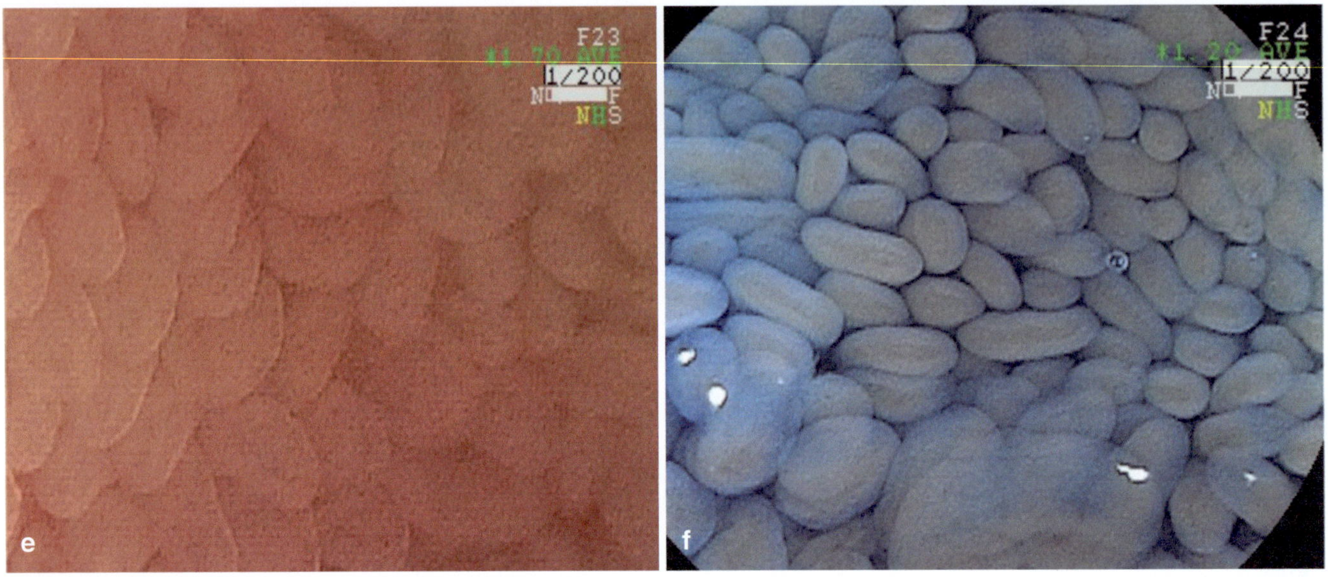

Fig. 6.1 (continued)

6.2.2 Various Findings of Inflammation

6.2.2.1 Aphthous Ulcer, Small Ulcer

Aphthous ulcer is the small and shallow ulcerous lesion of the intestine. Although aphthous ulcers are often observed in various inflammatory small bowel disorders, these are not specific findings. However, certain characteristics of aphthous ulcers, such as their arrangement and distribution, might be useful in diagnosing each disease (Fig. 6.2, 6.3, 6.4, and 6.5).

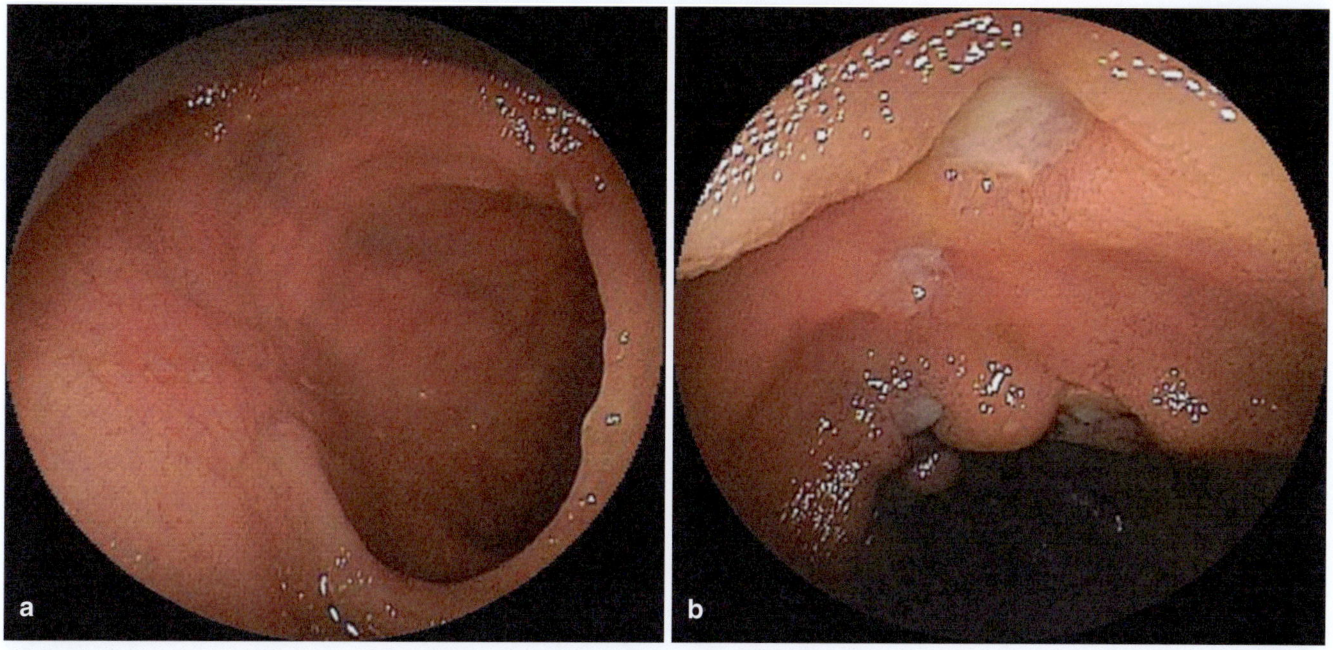

Fig. 6.2 Crohn's disease (the lower ileum, retrograde approach of DBE). (**a**) Multiple aphthous ulcers are arranged in a longitudinal direction. Typical small lesions of Crohn's disease (CD) show longitudinal arrangement. (**b**) The aphthous ulcers are relatively large and scattered densely in the ileal lumen. These types of aphthous ulcers are more likely to progress to the typical longitudinal ulcer (Reprinted **b** with permission from Hirai et al. [21]. Copyright 2009 by IGAKU-SHOIN Ltd)

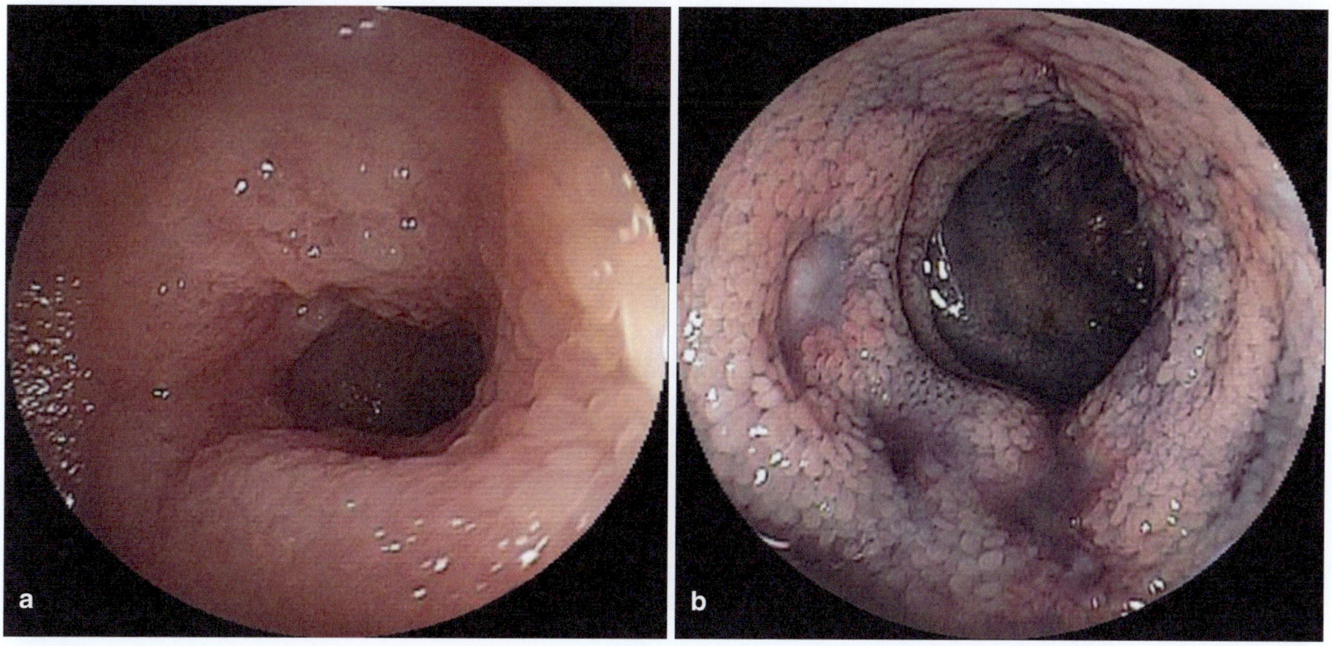

Fig. 6.3 NSAID-induced small bowel lesions (the mid ileum, retrograde approach). NSAID-induced small bowel lesions tend to show the circumferential arrangement. (**a**, **b**) Multiple aphthous ulcers are arranged in a transverse direction (**a** white light, **b** after dye spraying)

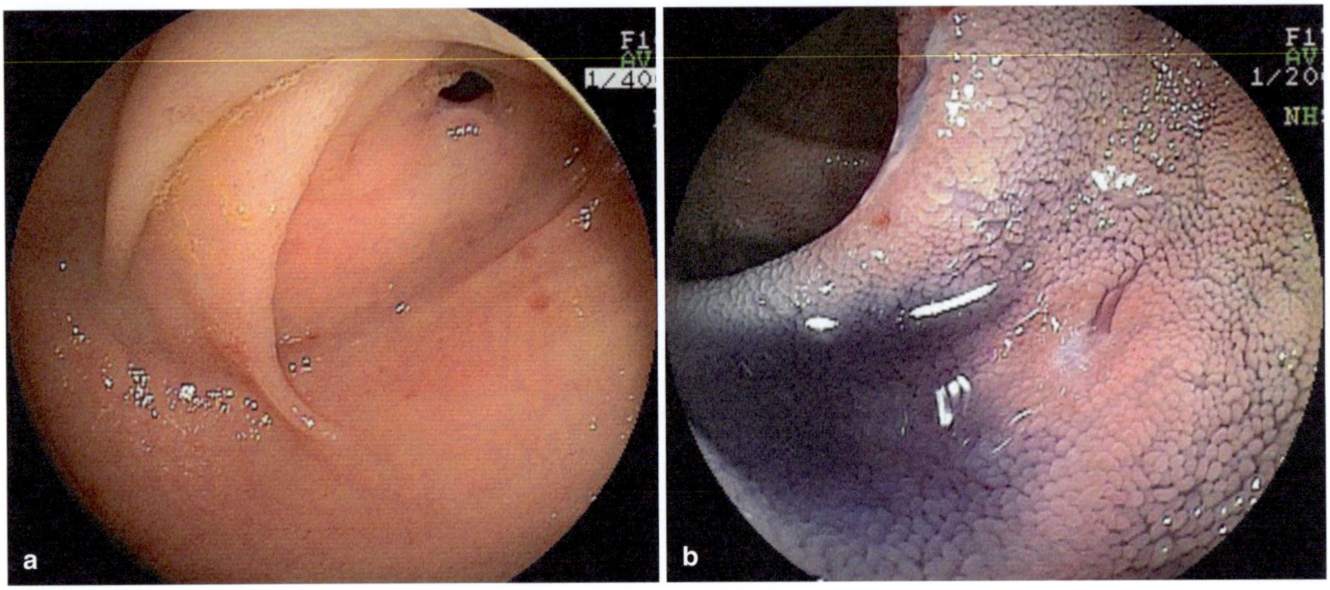

Fig. 6.4 Chronic nonspecific multiple ulcers of the small intestine (the lower ileum, retrograde approach). Chronic nonspecific multiple ulcers of the small intestine (CMUSI) are rare entity which manifest the chronic clinical course of iron deficiency anemia and hypoproteinemia resulting from occult blood loss from multiple ulcers of the small intestine. Small bowel lesions of CMUSI are usually located in the lower ileum without involving the terminal ileum and show various types of ulcers including aphthous ulcers. (**a**) A few small red aphthous ulcers are observed close to the ileal stricture. (**b**) An aphthous ulcer is seen close to the main shallow lineal ulcer with partial stenosis. Small lesions of CMUSI are usually located near the main lesions (Reprinted **b** with permission from Hirai et al. [21] Copyright 2009 by IGAKU-SHOIN Ltd)

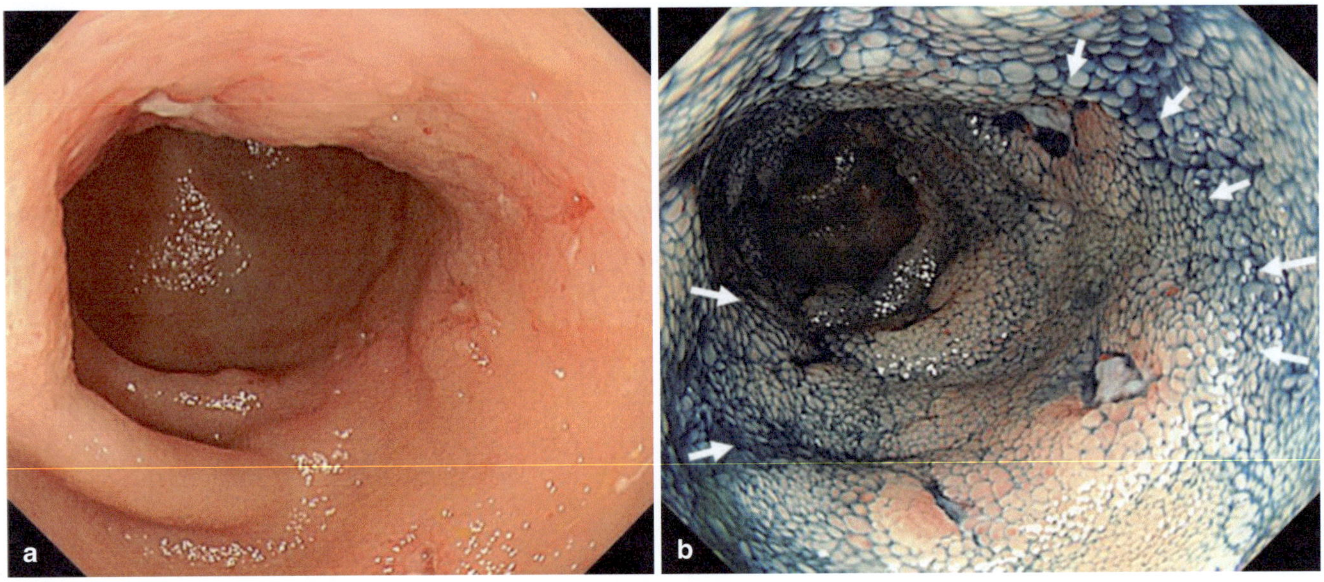

Fig. 6.5 Intestinal tuberculosis (the terminal ileum, retrograde approach). The small lesions of intestinal tuberculosis are typically seen in a Peyer's patch. These small ulcerous lesions usually tend to spread in a transverse or circumferential orientation relative to the long axis of the intestinal lumen. (**a**, **b**) Multiple aphthous ulcers are seen in a Peyer's patch (*arrows*) of the terminal ileum (**a** white light, **b** after dye spraying)

6.2.2.2 Ulcer, Ulcerous Lesion

Ulcer is the most popular lesion of small bowel inflammatory disorders. Various shapes, sizes, depths, and arrangement patterns of small bowel ulcers can be observed by BAE. These characteristics of ulcers are useful for the diagnosis of each disease (Fig. 6.6, 6.7, 6.8, 6.9, 6.10, 6.11, 6.12, and 6.13).

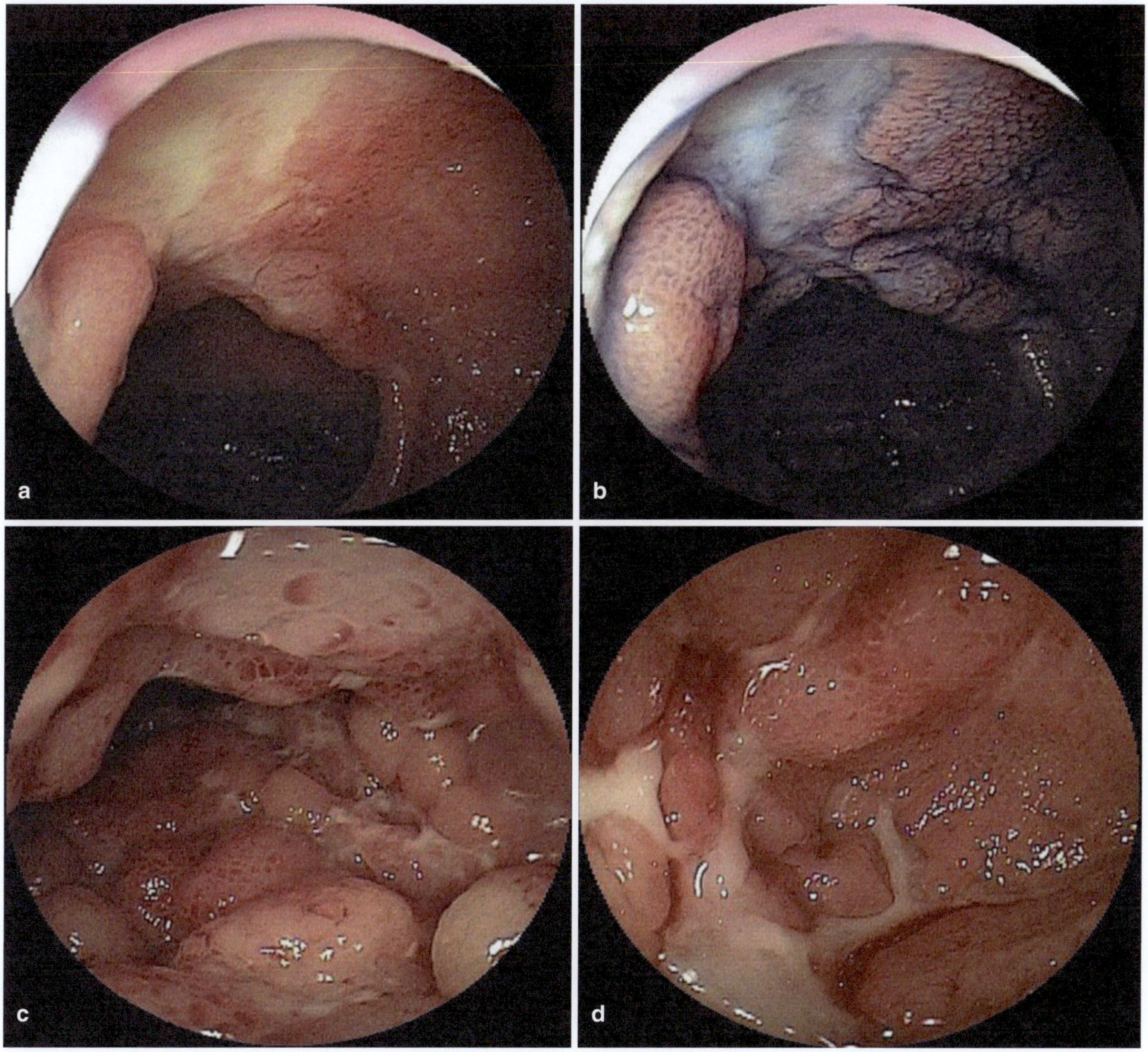

Fig. 6.6 Crohn's disease (the lower ileum, retrograde approach). (**a**, **b**) A typical longitudinal ulcer is seen in the mesenteric side of the ileal lumen (**a** white light, **b** after dye spraying). (**c**, **d**) Cobblestone appearance with longitudinal ulcers is seen in the ileum

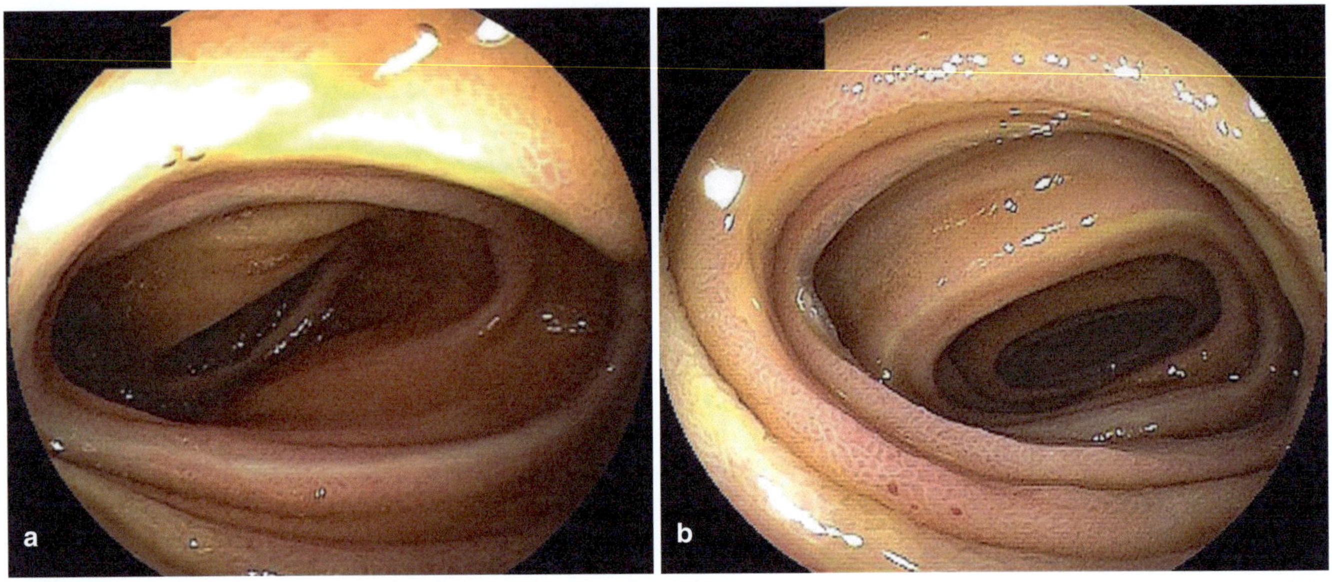

Fig. 6.7 NSAID-induced small bowel lesions (the mid jejunum, antegrade approach). Typical ulcers of NSAID-induced small bowel lesions are usually seen arranged circumferentially along the Kerckring's fold. (**a**, **b**) A narrow circumferential ulcer along the Kerckring's fold is seen in the jejunum (Reprinted **b** with permission from Hirai et al. [22]. Copyright 2007 by TOKYO IGAKUSHA LTD)

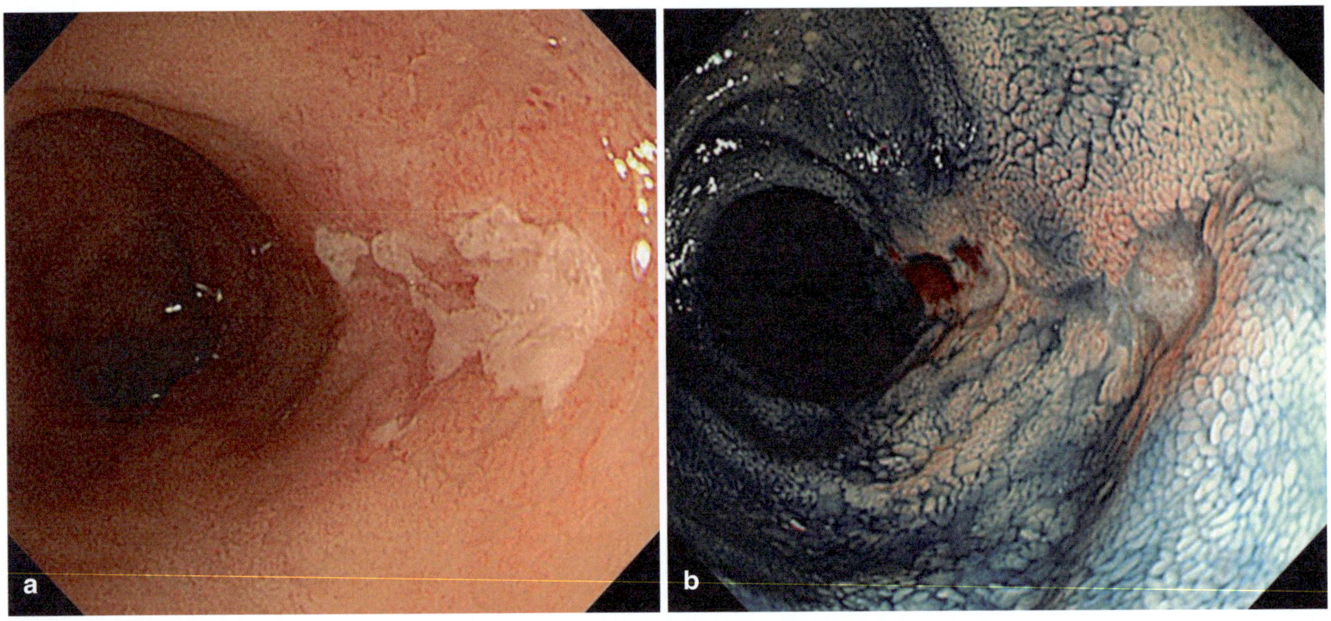

Fig. 6.8 Intestinal tuberculosis (the mid ileum, retrograde approach). (**a**, **b**) Geographically shaped ulcer is seen in a Peyer's patch in the lower ileum (**a** white light, **b** after dye spraying). (**c**, **d**) Irregularly shaped ulcers with exudate in the antimesenteric side of the ileal lumen (**a** white light, **b** after dye spraying)

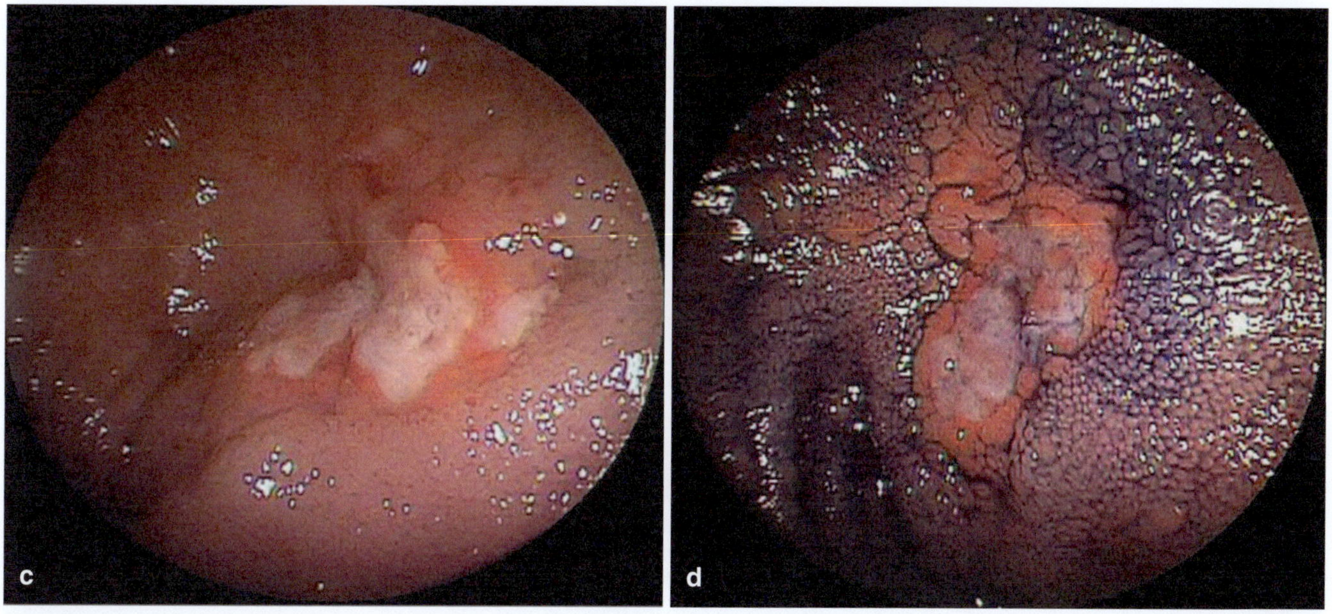

Fig. 6.8 (continued)

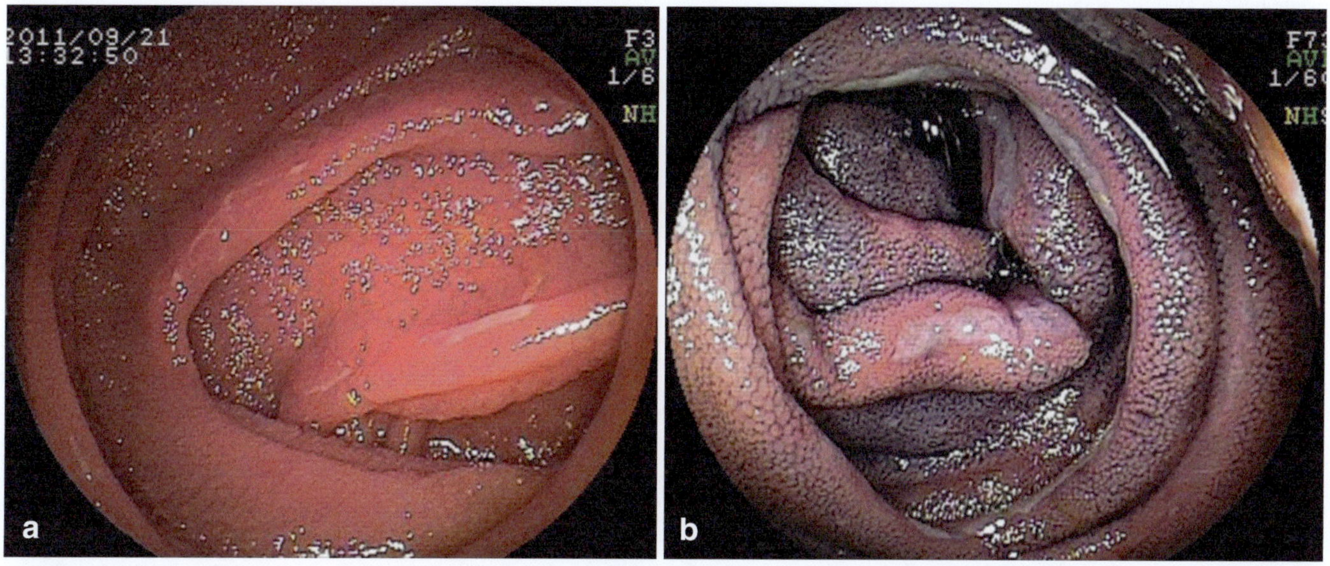

Fig. 6.9 Chronic nonspecific multiple ulcers of the small intestine (the lower ileum, retrograde approach). (**a**) A thin and linear ulcer is seen in a diagonal orientation relative to the long axis of the ileal lumen. (**b**) An ulcer with clear shape and margin in the lower ileum

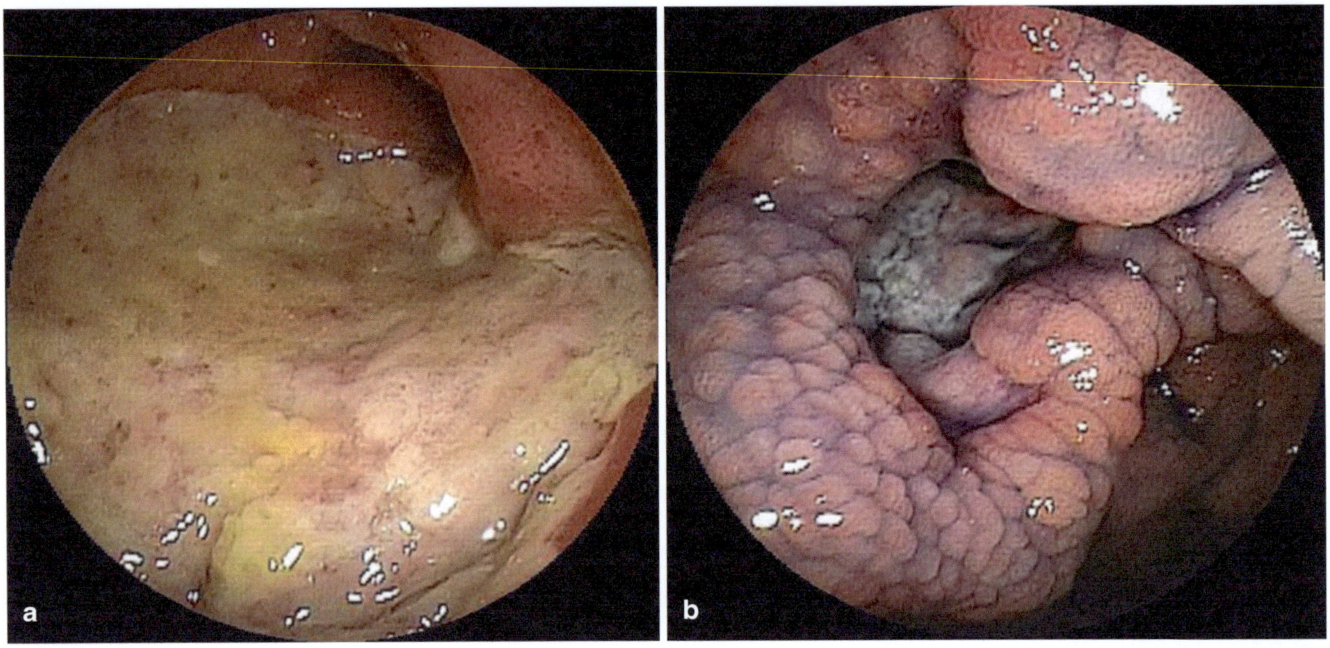

Fig. 6.10 Intestinal Behçet's disease (the terminal ileum, retrograde approach). (**a**, **b**) A sharply demarcated deep ulcer in the terminal ileum (**a** white light, **b** after dye spraying)

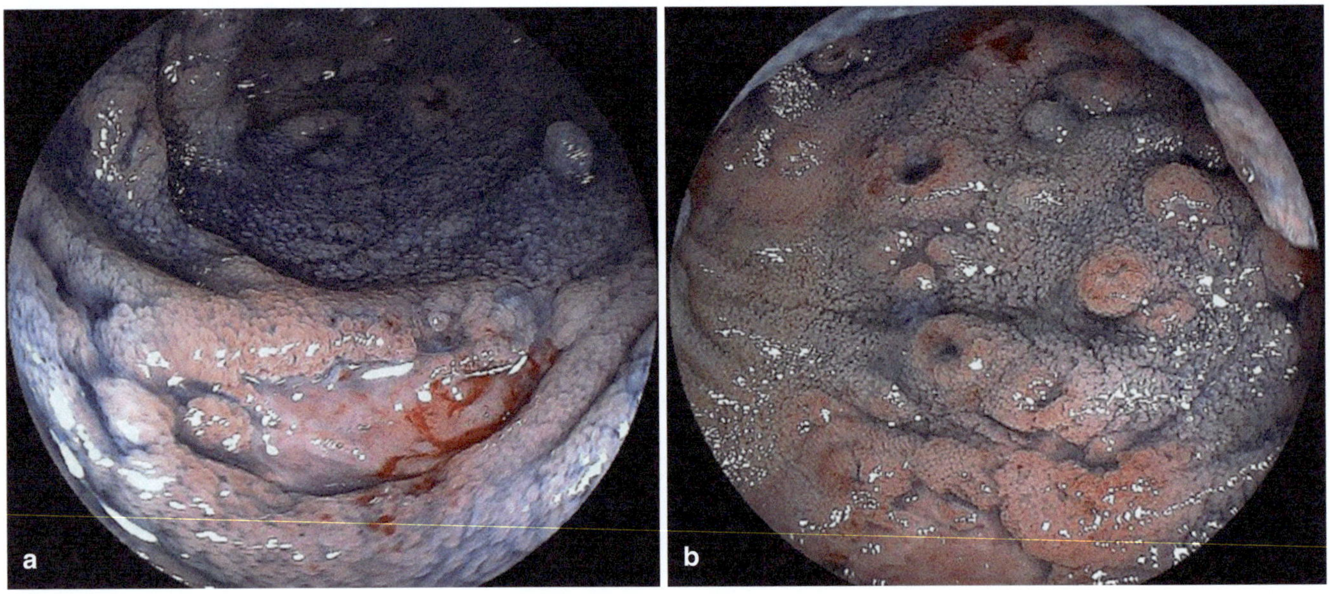

Fig. 6.11 Yersinia enteritis (the terminal ileum, retrograde approach). Infectious diseases frequently involve the small bowel. However, mainly because of the severe abdominal symptoms in acute phase, it is uncommon to be able to observe small bowel lesions endoscopically. The lesions of Yersinia enteritis are usually observed in the terminal ileum. The terminal ileal ulcerous lesions of this disease and the CD lesions are often very alike. Therefore, Yersinia enteritis is one of the important diseases which should be differentiated from CD. (**a**) A slightly irregularly shaped ulcer and aphthous ulcers with a longitudinal arrangement are seen in the terminal ileum (after dye spraying). (**b**) Lymphoid hyperplasia and aphthous ulcers are also seen (after dye spraying)

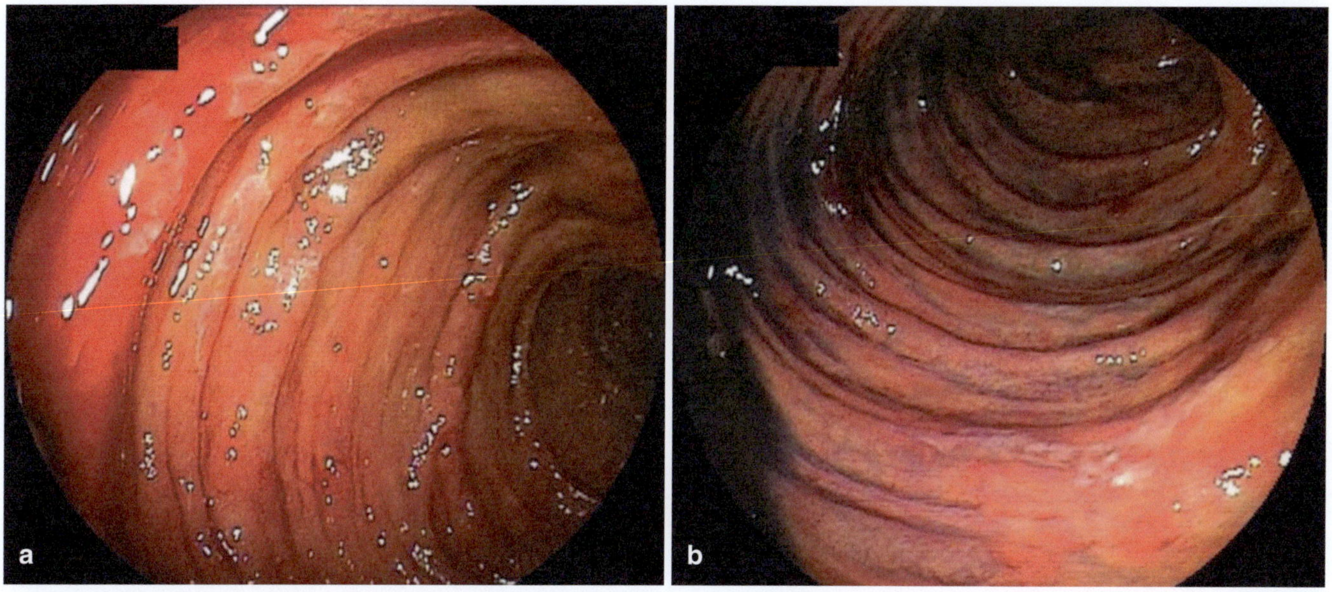

Fig. 6.12 Secondary amyloidosis (the upper jejunum, antegrade approach). Systemic diseases (e.g., amyloidosis, collagen disorder, endocrine metabolic disease, etc.) often have small bowel lesions. (**a**, **b**) Friability, redness, and erosions of the jejunum are observed in patients with secondary amyloidosis. In this case, AA-type amyloid was confirmed by pathological evaluation of the biopsy specimen from the jejunal lesion (**a** white light, **b** after dye spraying)

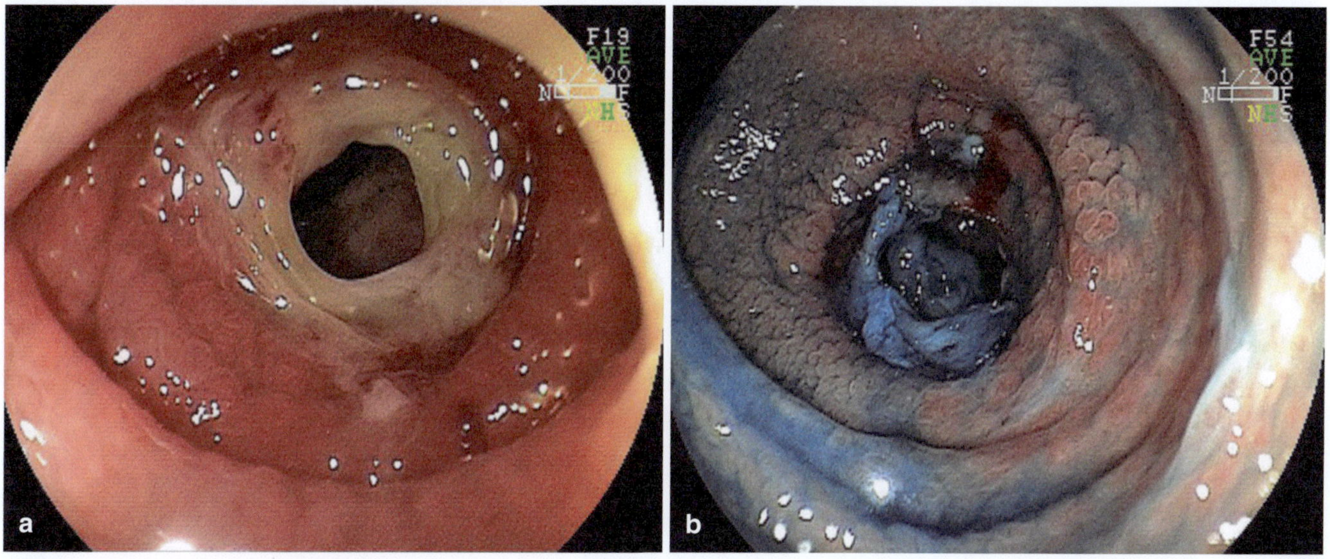

Fig. 6.13 Ischemic enteritis (the lower ileum, retrograde approach). Ischemic enteritis is a rare entity compared with ischemic colitis, although the cause of both diseases is ischemia of the intestine. Moreover, since ischemic enteritis is a more severe condition, in general, surgical intervention is necessary. (**a**, **b**) A girdle ulcer with mild luminal stricture of the ileum (**a** white light, **b** after dye spraying)

6.2.2.3 Strictures

Inflammatory intestinal disorders often cause strictures as the result of severe inflammation or regenerative process. Various types and degrees of strictures are seen in the small bowel by BAE (Fig. 6.14, 6.15, 6.16, and 6.17).

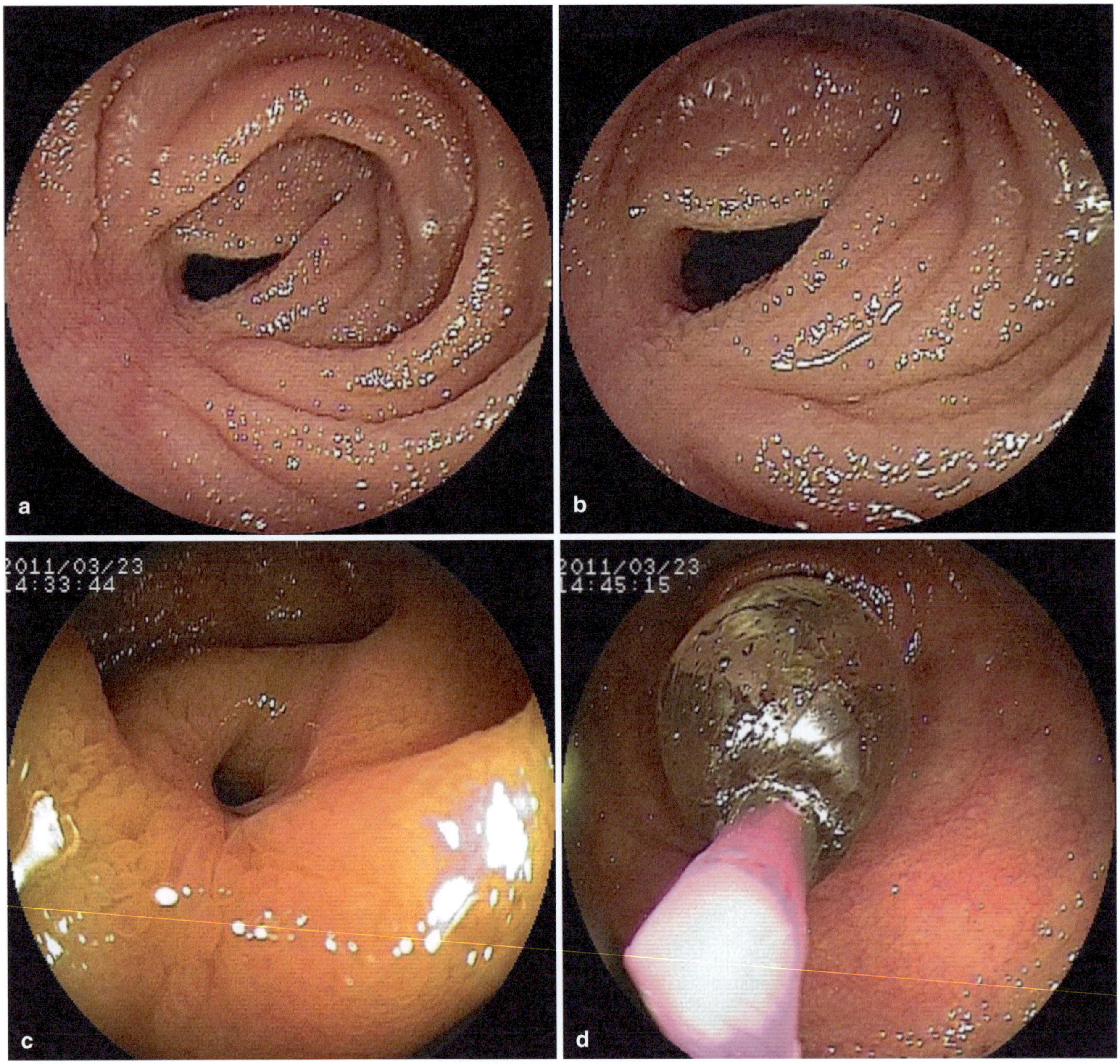

Fig. 6.14 Crohn's disease (the lower ileum, retrograde approach). CD is one of the most common diseases which cause benign intestinal strictures. Various degrees of strictures are seen in active or nonactive lesions of the naïve and the anastomosis sites of the small intestine. Endoscopic balloon dilation is frequently performed for inactive Crohn's strictures [23–24]. (**a**, **b**) A moderate stricture with deformity is seen in the ileum. There are no active lesions of CD. (**c**–**f**) A severe stricture of ileoileal anastomosis with pseudodiverticular formation is seen in the lower ileum. (**c**) During endoscopic balloon dilation (**d**), stricture site is seen through the balloon catheter. (**e**) Stricture site after endoscopic balloon dilation (**f**)

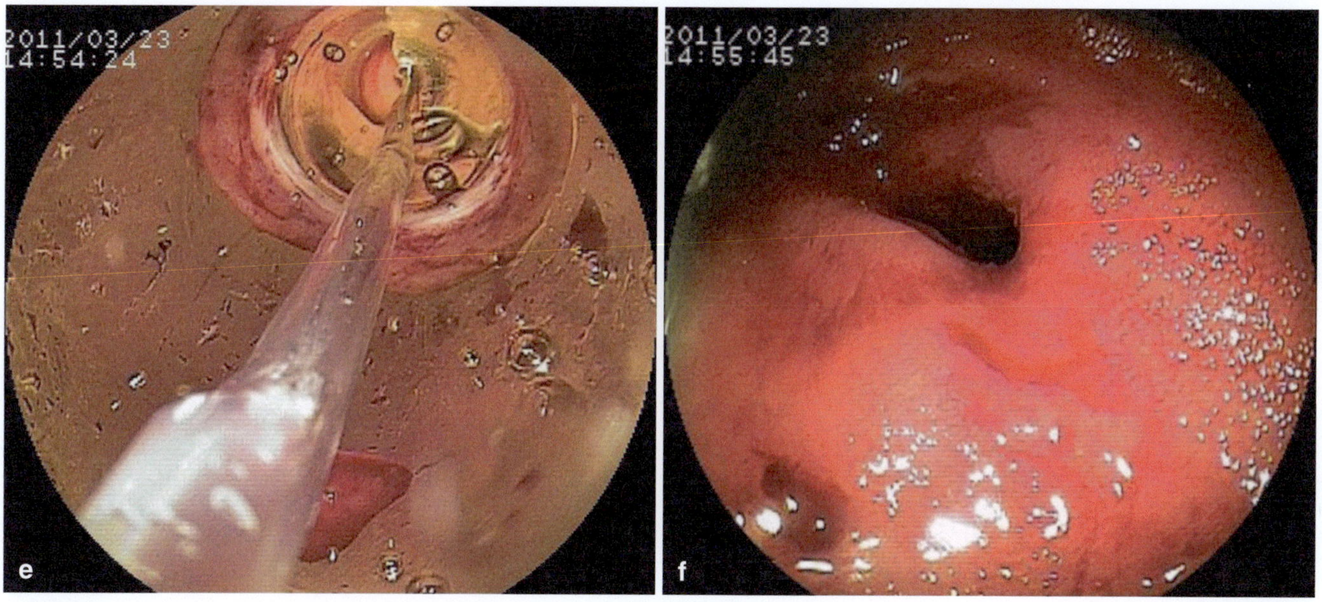

Fig. 6.14 (continued)

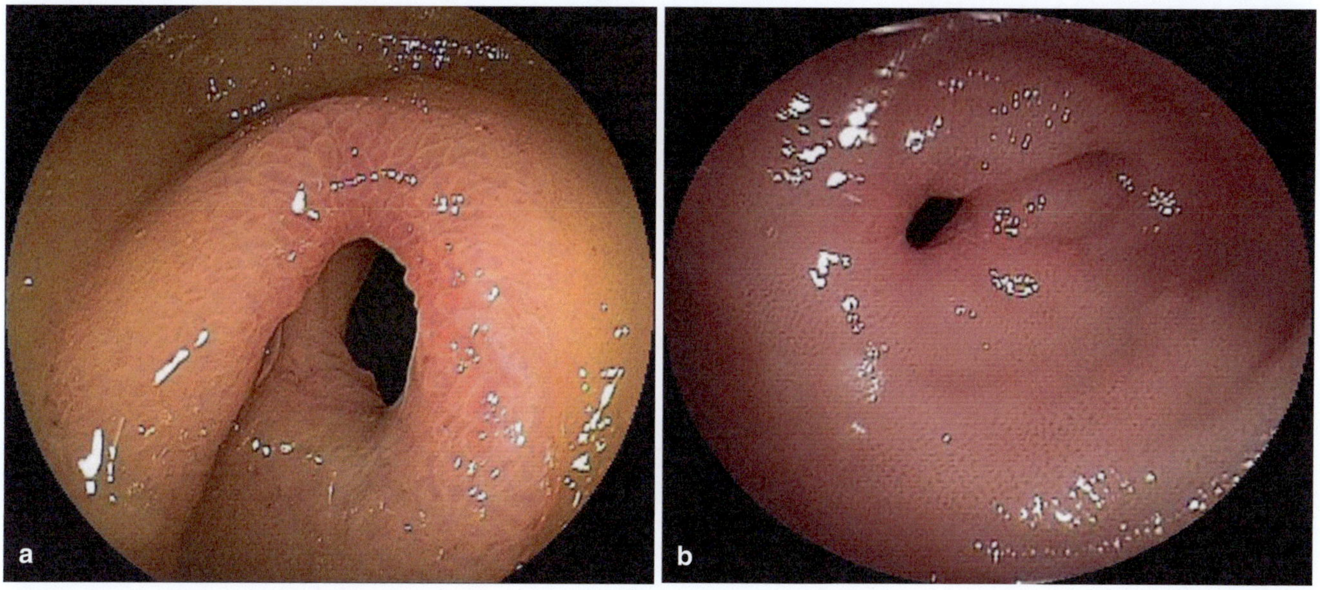

Fig. 6.15 NSAID-induced small bowel lesions (the mid jejunum, antegrade approach). (**a**) Moderate stricture with a circumferential ulcer scar is seen in the jejunum. (**b**) A severe stricture, the so-called diaphragm-like stricture of the jejunum

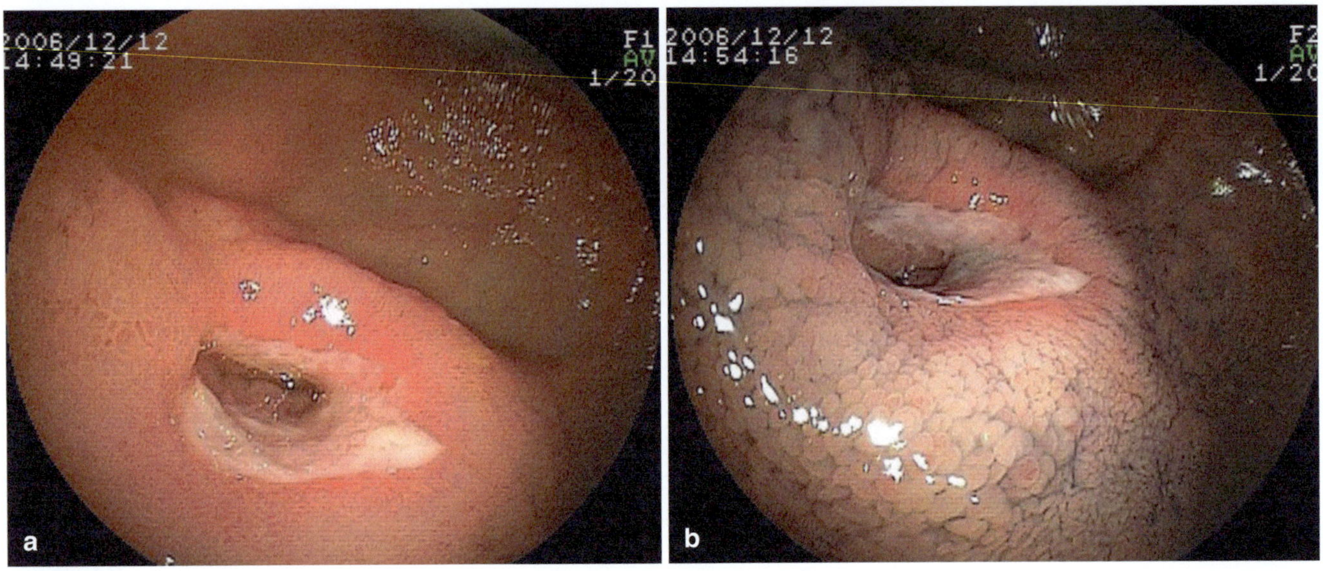

Fig. 6.16 Intestinal tuberculosis (the mid ileum, retrograde approach). (**a**, **b**) A moderate stricture with an irregularly shaped circumferential ulcer is seen in the lower ileum (**a** white light, **b** after dye spraying)

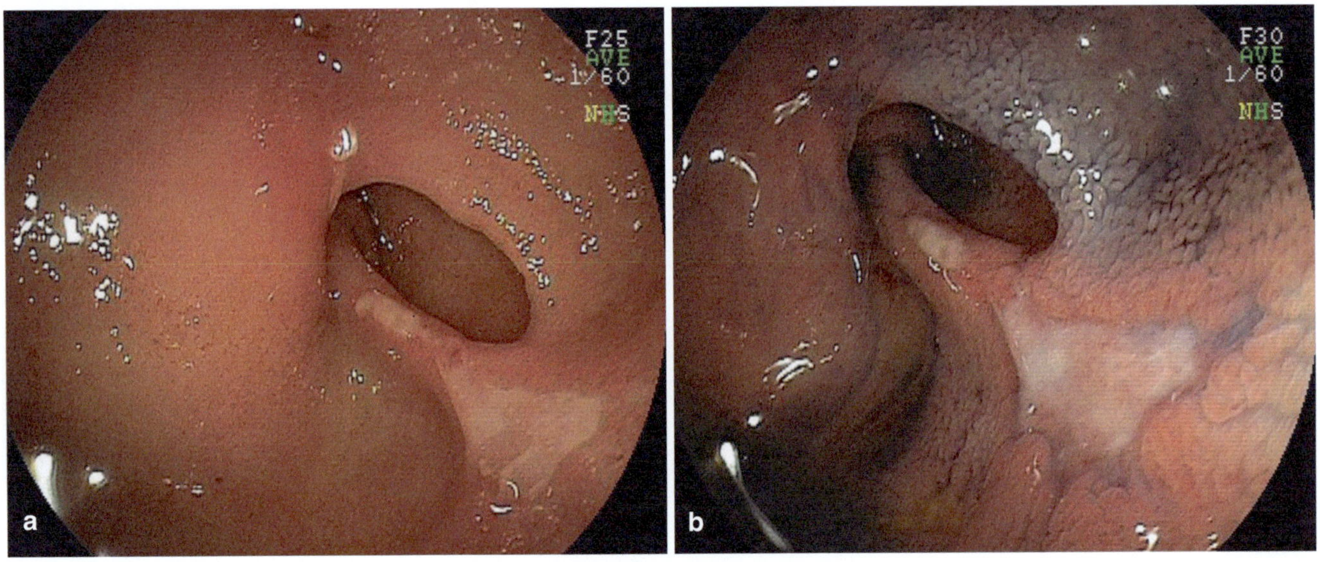

Fig. 6.17 Chronic nonspecific multiple ulcers of the small intestine (the lower ileum, retrograde approach). (**a**, **b**) A severe stricture with a shallow ulcer showing a diagonal orientation is seen in the lower ileum (**a** white light, **b** after dye spraying)

6.3 Capsule Endoscopy

6.3.1 Normal Findings

Figures 6.18 and 6.19.

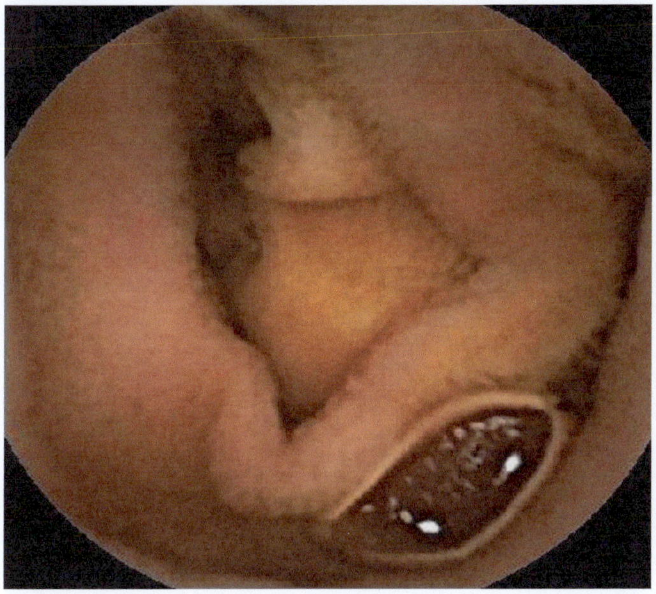

Fig. 6.18 Normal findings of the jejunum

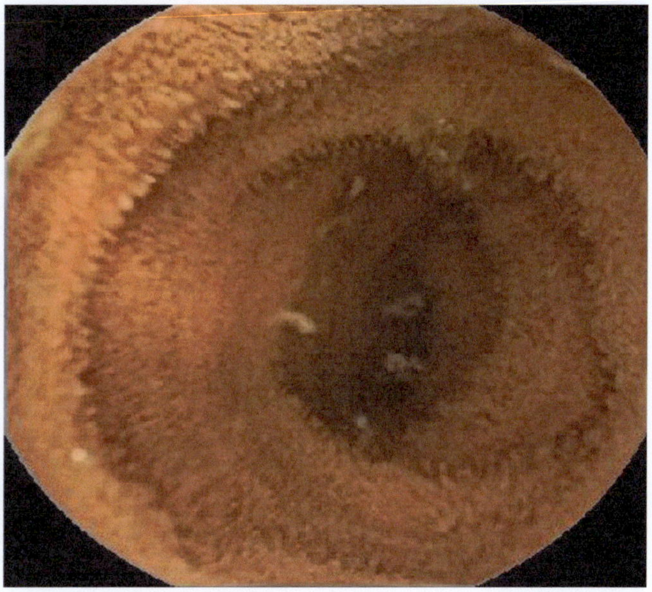

Fig. 6.19 Normal findings of the ileum

6.3.2 Various Findings of Inflammatory Disorders

Figures 6.20, 6.21, 6.22, 6.23, and 6.24.

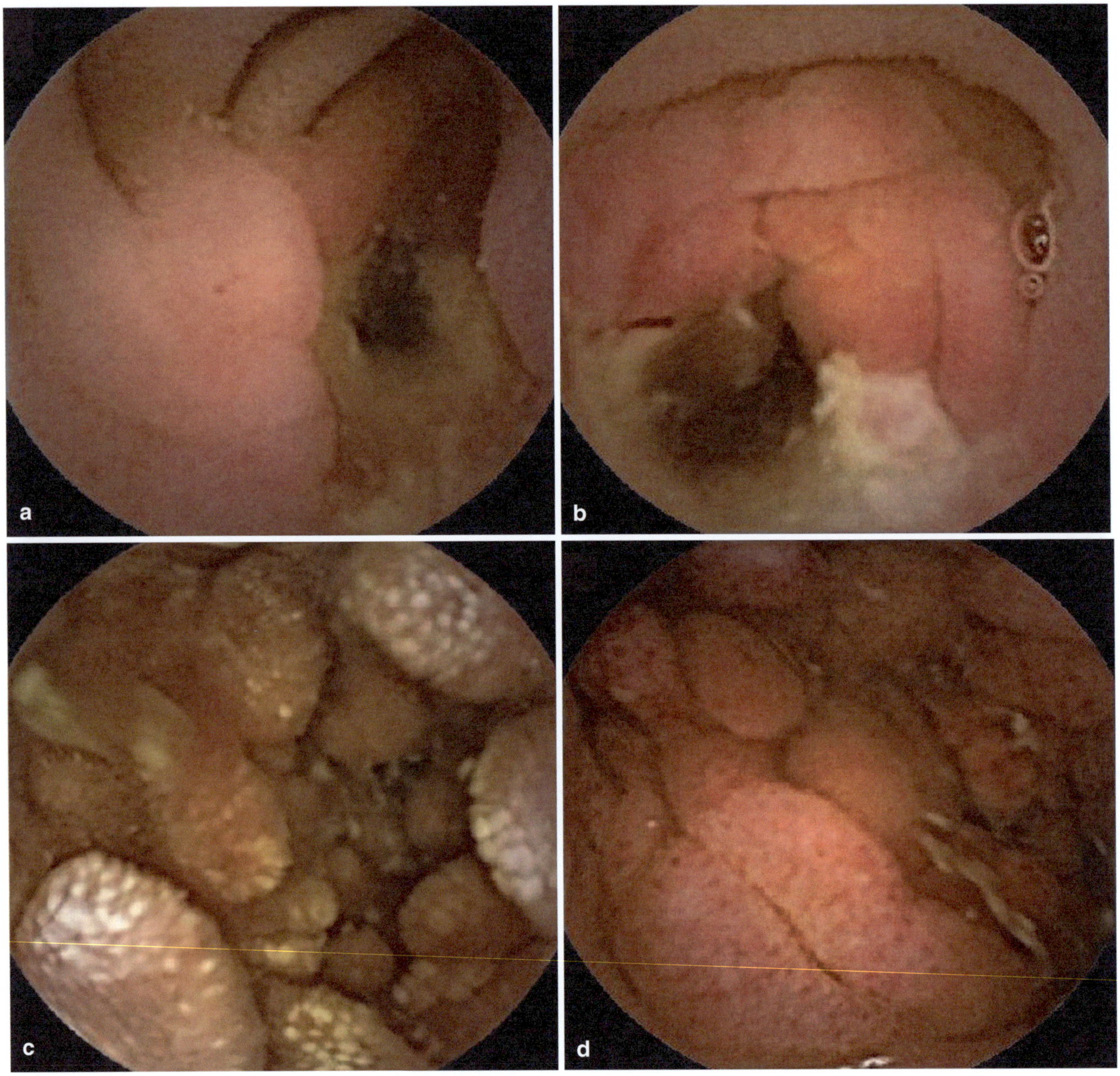

Fig. 6.20 Crohn's disease. In Western countries, confirmation of three to five or more ulcers of the small intestine by CE is thought to be the definition of CD. On the other hand, according to the Japanese guideline, the main findings of CD for diagnosis are longitudinal ulcer, cobblestone appearance, and epithelioid cell granuloma. However, it is not always easy to confirm the typical longitudinal ulcers or cobblestone appearance by CE. Moreover, high retention rate is an issue on the use of CE in patients with confirmed CD or suspected CD. The patency capsule should be performed precisely prior to CE. The obvious definition of CD using CE would be needed for the correct diagnosis in the future. (**a**, **b**) A typical longitudinal ulcer is seen in the ileum. (**c**, **d**) Cobblestone appearance with mild stricture is seen in the ileum. (**e**, **f**) Multiple small ulcers in a patient with CD that meet the Japanese diagnostic criteria. (**g**, **h**) Multiple aphthous ulcers with longitudinal arrangement in a patient with CD that meet the Japanese diagnostic criteria

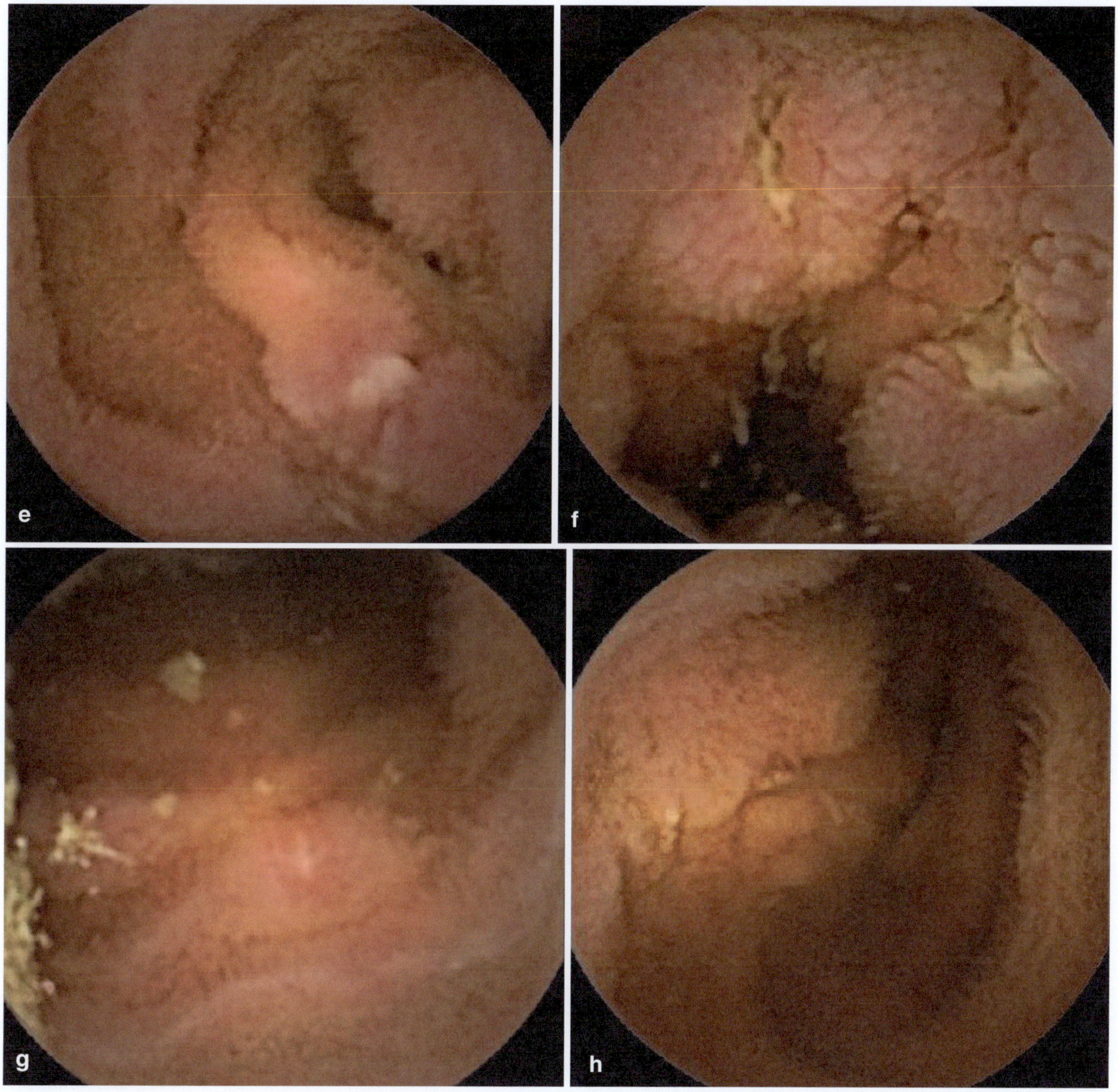

Fig. 6.20 (continued)

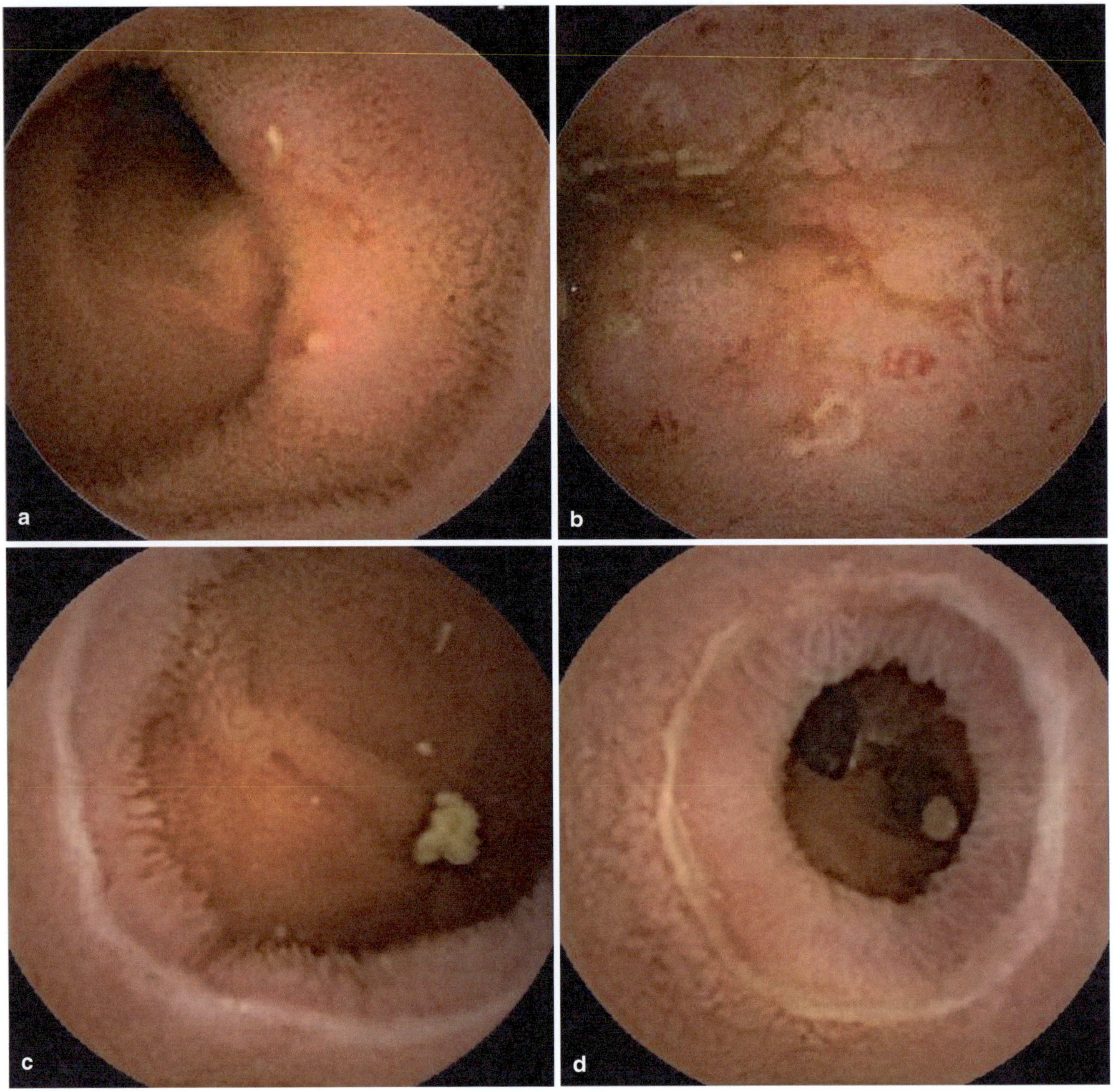

Fig. 6.21 NSAID-induced small bowel lesions. CE is a useful diagnostic modality for patients with obscure gastrointestinal bleeding (OGIB). NSAID users with OGIB have small bowel lesions frequently. In CE findings, various types of small bowel ulcerous lesions are seen in NSAID-induced small bowel lesions. (**a**, **b**) Multiple aphthous ulcers are seen in the ileum. Only these endoscopic findings are not confirmative for specific diseases such as CD, but nonspecific. (**c**, **d**) A shallow and narrow circumferential ulcer along the Kerckring's fold is seen in the ileum. (**e**, **f**) Linear ulcer scar in the ileum

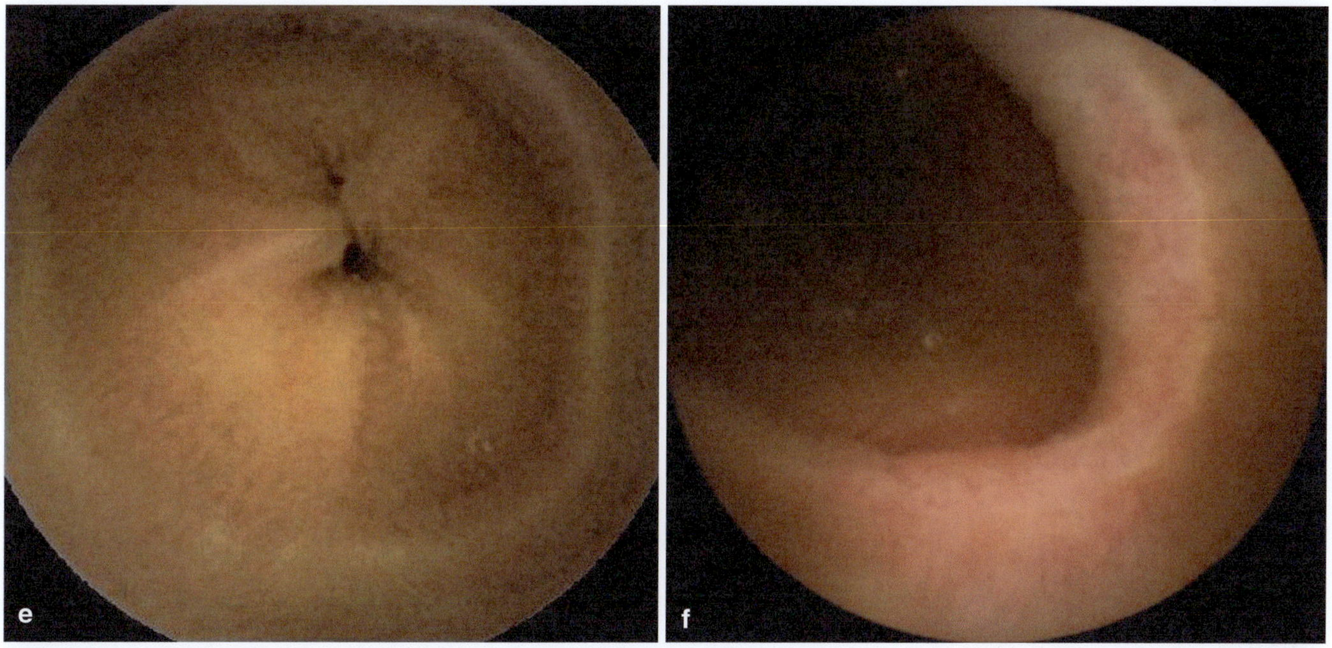

Fig. 6.21 (continued)

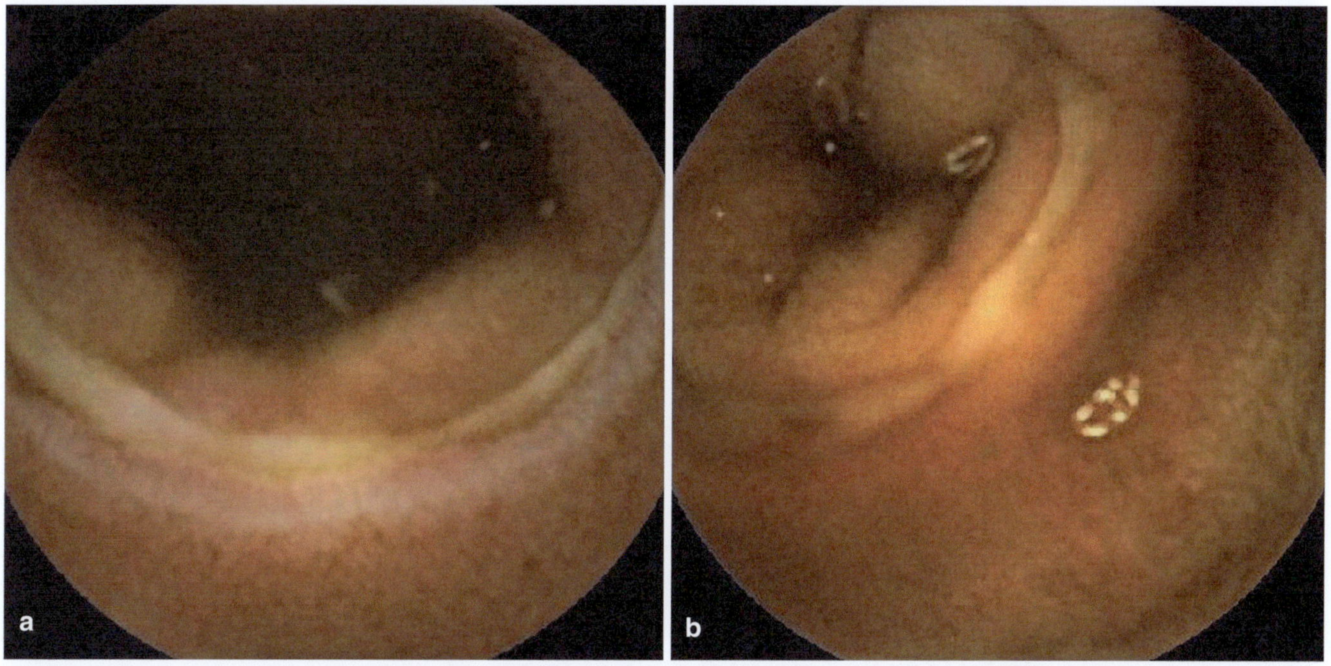

Fig. 6.22 Chronic nonspecific multiple ulcers of the small intestine. (**a**, **b**) A thin and linear ulcer is seen in the ileum. The ulcer shows a diagonal orientation relative to the long axis of the ileal lumen. (**c**, **d**) The edge of this ulcer is extremely sharp, and the mucosa surrounding the ulcer is normal

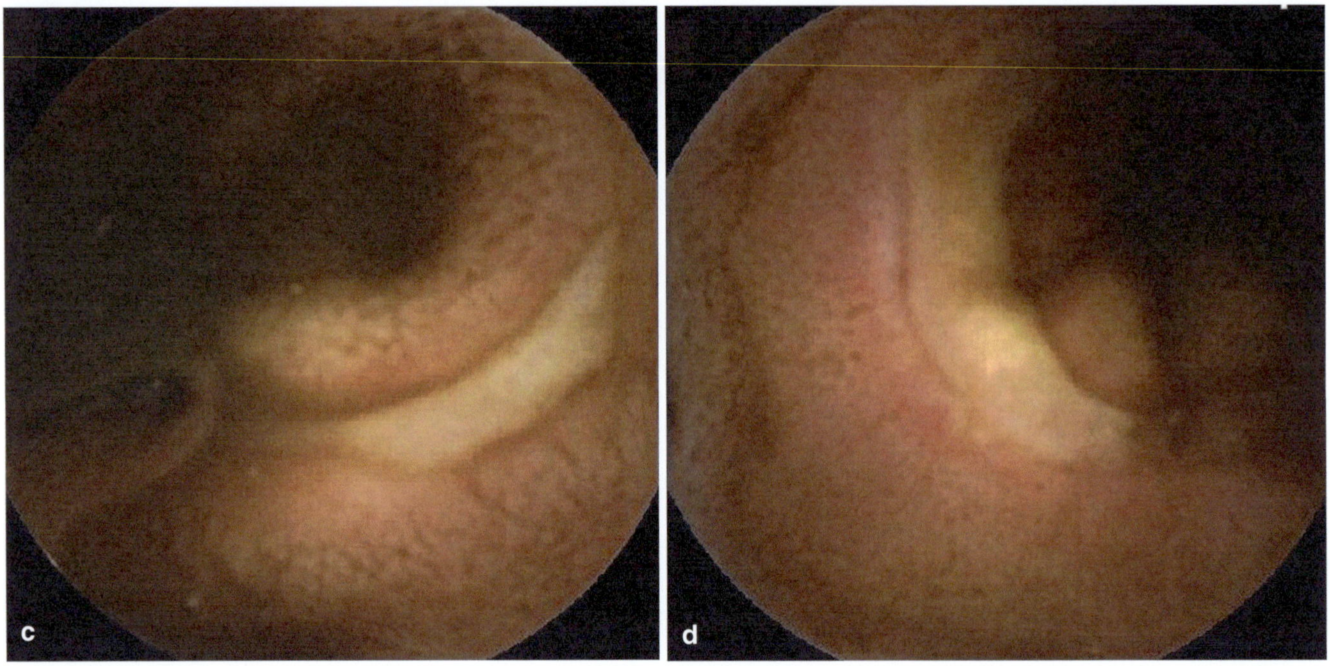

Fig. 6.22 (continued)

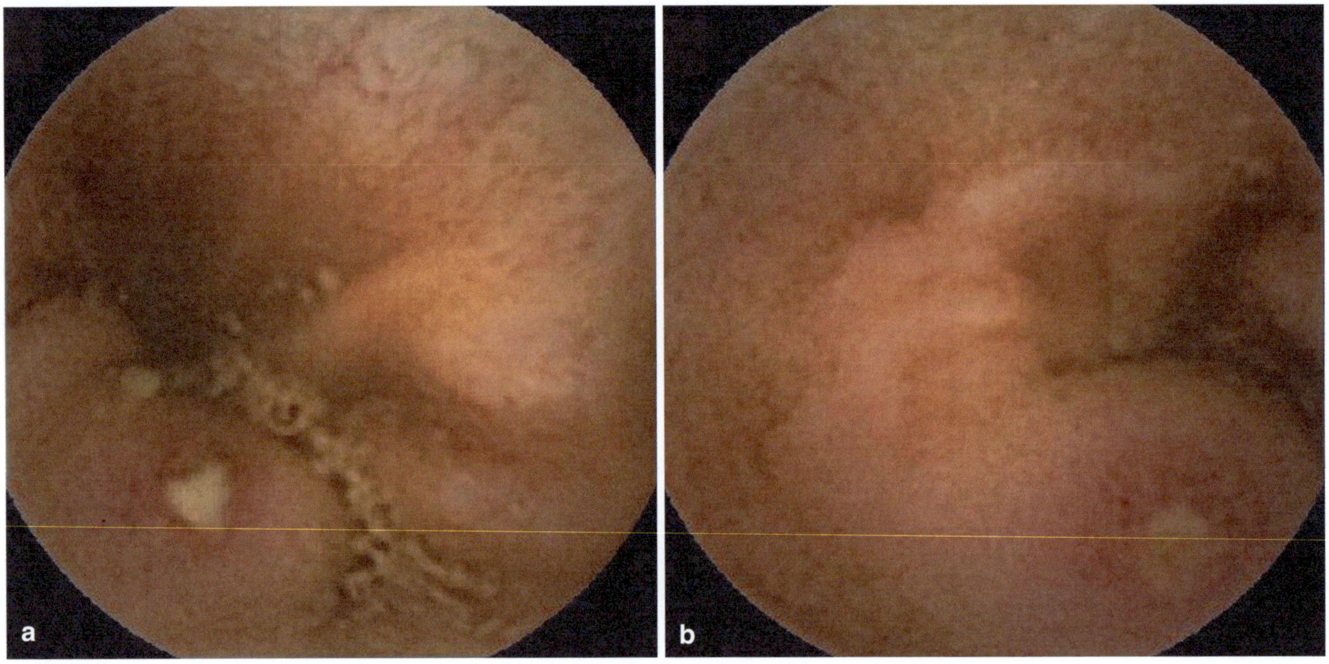

Fig. 6.23 Intestinal Behçet's disease (the terminal ileum, retrograde approach). (**a**, **b**) Small ileal ulcers are seen in a patient with intestinal Behçet's disease. These ulcers are thought to be the daughter lesions

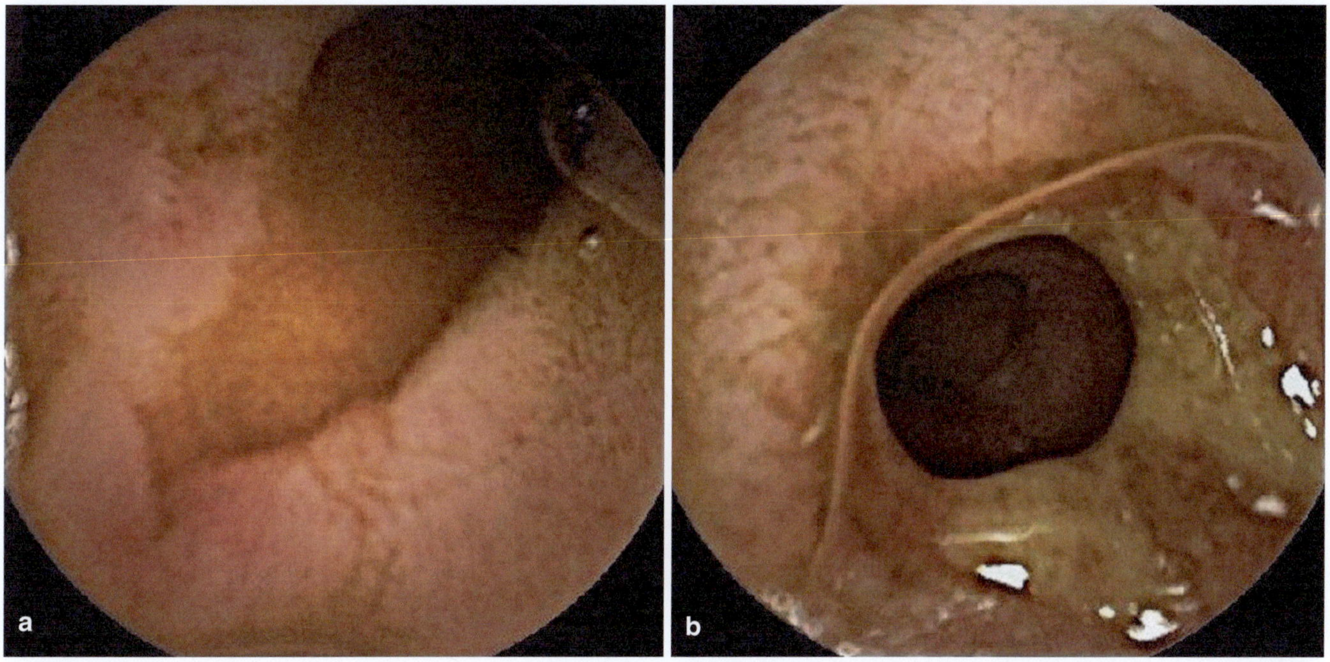

Fig. 6.24 Small bowel lesions induced by cytomegalovirus infection. In immunocompromised hosts, the reactivation of cytomegalovirus (CMV) occurs frequently. Cytomegalovirus infection can involve potentially all parts of the gastrointestinal tract. Although the colon and esophagus are the most common sites, small bowel lesions are sometimes observed by CE. (**a**) A clear shape of small ulcer is seen in the ileum of a patient with diabetes mellitus. (**b**) A geographically shaped large ulcer is seen in the lower ileum. In this case, inclusion body was confirmed by pathological findings of biopsy specimen from the ileal lesion

References

1. Yamamoto H, Kita H, Sunada K, Hayashi Y, Sato H, Yano T, Iwamoto M, Sekine Y, Miyata T, Kuno A, Ajibe H, Ido K, Sugano K. Clinical outcomes of double-balloon endoscopy for the diagnosis and treatment of small-intestinal diseases. Clin Gastroenterol Hepatol. 2004;2:1010–6.
2. Liao Z, Gao R, Xu C, Li ZS. Indications and detection, completion, and retention rates of small-bowel capsule endoscopy: a systematic review. Gastrointest Endosc. 2010;71:280–6.
3. Nakamura T, Terano A. Capsule endoscopy: past, present, and future. J Gastroenterol. 2008;43:93–9.
4. Van Assche G, Dignass A, Panes J, Beaugerie L, Karagiannis J, Allez M, Ochsenkühn T, Orchard T, Rogler G, Louis E, et al. The second European evidence-based consensus on the diagnosis and management of Crohn's disease: definitions and diagnosis. J Crohns Colitis. 2010;4:7–27.
5. Ueno F, Matsui T, Matsumoto T, Matsuoka K, Watanabe M, Hibi T, Guidelines Project Group of the Research Group of Intractable Inflammatory Bowel Disease subsidized by the Ministry of Health, Labour and Welfare of Japan and the Guidelines Committee of the Japanese Society of Gastroenterology. Evidence-based clinical practice guidelines for Crohn's disease, integrated with formal consensus of experts in Japan. J Gastroenterol. 2013;48:31–72.
6. Hisabe T, Hirai F, Matsui T, Watanabe M. Evaluation of diagnostic criteria for Crohn's disease in Japan. J Gastroenterol. 2014;49: 93–9.
7. Tsurumi K, Matsui T, Hirai F, Takatsu N, Yano Y, Hisabe T, Sato Y, Beppu T, Fujiwara S, Ishikawa S, Matsushima Y, Okado Y, Ono Y, Yoshizawa N, Nagahama T, Takaki Y, Yao K, Iwashita A. Incidence, clinical characteristics, long-term course, and comparison of progressive and nonprogressive cases of aphthous-type Crohn's disease: a single-center cohort study. Digestion. 2013;87:262–8.
8. Esaki M, Matsumoto T, Watanabe K, Arakawa T, Naito Y, Matsuura M, Nakase H, Hibi T, Matsumoto T, Nouda S, Higuchi K, Ohmiya N, Goto H, Kurokawa S, Motoya S, Watanabe M. Use of capsule endoscopy in patients with Crohn's disease in Japan: a multicenter survey. J Gastroenterol Hepatol. 2014;29:96–101.
9. Bourreille A, Ignjatovic A, Aabakken L, Loftus EV, Eliakim R, Pennazio M, Bouhnik Y, Seidman E, Keuchel M, Albert JG, et al. Role of small-bowel endoscopy in the management of patients with inflammatory bowel disease: an international OMED-ECCO consensus. Endoscopy. 2009;41:618–37.
10. Legnani P, Abreu MT. Use of capsule endoscopy for established Crohn's disease. Gastrointest Endosc Clin N Am. 2006;16: 299–306.
11. Dionisio PM, Gurudu SR, Leighton JA, Leontiadis GI, Fleischer DE, Hara AK, Heigh RI, Shiff AD, Sharma VK. Capsule endoscopy has a significantly higher diagnostic yield in patients with suspected and established small-bowel Crohn's disease: a meta-analysis. Am J Gastroenterol. 2010;105:1240–8. quiz 1249.
12. Tharian B, Caddy G, Tham TC. Enteroscopy in small bowel Crohn's disease: a review. World J Gastrointest Endosc. 2013;5: 476–86.
13. Matsumoto T, Kudo T, Esaki M, Yano T, Yamamoto H, Sakamoto C, Goto H, Nakase H, Tanaka S, Matsui T, Sugano K, Iida M. Prevalence of non-steroidal anti-inflammatory drug-induced enteropathy determined by double-balloon endoscopy. Scand J Gastroenterol. 2008;43:490–6.
14. Lang J, Price AB, Levi AJ, Burke M, Gumpel JM, Bjarnason I. Diaphragm disease: pathology of disease of the small intestine induced by non-steroidal anti-inflammatory drugs. J Clin Pathol. 1988;41:516–26.
15. Almadi MA, Ghosh S, Aljebreen AM. Differentiating intestinal tuberculosis from Crohn's disease: a diagnostic challenge. Am J Gastroenterol. 2009;104:1003–12.
16. Pulimood AB, Amarapurkar DN, Ghoshal U, Phillip M, Pai CG, Reddy DN, Nagi B, Ramakrishna BS. Differentiation of Crohn's disease from intestinal tuberculosis in India in 2010. World J Gastroenterol. 2011;17:433–43.
17. Lee YJ, Yang SK, Byeon JS, Myung SJ, Chang HS, Hong SS, Kim KJ, Lee GH, Jung HY, Hong WS, Kim JH, Min YI, Chang SJ, Yu CS. Analysis of colonoscopic findings in the differential diagnosis between intestinal tuberculosis and Crohn's disease. Endoscopy. 2006;38:592–7.
18. Hisamatsu T, Ueno F, Matsumoto T, Kobayashi K, Koganei K, Kunisaki R, Hirai F, Nagahori M, Matsushita M, Kobayashi K, Kishimoto M, Takeno M, Tanaka M, Inoue N, Hibi T. The 2nd edition of consensus statements for the diagnosis and management of intestinal Behçet's disease: indication of anti-TNFα monoclonal antibodies. J Gastroenterol. 2014;49:156–62.
19. Matsumoto T, Nakamura S, Esaki M, Yada S, Koga H, Yao T, Iida M. Endoscopic features of chronic nonspecific multiple ulcers of the small intestine: comparison with nonsteroidal anti-inflammatory drug-induced enteropathy. Dig Dis Sci. 2006;51: 1357–63.
20. Matsumoto T, Kubokura N, Matsui T, Iida M, Yao T. Chronic nonspecific multiple ulcer of the small intestine segregates in offspring from consanguinity. J Crohns Colitis. 2011;5:559–65.
21. Hirai F, et al. Endoscopic diagnosis for small lesions of the small intestine (in Japanese). Stomach Intestine. 2009;44:983–93.
22. Hirai F, et al. Endoscopic balloon dilation using double balloon endoscope for benign small bowel strictures of inflammatory bowel diseases except Crohn's disease (in Japanese). Endoscop Dig. 2007;19:1571–5.
23. Hirai F, Beppu T, Sou S, Seki T, Yao K, Matsui T. Endoscopic balloon dilatation using double-balloon endoscopy is a useful and safe treatment for small intestinal strictures in Crohn's disease. Dig Endosc. 2010;22:200–4.
24. Ono Y, Hirai F, Matsui T, Beppu T, Yano Y, Takatsu N, Takaki Y, Nagahama T, Hisabe T, Yao K, Higashi D, Futami K. Value of concomitant endoscopic balloon dilation for intestinal stricture during long-term infliximab therapy in patients with Crohn's disease. Dig Endosc. 2012;24:432–8.

Esophagogastroduodenoscopy (EGD)

7

Dong Il Park

Endoscopic evaluation of the upper gastrointestinal (GI) tract in inflammatory bowel disease (IBD) is performed either for IBD-related indications or for the evaluation of symptoms that may not be directly related to IBD. Because direct involvement of the upper GI tract usually does not occur with ulcerative colitis, the focus of this chapter will be on upper GI Crohn's disease (CD). CD is a chronic, idiopathic, inflammatory disease generally involving the ileum and/or colon. It can also affect the whole GI tract from mouth to anus. While involvement of the lower GI tract has been studied in detail, that related to the upper GI tract has not been fully evaluated.

The definition of upper GI involvement in CD is controversial. Some suggests a more stringed classification in terms of the mucosal alterations compatible with upper GI CD. On the other hand, according to other recommendations, a wider spectrum of microscopic lesions should be considered evidence of upper GI CD. A general consensus is also lacking concerning definitions of the macroscopic upper GI involvement; hence, the clinical interpretation of findings, at endoscopy, is challenging. At present, the macroscopic minimum criteria for CD involvement are evidence of ulceration or the presence of aphthous lesions. The finding of erythema and/or edema does not necessarily mean that the tract is affected by CD. Likewise, a histological evaluation, nonspecific inflammation, or inflammatory changes that could be otherwise explained cannot be classified as having CD. The histology of gastric mucosa in CD patients has yet to be fully elucidated. Gastric mucosal biopsy specimens are usually difficult to interpret. The occurrence of non-caseating granulomas is still considered the histological hallmark of gastric CD, but the chance to detect these in gastric biopsy specimens is very low. *Helicobacter pylori*-negative focally active chronic gastritis represents a pattern of inflammation that is, more likely, suggestive of CD [1]. Nugent and Roy [2] have proposed that to establish a diagnosis of upper GI CD, one of the following two criteria must be met: (1) on pathology, the finding of non-caseating granulomatous inflammation of the upper GI tract with or without coexisting CD at other GI sites and without an alternative systemic granulomatous disorder or (2) clearly documented CD at another GI site and endoscopic/radiologic evidence of diffuse inflammatory changes suggestive of CD.

The prevalence of upper GI involvement is much higher in prospective studies than in retrospective series. Most of the data available in the adult population come from retrospective studies. These retrospective investigations carried out in CD patients with symptoms suggesting upper GI involvement have reported that the uncommon occurrence rate of upper GI involvement ranges from 1 % to 5 % [2, 3]. On the other hand, prospective studies, in which patients with CD underwent routine endoscopic evaluation with biopsies, revealed a much higher frequency of endoscopic (30–75 %) [4, 5] and histologic abnormalities (up to 70 %). Since *Helicobacter pylori* is the most frequent cause of gastritis and the most important etiologic factor in peptic ulcer disease, it is important to assess the contribution of *Helicobacter pylori* in the interpretation of the abnormalities observed in the upper GI tract in patients with CD.

Upper GI CD most commonly involves the stomach, followed by the duodenum and the esophagus, and the most observed mucosal abnormalities includes edema, erythema, and nodularity of the mucosa followed by ulcers and aphthous ulcers [6]. CD involving the upper GI tract is nearly invariably accompanied by small or large bowel involvement.

In routine practice, EGD is performed in CD patients with symptoms suggesting upper GI disease and recommended in patients with an indeterminate colitis, since focally active gastritis, in the absence of a macroscopic finding, may be a feature of gastric CD and, therefore, EGD is possibly helpful in establishing the diagnosis of CD. However, the

D.Il. Park
Department of Internal Medicine,
Kangbuk Samsung Hospital, Sungkyunkwan University, School of Medicine,
Seoul, South Korea
e-mail: diksmc.park@samsung.com

W.H. Kim, J.H. Cheon (eds.), *Atlas of Inflammatory Bowel Diseases*,
DOI 10.1007/978-3-642-39423-2_7, © Springer-Verlag Berlin Heidelberg 2015

European Crohn's and Colitis Organisation (ECCO) guideline recommends an examination of the location and extent in CD in the upper GI tract, irrespective of the findings at ileocolonoscopy. Indeed, levels of evidence and grades of recommendation, for this statement, are very low, since they are based only upon expert opinion in the lack of consistent and conclusive studies [7]. Data from a pediatric population study suggested the usefulness of EGD in differentiating CD from UC when inflammation is confined to the colon.

Esophageal CD is thought to be relatively uncommon, with the prevalence of disease below 2 % in adult population. Over 80 % of patients with esophageal CD have CD in other GI sites [8]. Esophageal involvement is usually seen in seriously ill patients presenting with heartburn and chest and epigastric pain which are often identical to those patients with gastroesophageal reflux disease. Odynophagia is likely more common in patients with a large discrete ulcer in the esophagus (Fig. 7.1). Severe involvement of the esophagus with ulceration followed by fibrosis may lead to progressive dysphagia. Endoscopic findings are generally nonspecific and include granularity, aphthous ulcers, friability, cobblestoning, ulceration, and stricture formation. Huchzermeyer et al. [9] described two different stages of esophageal involvement in CD. The first stage is that of inflammatory involvement of the esophagus. It may start with merely erythema and edema, possibly earlier form of the disease. This may progress to erosions and aphthous ulcerations with intervening normal mucosa. When the changes extend over a larger area, the endoscopic appearance may be similar to CD in the colon with flat, extending ulcerations and granularity. The second stage that these authors described is characterized by esophageal stricturing and stenosis. The pattern of distribution is that of the distal esophagus with some extension into the mid-esophagus.

The incidence of gastric and duodenal CD varies greatly in series of patients with CD, ranging from 0.5 % to 4 %. Many patients do not have endoscopically detectable lesions in the stomach and duodenum, although examination of biopsies for normal-looking mucosa does reveal histopathologic changes suggestive of CD. Gastroduodenal involvement often leads to symptoms similar to peptic ulcer disease or non-ulcer dyspepsia, such as epigastric pain and anorexia and sometimes signs of gastric outlet obstruction. Compared with distal CD, abdominal pain, cramping, and general malaise are more frequent with proximal disease.

There are a range of endoscopic findings reported in association with gastroduodenal CD. Danzi et al. [10] described patchy erythema, mucosal nodularity, aphthous lesion (Fig. 7.2a), ulceration, cobblestoning, and strictures (Fig. 7.2b, c) in their series of 14 patients. A bamboo-joint-like (BJL) appearance is an endoscopic finding characterized by swollen longitudinal folds transversed by erosive fissures or linear furrows, which seems to be associated with CD (Fig. 7.2d, e) [11, 12].

The ulcerations in gastroduodenal CD were much more likely to be serpiginous or longitudinal (Fig. 7.3a, b) than round or oval. The round or oval ulcerations are felt to be suggestive of acid peptic disease. Gastroduodenal disease tends to be contiguous. In the series reported by Nugent and Roy [2], 60 % of patients had contiguous involvement of the antrum and duodenum. Forty percent had duodenal involvement only. Gastric CD usually involves the antrum. In isolated duodenal disease, any part of the duodenum can be involved, but the second part is most frequently affected, with typical mucosal defects on top of Kerckring's folds (Fig. 7.3c, d), called "notching." In the duodenum, stricturing may also occur. Upper endoscopy may lend itself to potential therapeutic intervention in patients with gastroduodenal CD. In case of stricturing with obstructive symptoms, there have been some reports on the successful balloon dilatation of strictures (Fig. 7.3e–g) [13].

It is noteworthy that symptoms of upper GI involvement can be relieved by conventional anti-inflammatory and antisecretory agents (especially proton pump inhibitors) but that the lesions rarely disappear upon endoscopic follow-up.

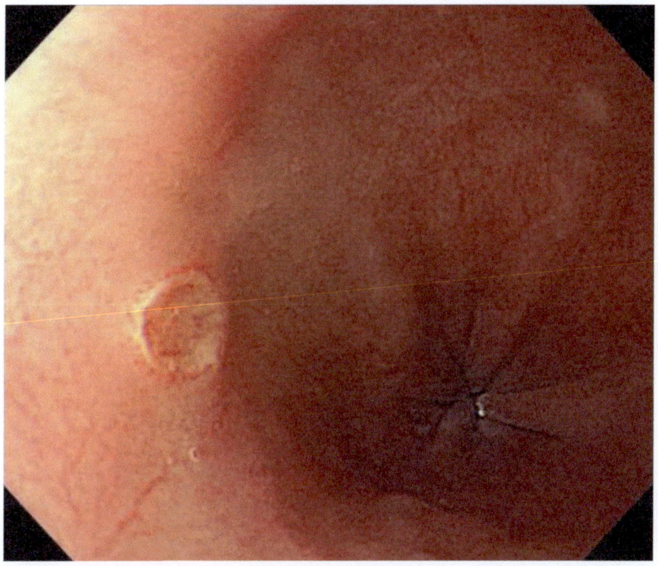

Fig. 7.1 A discrete esophageal ulcer in a patient with Crohn's disease

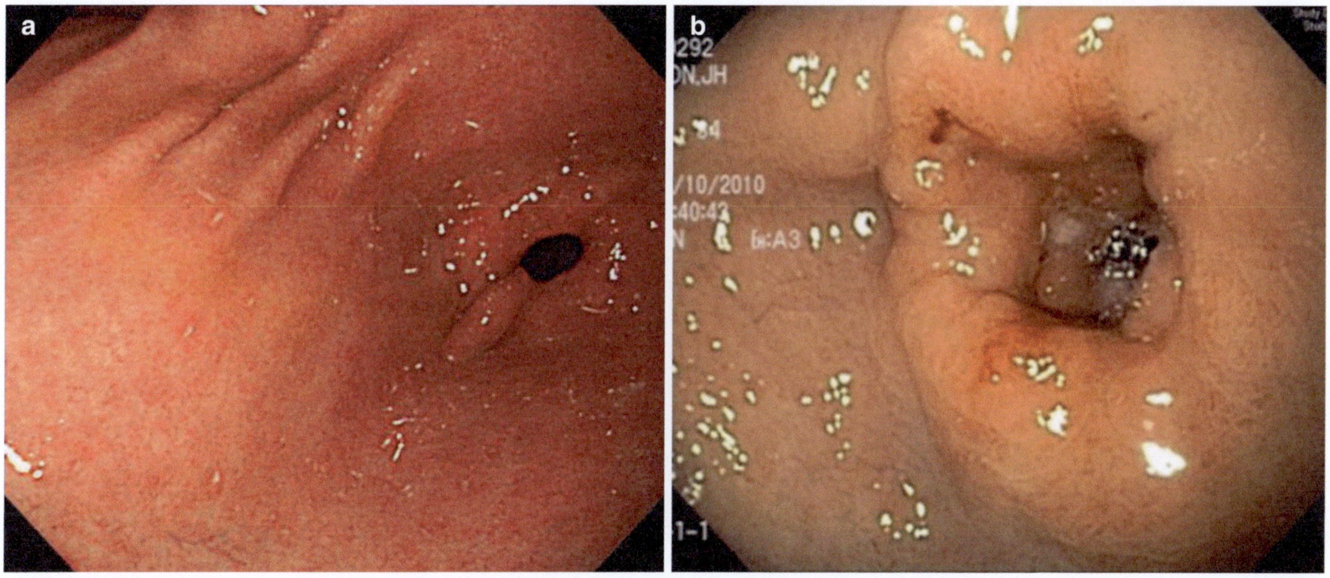

Fig. 7.2 Endoscopic findings of gastroduodenal Crohn's disease. (**a**) Multiple aphthous lesions in the antrum. (**b**) Pyloric stricture associated with gastroduodenal Crohn's disease. A patient presented with vomiting, epigastric pain, and weight loss. (**c**) Gastroduodenal disease tends to be contiguous. (**d**) Bamboo-joint-like appearance on the cardia. (**e**) Swollen longitudinal folds transversed by linear furrows (after indigo carmine spray)

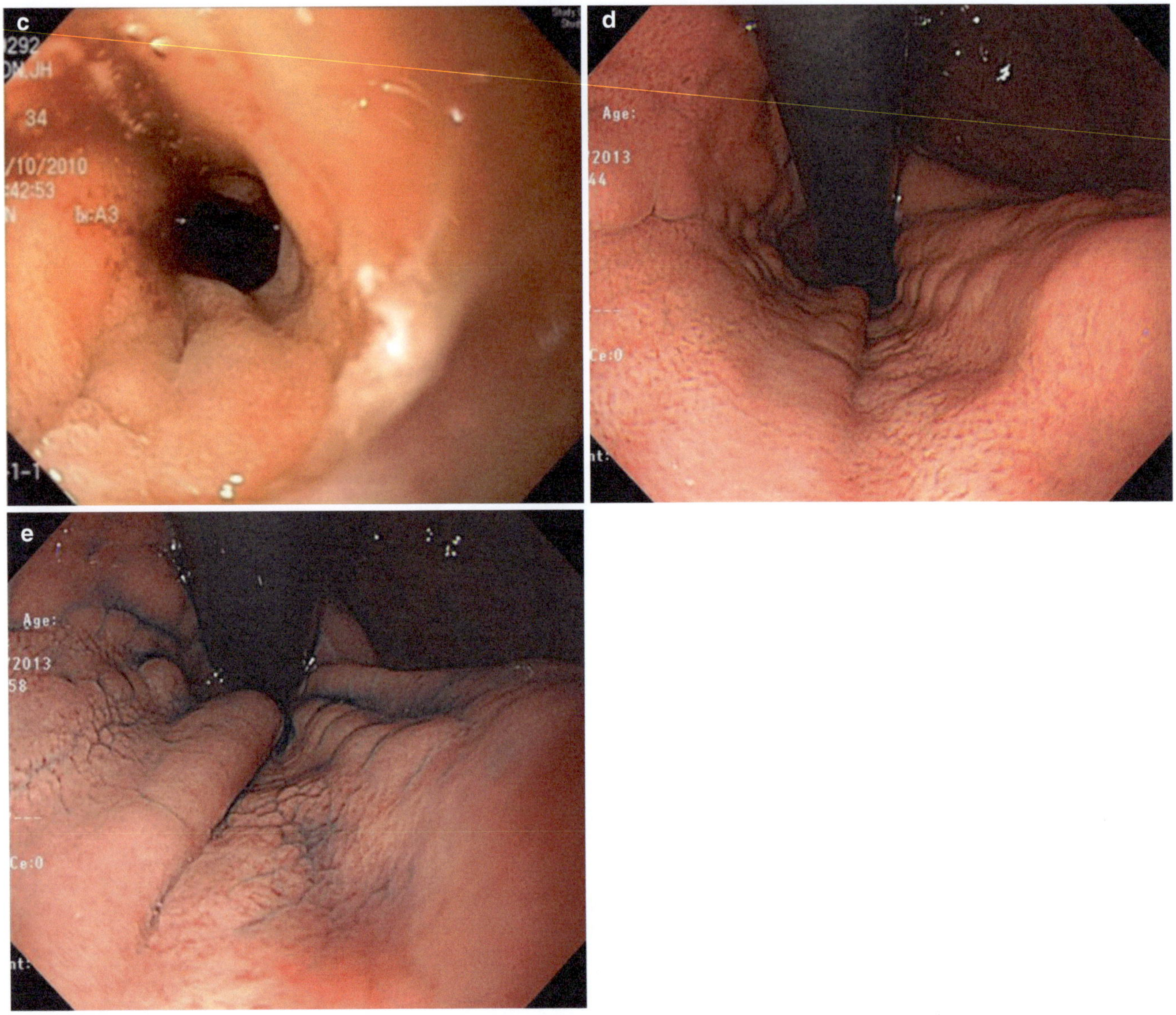

Fig. 7.2 (continued)

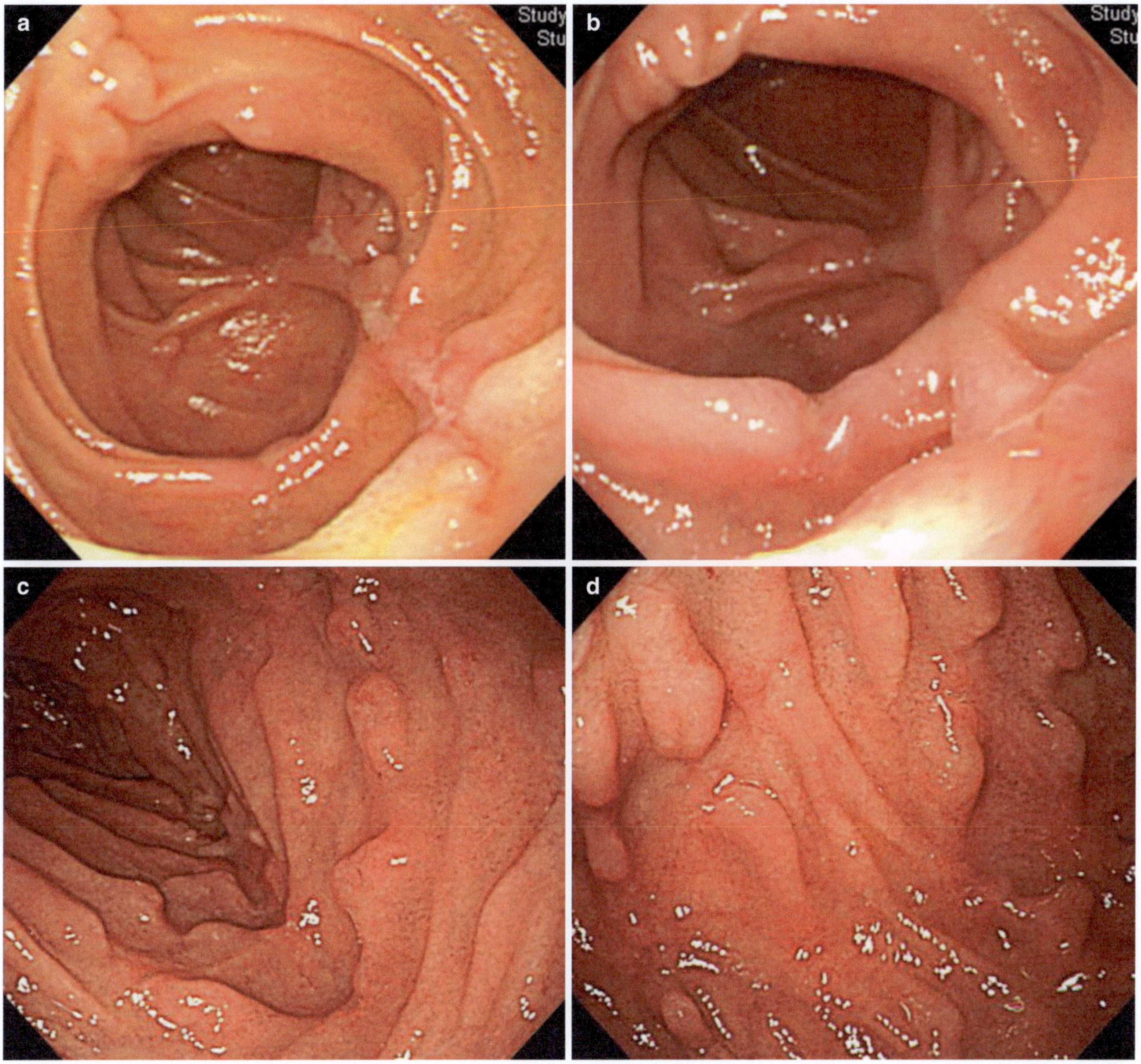

Fig. 7.3 Endoscopic findings of duodenal Crohn's disease. (**a**, **b**) Longitudinal ulcer in the second portion of duodenum before and after treatment. (**c**, **d**) Typical mucosal defects on top of Kerckring's folds, called "notching." (**e**) Partial obstruction on the duodenal bulb. (**f**) TTS (through the scope) balloon dilatation. (**g**) Cobblestone appearance was detected prominently after the relief of luminal narrowing

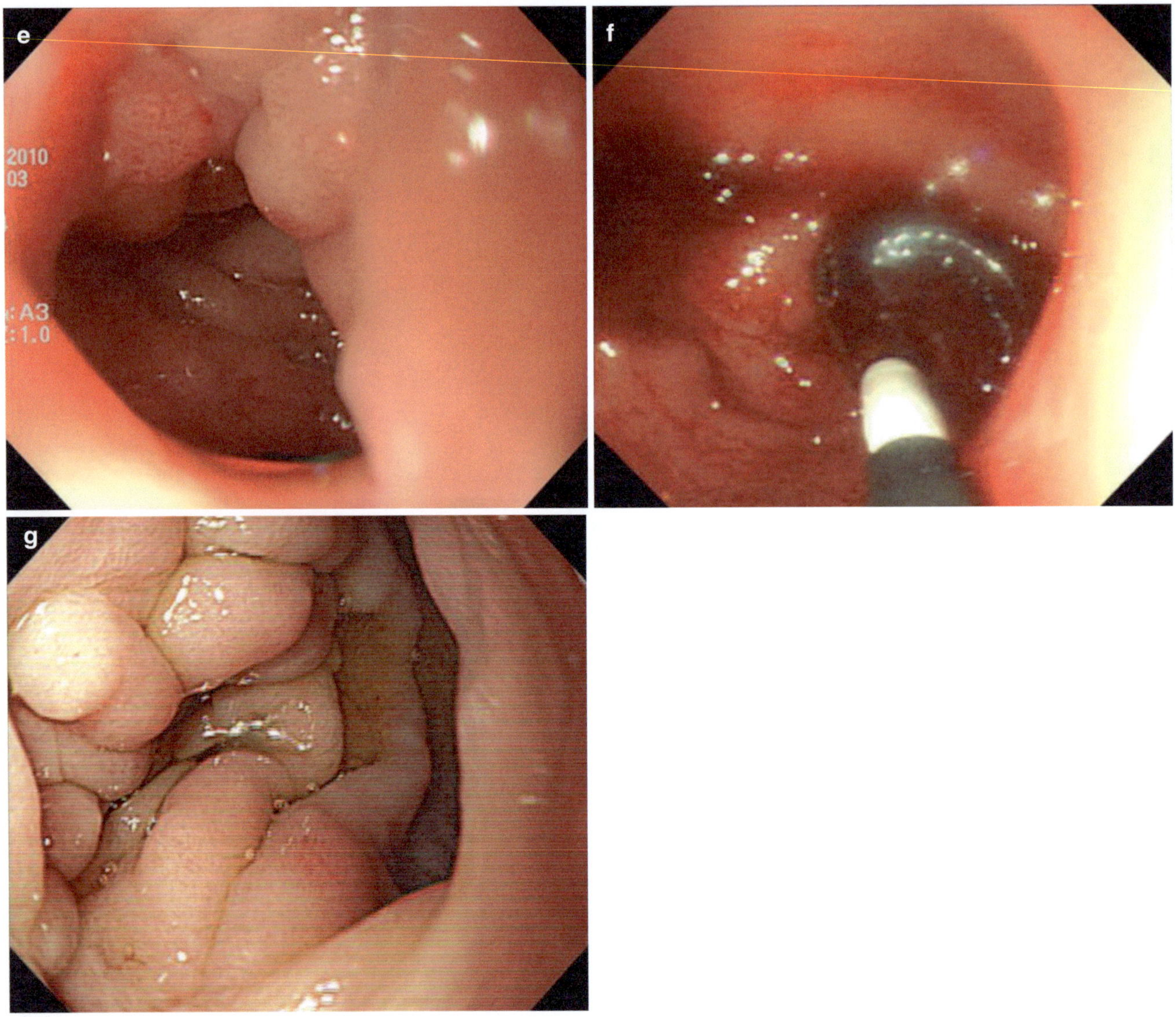

Fig. 7.3 (continued)

References

1. Oberhuber G, Püspök A, Oesterreicher C, Novacek G, Zauner C, Burghuber M, Vogelsang H, Pötzi R, Stolte M, Wrba F. Focally enhanced gastritis: a frequent type of gastritis in patients with Crohn's disease. Gastroenterology. 1997;112:698–706.
2. Nugent FW, Roy MA. Duodenal Crohn's disease: an analysis of 89 cases. Am J Gastroenterol. 1989;84:249–54.
3. Rutgeerts P, Onette E, Vantrappen G, Geboes K, Broeckaert L, Talloen L. Crohn's disease of the stomach and duodenum: a clinical study with emphasis on the value of endoscopy and endoscopic biopsies. Endoscopy. 1980;12:288–94.
4. Kuriyama M, Kato J, Morimoto N, Fujimoto T, Okada H, Yamamoto K. Specific gastroduodenoscopic findings in Crohn's disease: Comparison with findings in patients with ulcerative colitis and gastroesophageal reflux disease. Dig Liver Dis. 2008;40(6): 468–75.
5. Annunziata ML, Caviglia R, Papparella LG, Cicala M. Upper gastrointestinal involvement of Crohn's disease: a prospective study on the role of upper endoscopy in the diagnostic work-up. Dig Dis Sci. 2012;57(6):1618–23.
6. Witte AM, Veenendaal RA, Van Hogezand RA, Verspaget HW, Lamers CB. Crohn's disease of the upper gastrointestinal tract: the value of endoscopic examination. Scand J Gastroenterol Suppl. 1998;225:100–5.
7. Van Assche G, Dignass A, Panes J, Beaugerie L, Karagiannis J, Allez M, Ochsenkühn T, Orchard T, Rogler G, Louis E, Kupcinskas L, Mantzaris G, Travis S, Stange E, European Crohn's and Colitis Organisation (ECCO). The second European evidence-based consensus on the diagnosis and management of Crohn's disease: definitions and diagnosis. J Crohns Colitis. 2010;4: 7–27.
8. Isaacs KL. Upper gastrointestinal tract endoscopy in inflammatory bowel disease. Gastrointest Endosc Clin N Am. 2002;12: 451–62.
9. Huchzermeyer H, Paul F, Seifert E, Fröhlich H, Rasmussen CW. Endoscopic results in five patients with Crohn's disease of the esophagus. Endoscopy. 1977;8:75–81.
10. Danzi JT, Farmer RG, Sullivan Jr BH, Rankin GB. Endoscopic features of gastroduodenal Crohn's disease. Gastroenterology. 1976;70:9–13.
11. Yokota K, Saito Y, Einami K, Ayabe T, Shibata Y, Tanabe H, Watari J, Ohtsubo C, Miyokawa N, Kohgo Y. A bamboo joint-like appearance of the gastric body and cardia: possible association with Crohn's disease. Gastrointest Endosc. 1997;46:268–72.
12. Kang MS, Park DI, Park JH, Kim HJ, Cho YK, Sohn CI, Jeon WK, Kim BI. Bamboo joint-like appearance of stomach in Korean patients with Crohn's disease. Korean J Gastroenterol. 2006;48: 395–400.
13. Endo K1, Takahashi S, Shiga H, Kakuta Y, Kinouchi Y, Shimosegawa T. Short and long-term outcomes of endoscopic balloon dilatation for Crohn's disease strictures. World J Gastroenterol. 2013;19(1):86–91.

8 Radiology

Joon Seok Lim

8.1 Radiological Features of Inflammatory Bowel Disease

8.1.1 Crohn's Disease

Crohn's disease tends to be transmural, segmental, and usually discontinuous. Multifocal small bowel diseases may present with areas of different activity, some areas with acute inflammatory, and others with fibrostenosing disease [1–3]. The characteristic radiological features of Crohn's disease on barium study include aphthoid or deep ulcerations, cobblestone appearance, sinus tract, and fistula with discontinuous and asymmetric involvement (Figs. 8.1, 8.2, and 8.3).

Crohn's disease also has a variety of appearances at CT or MR depending on whether the activity is acute inflammatory or chronic fibrostenosing and whether there are complications such as fistula or abscess. The optimal distension of the small bowel loops is important for the accurate evaluation of the bowel wall because collapsed bowel can hide or mimic disease. CT or MR which is performed after oral contrast ingestion to achieve small bowel distension is called CT or MR enterography. The negative oral contrast agents, such as polyethylene glycol solution (PEG), suspension of 0.1 % barium sulfate (Volumen), and water-methylcellulose solution, are preferred because they allow better depiction of bowel wall enhancement [1].

On CT or MR, enteric findings such as mural hyperenhancement, bowel wall thickening, mural stratification, and extraenteric findings such as engorged vasa recta ("comb sign") [4] and increased attenuation of the mesenteric fat are features of active inflammatory small bowel Crohn's disease (Figs. 8.4 and 8.5) [3, 5]. Among these findings, combinations of mural hyperenhancement and bowel wall thickening are the most sensitive findings suggesting the presence of active inflammation [5]. It is important to differentiate active inflammatory small bowel strictures from fibrotic strictures in patients with Crohn's disease because the former are mostly managed medically, whereas the latter may require endoscopic or surgical interventions (e.g., balloon dilation, strictureplasty, or bowel resection) [6]. In fibrostenosing Crohn's disease (Figs. 8.6 and 8.7), mural stratification may be absent because of the transmural fibrosis and/or muscular hypertrophy and collagen deposition leading to a homogeneous and less-intense enhancement [7] (Table 8.1). Low-signal intensity of the stricture site on T2-weighted MR imaging may be helpful for diagnosing fibrostenotic Crohn's disease [8]. However, active inflammation and fibrosis often coexist in the same patient or even in the same affected bowel segments in Crohn's disease.

CT or MR has an important role in evaluating extraenteric complications of Crohn's disease. The most common extraenteric complications include fistula, sinus tract, and abscess [9–11]. On CT or MR, sinuses or fistulas are demonstrated as tethering of bowel loops and visualization of linear enhancing tracts with or without communication with adjacent structures such as peritoneal or retroperitoneal spaces, skin or adjacent organs, or bowel, respectively (Figs. 8.8, 8.9, and 8.10) [12]. Abscesses are usually contiguous to the diseased bowel segment and are seen in the mesentery or retroperitoneal space (Fig. 8.11) [3]. The accurate detection of abscesses and fistulas has high importance because it affects the decision to treat medically or surgically. Particularly, in the identification of perianal fistula tracts, MR imaging is useful because of its better multiplanar imaging capability and soft tissue contrast than those of CT (Fig. 8.10). Bowel perforation can be developed in Crohn's disease. It is associated with bowel distension with increased intraluminal pressure proximal to an obstruction or ischemic hypothesis (Fig. 8.12) [13]. Other extraenteric manifestations of Crohn's disease, such as mesenteric lymphadenopathy, cholelithiasis, nephrolithiasis, sacroiliitis, and primary sclerosing cholangitis, can also be evaluated [3].

J.S. Lim
Department of Radiology,
Yonsei University College of Medicine,
Severance Hospital, Seoul, South Korea
e-mail: jslim1@yuhs.ac

W.H. Kim, J.H. Cheon (eds.), *Atlas of Inflammatory Bowel Diseases*,
DOI 10.1007/978-3-642-39423-2_8, © Springer-Verlag Berlin Heidelberg 2015

Radiation concern is an important issue in CT because patients with Crohn's disease are relatively younger and are expected to undergo multiple follow-up CT studies [14]. In terms of radiation issue, MR enterography is an emerging diagnostic tool for evaluating patients with known or suspected Crohn's disease by virtue of its ability to help physician confirm the diagnosis, assess its extent and inflammatory activity, and detect extraintestinal complications (Figs. 8.9 and 8.10). Major MR enterographic findings of Crohn's disease are not different from those of CT. The two diagnostic modalities appear to be similar in terms of detecting active inflammation, fibrosis, and extraenteric complications [15]. However, CT is preferred in elderly patients because MRI is more time consuming and sometimes requires breath-holding technique [16]. Moreover, CT should be preferred in emergency settings such as suspicious bowel perforation or obstruction.

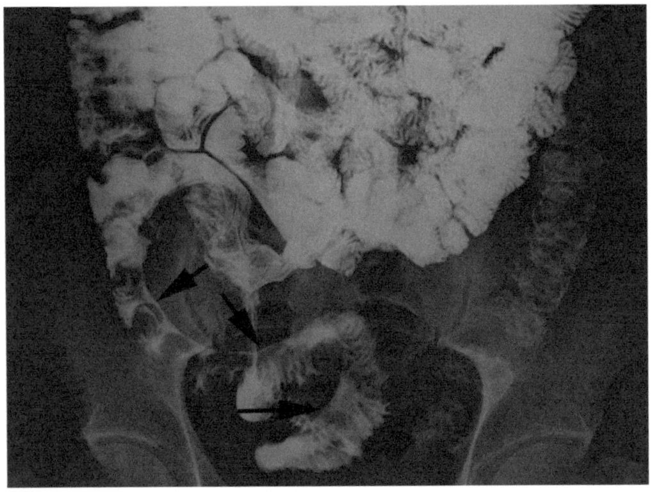

Fig. 8.1 Barium study for Crohn's disease. Multisegmental longitudinal ulcers (*arrows*) are seen in the mesenteric side throughout ileal loops with discontinuous and asymmetric pattern

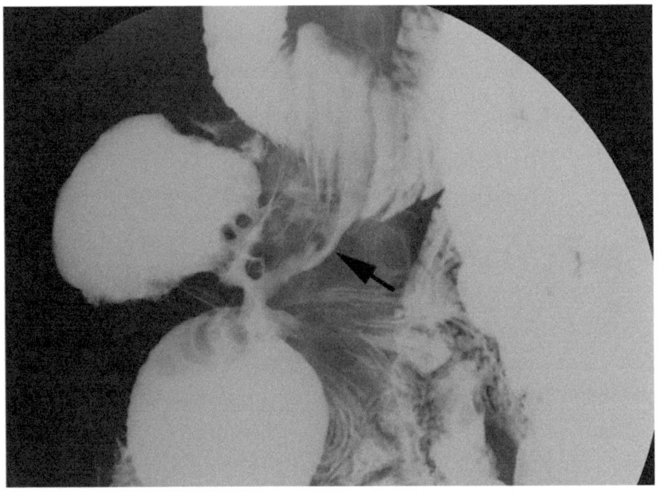

Fig. 8.3 Barium study for Crohn's disease. Fistula (*arrow*) between the duodenum and ascending colon is demonstrated

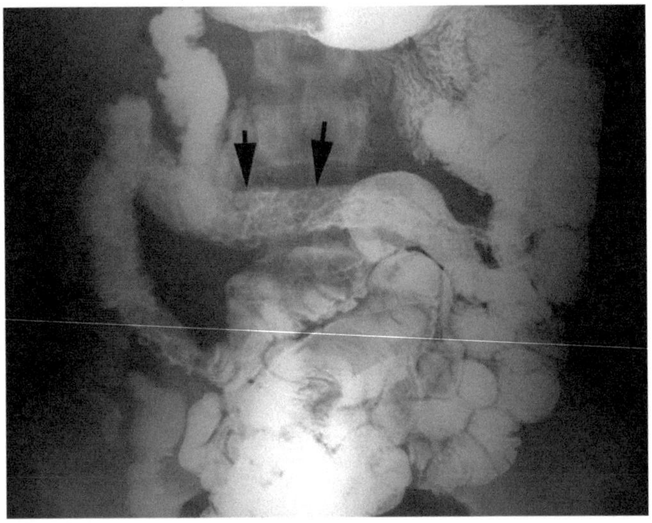

Fig. 8.2 Barium study for Crohn's disease. Longitudinal and transverse ulcers of the distal ileal loop produce a cobblestone appearance (*arrows*)

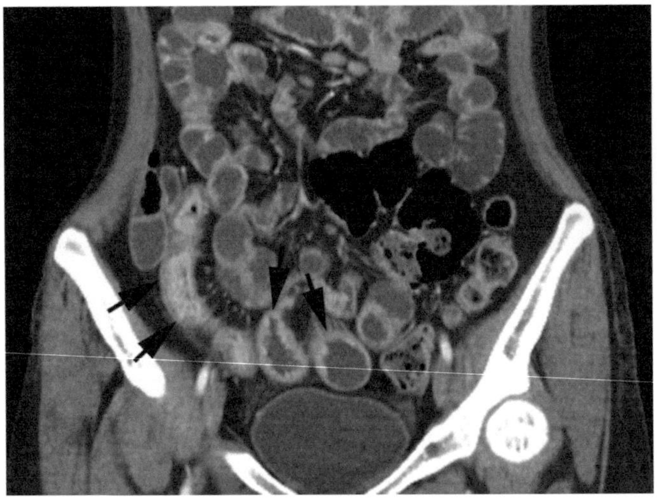

Fig. 8.4 Active Crohn's disease. Coronal CT image demonstrates multifocal segmental mural hyperenhancement and layered mural stratification in the ileum (*arrows*), suggesting active disease. Increased perienteric fat attenuation is also seen

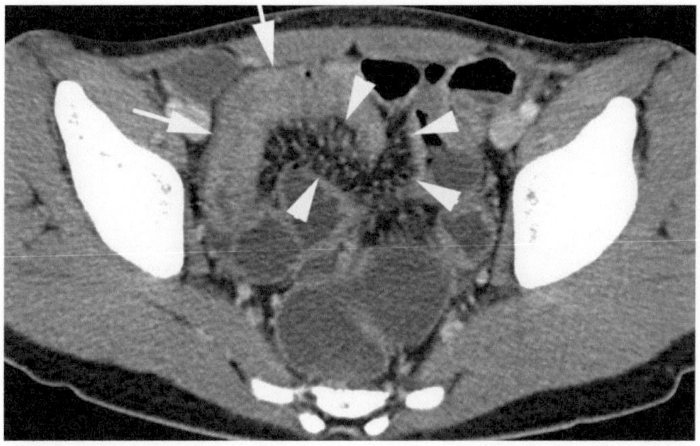

Fig. 8.5 Active Crohn's disease. Axial CT image demonstrates multifocal segmental mural thickenings with hyperenhancement (*arrows*) with engorged vasa recta (positive comb sign) (*arrow heads*)

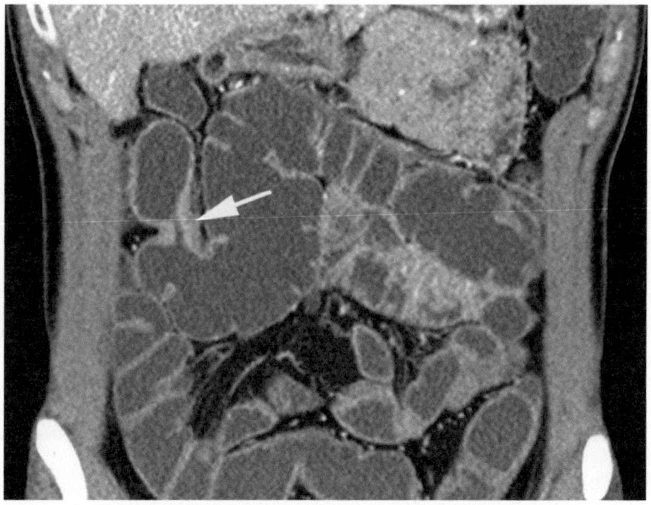

Fig. 8.6 Fibrostenotic Crohn's disease. Coronal CT image shows segmental stricture with homogeneous mural thickening at anastomosis site of right hemicolectomy. Less-intense enhancement without stratification is characteristic of fibrostenosing disease

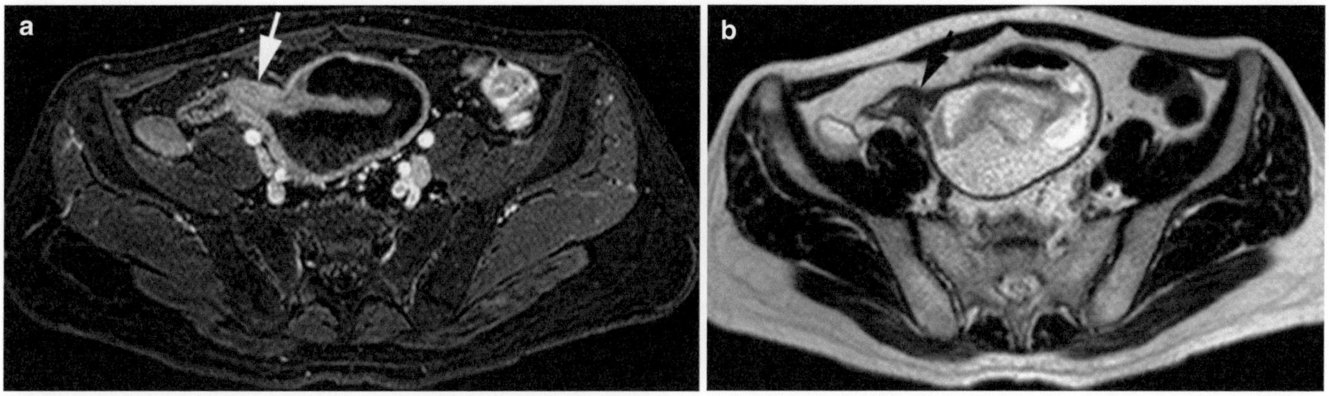

Fig. 8.7 Fibrostenotic Crohn's disease. MR image shows a homogeneous, less-enhancing strictured bowel segment (*arrow*) on T1-weighted contrast-enhanced axial image (**a**) and low signal intensity of the corresponding segment (*arrow*) on T2-weighted axial image (**b**)

Table 8.1 Differential diagnosis of inflammatory stricture and fibrotic stricture in Crohn's disease on cross-sectional imaging

	Inflammatory stricture	Fibrotic stricture
Mural thickening	More severe	Less severe
Mural hyperenhancement	More strong	Less enhancement
Mural stratification	Frequent	Homogeneous without stratification
Submucosal fat deposition	Rare	More frequent
Signal intensity on T2-weighted MR imaging	Mild to moderate high SI	More low signal intensity

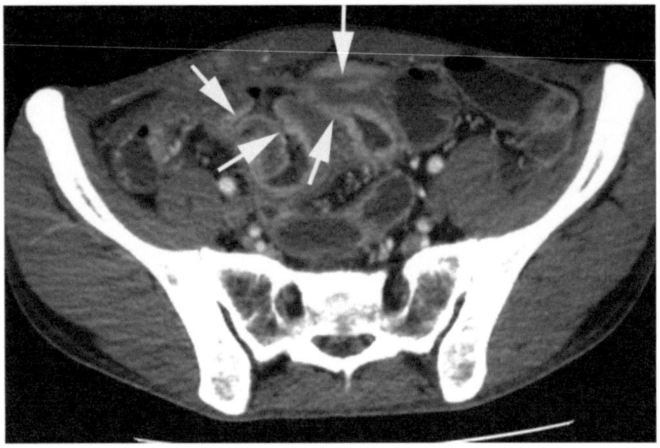

Fig. 8.8 Fistula. Axial CT image shows multiple enteroenteric fistulas (*arrows*) between the ileal loops

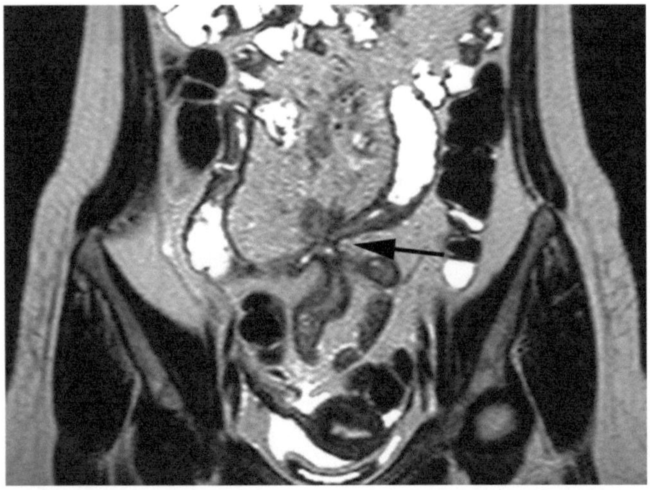

Fig. 8.9 Fistula. Coronal single shot FSE T2-weighted MR image shows multiple enteroenteric fistulas (*arrows*) between the ileal loops

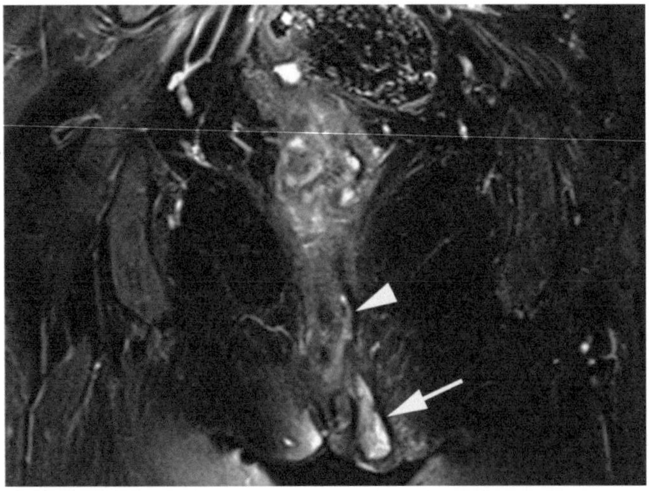

Fig. 8.10 Perianal fistula with abscess. Coronal T2-weighted fat-suppressed MR image shows intersphincteric type fistula (*arrowhead*) with abscess (*arrow*) in the perianal area

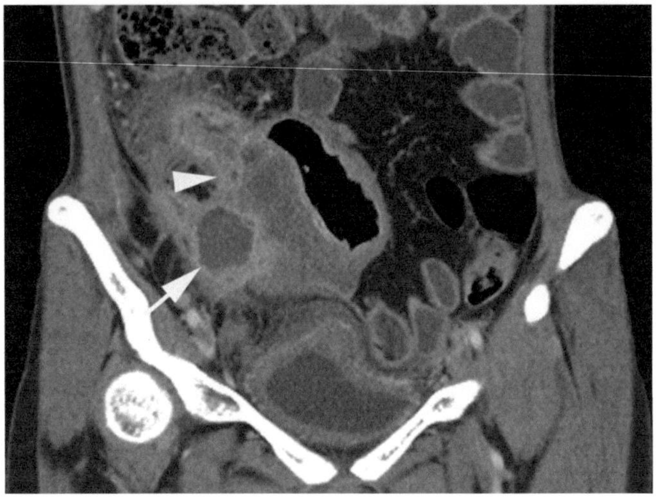

Fig. 8.11 Abscess. Coronal CT image demonstrates a mesenteric abscess (*arrow*) adjacent to the terminal ileum. Fistula (*arrowhead*) is seen between the cecum and abscess

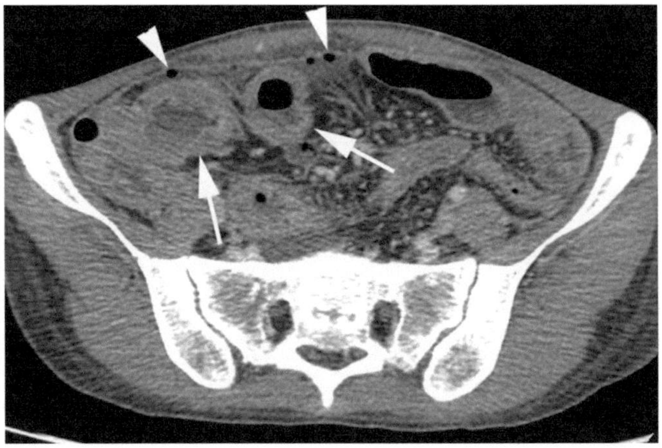

Fig. 8.12 Small bowel perforation. Several focal-free air foci are noted within the peritoneal cavity on axial CT image (*arrowheads*), suggesting intestinal perforation. Inflamed ileal loops are also seen (*arrows*)

8.1.2 Intestinal Tuberculosis

The most frequent site of intestinal tuberculosis involvement is the ileocecal area (approximately 90 % in case of gastrointestinal tuberculosis) (Figs. 8.13 and 8.14). Barium study may show contour deformity involving the ileocecal valve with stellate ulcers. In advanced stage, the cecum becomes conical and shrunken with wide opening of the ileocecal valve and the narrowed terminal ileum [17]. CT findings may show short segmental circumferential wall thickening related with the circumferential distribution of superficial ulcers in the cecum and terminal ileum (Figs. 8.14, 8.15, and 8.16) [18]. Central necrotic lymph nodes on CT are a specific finding for tuberculosis (Fig. 8.15).

CT findings that may be helpful for differentiating intestinal tuberculosis from Crohn's disease include short segmental enhancing wall thickening in tuberculosis, while Crohn's disease demonstrates relatively long segmental wall thickening (Table 8.2). In addition, incompetence of the ileocecal valve appears to be common in tuberculosis but uncommon in Crohn's disease. Mural stratification is known to be more frequent in Crohn's disease [19]. Among extraintestinal findings, fibrofatty proliferation, positive comb sign by increased mesenteric vascularity, and internal/perianal fistula suggest the possibility of Crohn's disease rather than intestinal tuberculosis. However, the differentiation between intestinal TB and Crohn's disease may be difficult because they sometimes share similar radiologic findings.

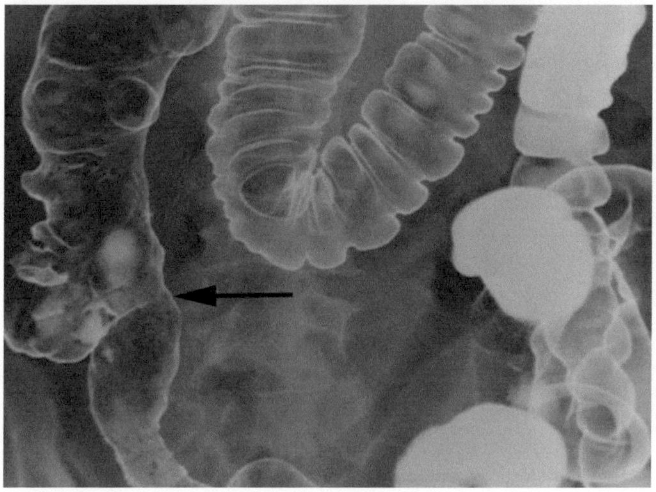

Fig. 8.13 Barium study of ileocecal tuberculosis. Barium study shows the characteristic abnormality of ileocecal tuberculosis such as loss of anatomic demarcation between the terminal ileum and the contracted cecum (*arrow*) and gapping of the ileocecal valve

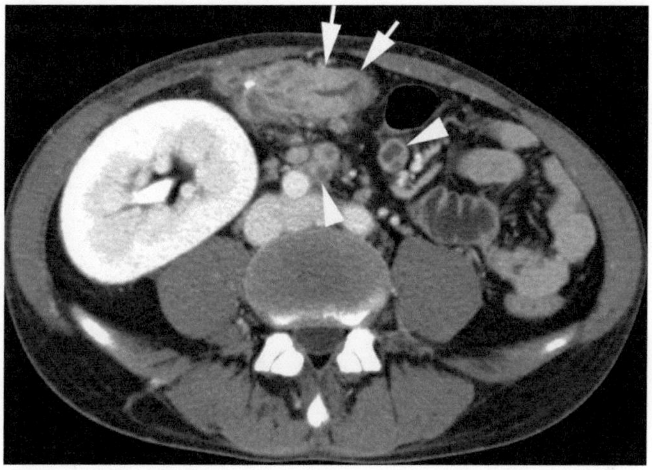

Fig. 8.15 CT findings of intestinal tuberculosis. Short segmental mural wall thickening with homogeneous mural enhancement is noted in the terminal ileum without mural stratification (*arrows*). Multiple central necrotic lymph node enlargements are seen in the mesentery (*arrowheads*)

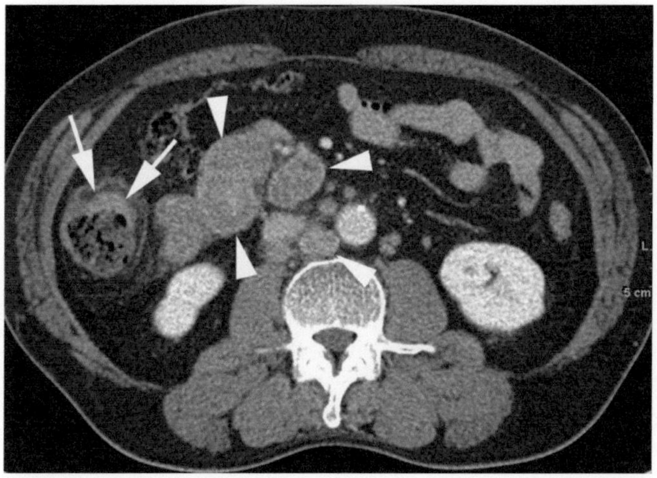

Fig. 8.14 CT findings of ileocecal tuberculosis. CT shows circumferential enhancing wall thickening in the cecum (*arrows*). Multiple low-attenuated lymph node enlargements, suggesting caseous necrosis, are seen in the ileocecal mesentery (*arrowhead*)

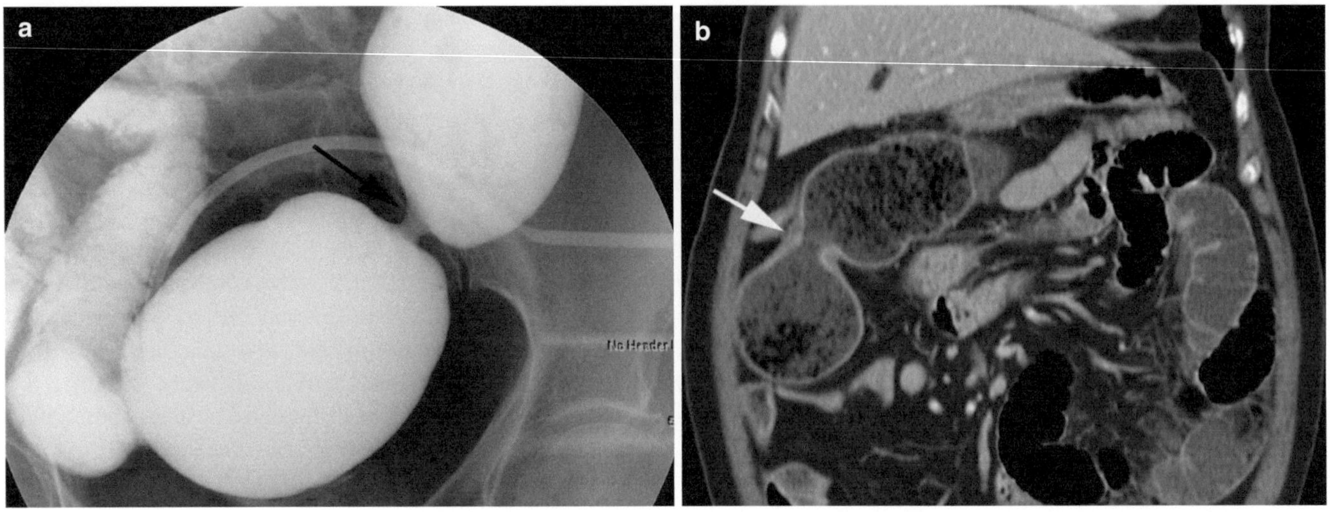

Fig. 8.16 Small bowel tuberculosis. Barium study (**a**) and CT (**b**) show short segmental bowel stricture at the level of the distal jejunal loop (*arrows*). Associated prestenotic bowel dilatation is also seen

Table 8.2 Differential diagnosis of Crohn's disease, intestinal tuberculosis, and intestinal Behçet's disease by radiologic imaging studies

	Crohn's disease	Intestinal tuberculosis	Behçet's disease
Involvement of ileocecal area	May spare	Common	Common
Stratification	Frequent	Rare	Possible
Distribution pattern and symmetry	Long eccentric involvement of thickening (mesenteric border) with antimesenteric pseudosacculation	Short circumferential thickening	Single or multiple deep penetrating ulcers (larger and deeper)
Mesenteric fibrofatty proliferation	Frequent	Rare	Rare
Positive comb sign	Frequent	Rare	Possible
Central necrosis of lymphadenopathy	–	Possible and specific	–
Complications	Frequent perianal internal fistula	Rare perianal internal fistula	Common perforation, fistula, and thrombophlebitis

8.1.3 Behçet's Disease

The most common site of involvement in the small intestine is the terminal ileum, and there is often simultaneous involvement of the proximal cecum (Figs. 8.17, 8.18, and 8.19). Behçet's disease involving the ileocecal region is commonly manifested as geographic, relatively large, and deep penetrating ulcers with bowel wall thickening and mural hyperenhancement (Table 8.1) [20]. The frequency of postoperative recurrence is high, and the most common type of the recurrent pattern is one or two deep ulcers at or near the anastomosis site (Fig. 8.20).

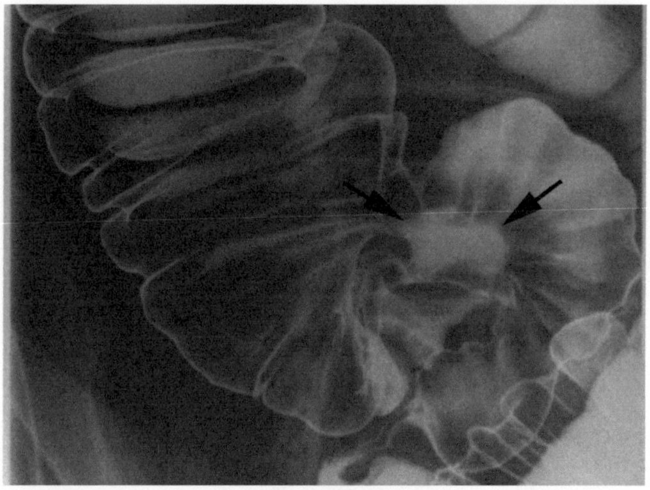

Fig. 8.17 Barium study of intestinal Behçet's disease. Image from a double-contrast barium enema study shows a large geographic ulcer (*arrows*) in the terminal ileum with convergence of thickened mucosal folds

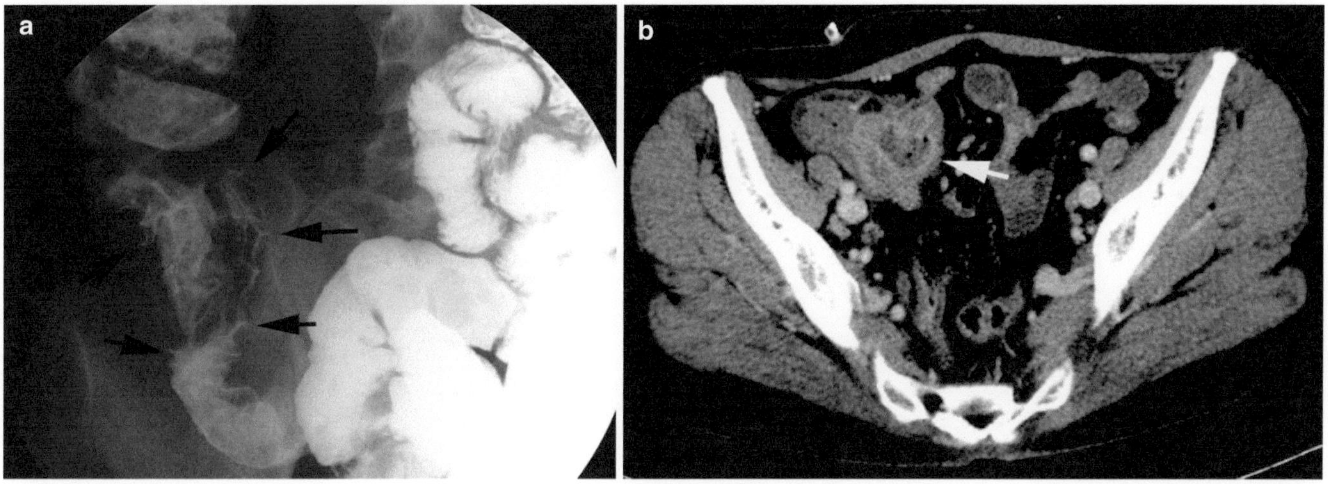

Fig. 8.18 Behçet's disease. Mucosal fold thickening is seen in the cecum and terminal ileum with multiple small penetrating ulcers in the terminal ileal loop (*arrows*) (**a**). After 3 years, large penetrating ulcer developed in the terminal ileal loop (*arrow*) (**b**)

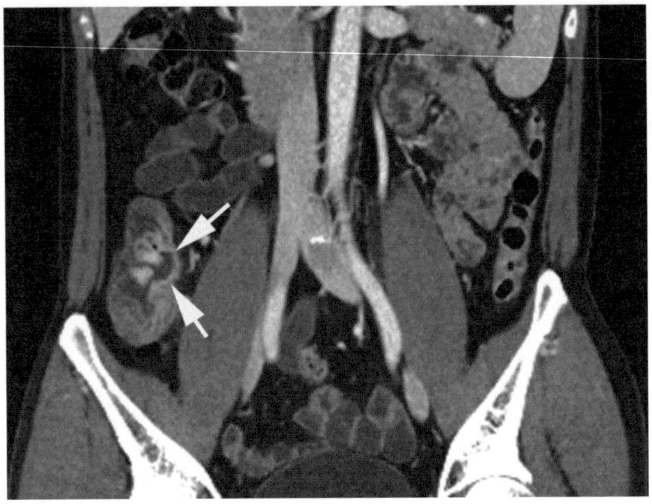

Fig. 8.19 CT of intestinal Behçet's disease. CT shows a penetrating ulcer with mural enhancement (*arrows*) in ileocecal area

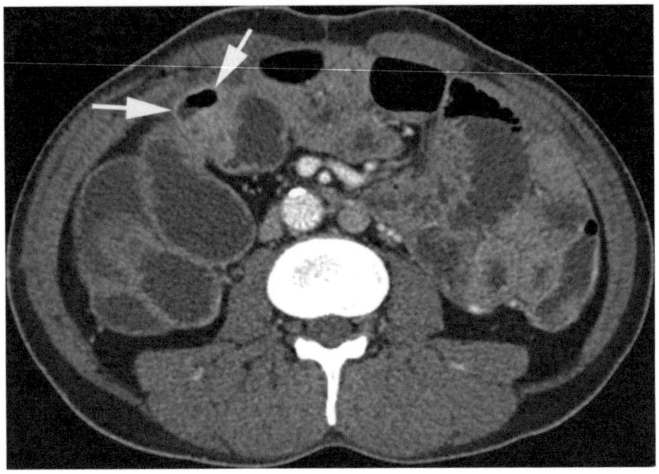

Fig. 8.20 Recurrent intestinal Behçet's disease. Axial CT image shows a penetrating ulceration with peripheral enhancement at the anastomosis of right hemicolectomy

8.1.4 Ulcerative Colitis

Rectal involvement is present in 95 % of cases, with variable degrees of contiguous, circumferential, and proximal extension throughout the large intestine. Small-bowel disease is rare. Barium study shows mucosal granularity/stippling, collar button ulcers, haustral thickening/loss, and inflammatory polyps on acute phase (Fig. 8.21) and luminal narrowing, loss of rectal valves, widened presacral space, and postinflammatory polyps on chronic phase (Figs. 8.22 and 8.23) [21]. Diffuse symmetric colonic mural thickening on CT is a common finding with target or halo sign (Fig. 8.24). Generally, ulcerative colitis produces less wall thickening than does Crohn's disease [22]. Toxic megacolon is the most severe life-threatening complication of inflammatory bowel disease and an indication for emergency surgery. It occurs more commonly in ulcerative colitis rather than Crohn's disease (Fig. 8.25). Ulcerative colitis is also associated with primary sclerosing cholangitis, a chronic cholestatic liver disease characterized by inflammation and scarring of the bile ducts (Fig. 8.26) [23].

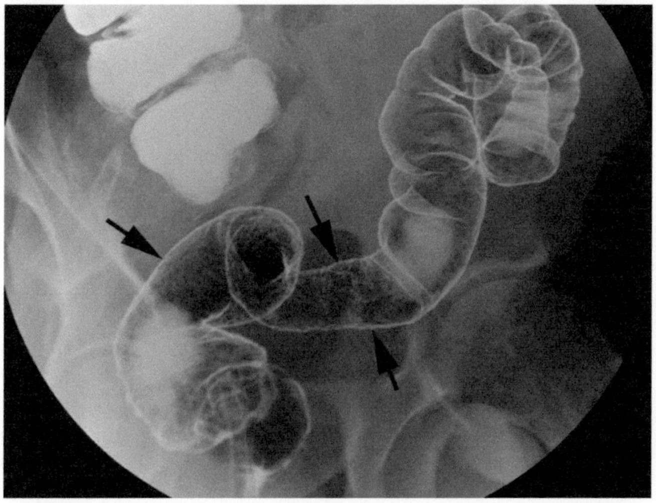

Fig. 8.21 Acute phase of ulcerative colitis. Double-contrast barium enema study shows mucosal granularity and stippling (crypt abscess) (*arrows*) in the rectum and sigmoid colon, suggesting early stage of ulcerative colitis

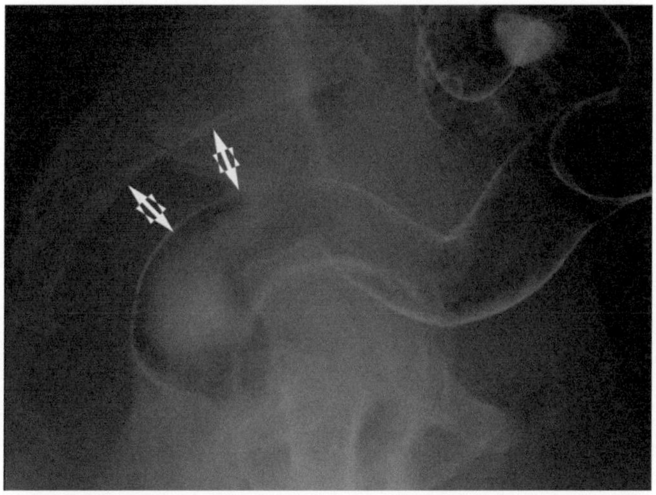

Fig. 8.22 Chronic phase of ulcerative colitis. Lateral rectal view shows widened presacral space (*arrows*). A distance greater than 1.5 cm is considered abnormal. The rectal lumen is also narrowed with the absent valves of Houston

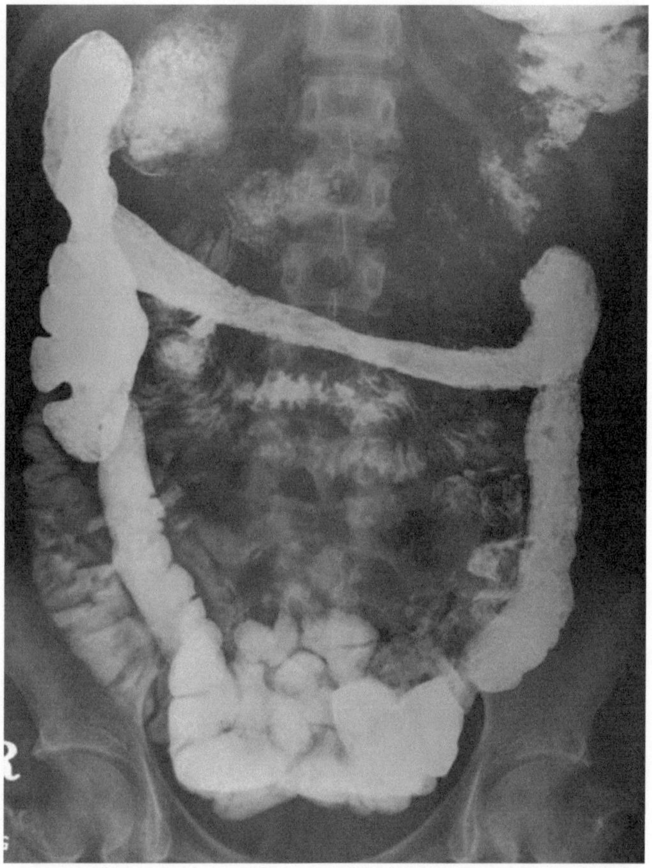

Fig. 8.23 Chronic phase of ulcerative colitis. Barium study shows chronic ulcerative pancolitis with diffuse luminal narrowing, blunting, and lost haustra in the near entire colon and rectum

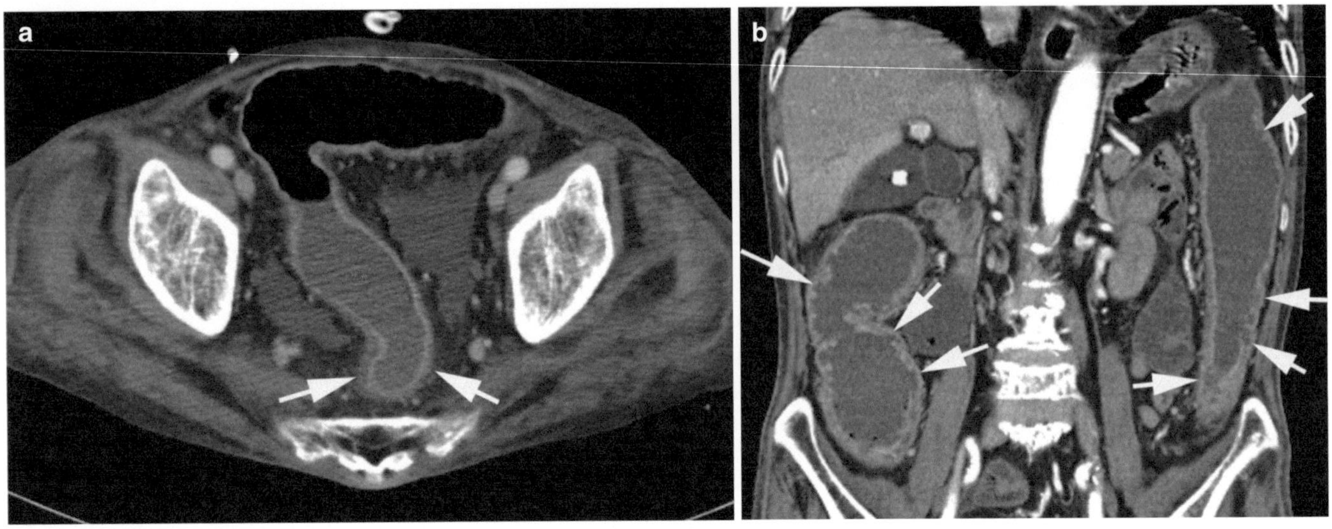

Fig. 8.24 CT of ulcerative colitis. (**a**) Axial CT image shows mural thickening with stratification in the rectum and sigmoid colon, suggesting acute inflammation. (**b**) Coronal CT image shows multiple ulcerations, corresponding to collar button ulcers in the ascending and descending colon with layered mural thickening

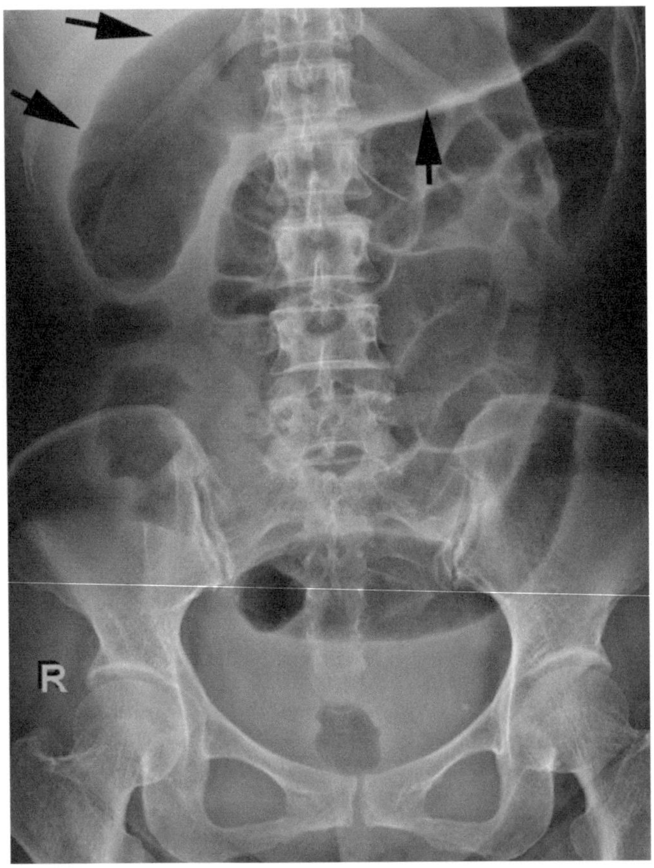

Fig. 8.25 Toxic megacolon. Toxic megacolon is the most severe life-threatening complication of inflammatory bowel disease. It occurs more frequently in ulcerative colitis than in Crohn's disease. It is an indication for emergency surgery. Simple abdomen film shows prominent dilatation of the transverse colon (*arrows*). Dilatation greater than 5 cm is considered abnormal

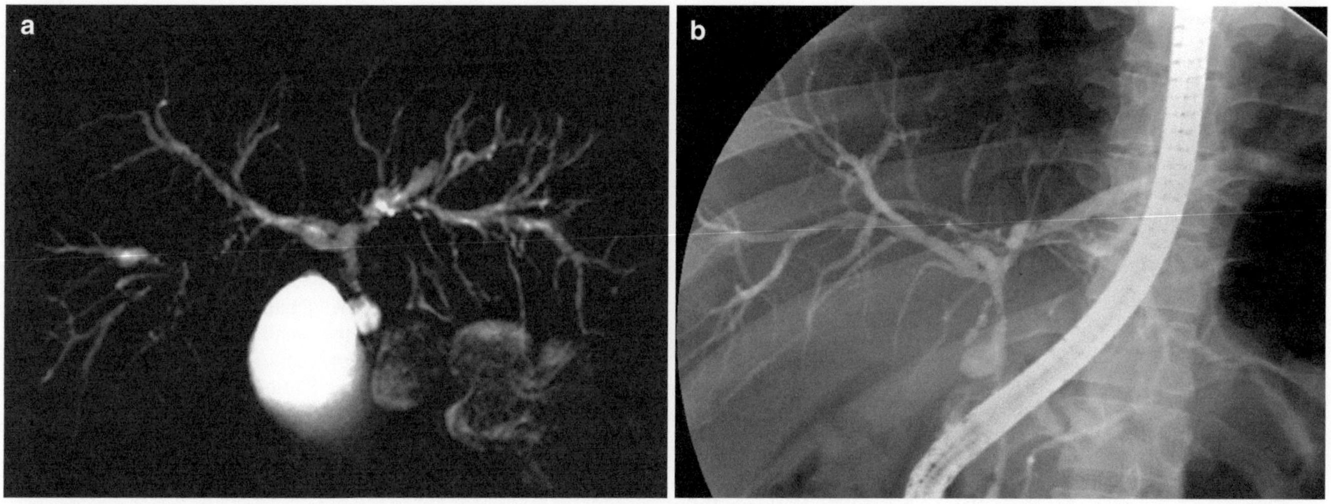

Fig. 8.26 Primary sclerosing cholangitis. Two-dimensional MR cholangiography (**a**) and endoscopic retrograde cholangiography (**b**) show intrahepatic biliary ducts with irregular and multifocal strictures with alternating segments of dilation, creating a beaded appearance of bile ducts

References

1. Park MJ, Lim JS. Computed tomography enterography for evaluation of inflammatory bowel disease. Clin Endosc. 2013;46(4): 327–66. doi:10.5946/ce.2013.46.4.327.
2. Furukawa A, Saotome T, Yamasaki M, Maeda K, Nitta N, Takahashi M, Tsujikawa T, Fujiyama Y, Murata K, Sakamoto T. Cross-sectional imaging in Crohn disease 1. Radiographics. 2004;24(3):689–702. doi:10.1148/rg.243035120.
3. Paulsen SR, Huprich JE, Fletcher JG, Booya F, Young BM, Fidler JL, Johnson CD, Barlow JM, Earnest F. CT enterography as a diagnostic tool in evaluating small bowel disorders: review of clinical experience with over 700 cases 1. Radiographics. 2006;26(3):641–57. doi:10.1148/rg.263055162.
4. Meyers MA, McGuire PV. Spiral CT demonstration of hypervascularity in Crohn disease: "vascular jejunization of the ileum" or the "comb sign". Abdom Imaging. 1995;20(4):327–32.
5. Booya F, Fletcher JG, Huprich JE, Barlow JM, Johnson CD, Fidler JL, Solem CA, Sandborn WJ, Loftus Jr EV, Harmsen WS. Active Crohn disease: CT findings and interobserver agreement for enteric phase CT enterography. Radiology. 2006;241(3):787–95. doi:10.1148/radiol.2413051444.
6. Maglinte DD, Sandrasegaran K, Lappas JC, Chiorean M. CT enteroclysis. Radiology. 2007;245(3):661–71. doi:10.1148/radiol.2453060798.
7. Madureira AJ. The comb sign. Radiology. 2004;230(3):783–4. doi:10.1148/radiol.2303020645.
8. Tolan DJ, Greenhalgh R, Zealley IA, Halligan S, Taylor SA. MR enterographic manifestations of small bowel Crohn disease. Radiographics. 2010;30(2):367–84. doi:10.1148/rg.302095028.
9. Maglinte DD, Gourtsoyiannis N, Rex D, Howard TJ, Kelvin FM. Classification of small bowel Crohn's subtypes based on multimodality imaging. Radiol Clin North Am. 2003;41(2):285–303.
10. Vogel J, da Luz MA, Baker M, Hammel J, Einstein D, Stocchi L, Fazio V. CT enterography for Crohn's disease: accurate preoperative diagnostic imaging. Dis Colon Rectum. 2007;50(11):1761–9. doi:10.1007/s10350-007-9005-6.
11. Schwartz DA, Loftus Jr EV, Tremaine WJ, Panaccione R, Harmsen WS, Zinsmeister AR, Sandborn WJ. The natural history of fistulizing Crohn's disease in Olmsted county, Minnesota. Gastroenterology. 2002;122(4):875–80.
12. Bruining DH, Siddiki HA, Fletcher JG, Tremaine WJ, Sandborn WJ, Loftus Jr EV. Prevalence of penetrating disease and extraintestinal manifestations of Crohn's disease detected with CT enterography. Inflamm Bowel Dis. 2008;14(12):1701–6. doi:10.1002/ibd.20529.
13. Greenstein AJ, Mann D, Sachar DB, Aufses Jr AH. Free perforation in Crohn's disease: I. A survey of 99 cases. Am J Gastroenterol. 1985;80(9):682–9.
14. Ghonge NP, Aggarwal B, Gothi R. CT enterography: state-of-the-art CT technique for small bowel imaging. Indian J Gastroenterol. 2013. doi:10.1007/s12664-013-0307-4.
15. Lee SS, Kim AY, Yang SK, Chung JW, Kim SY, Park SH, Ha HK. Crohn disease of the small bowel: comparison of CT enterography, MR enterography, and small-bowel follow-through as diagnostic techniques. Radiology. 2009;251(3):751–61. doi:10.1148/radiol.2513081184.
16. Masselli G, Gualdi G. CT and MR enterography in evaluating small bowel diseases: when to use which modality? Abdom Imaging. 2013;38(2):249–59. doi:10.1007/s00261-012-9961-8.
17. Akhan O, Pringot J. Imaging of abdominal tuberculosis. Eur Radiol. 2002;12(2):312–23. doi:10.1007/s003300100994.
18. Pereira JM, Madureira AJ, Vieira A, Ramos I. Abdominal tuberculosis: imaging features. Eur J Radiol. 2005;55(2):173–80. doi:10.1016/j.ejrad.2005.04.015.
19. Makanjuola D. Is it Crohn's disease or intestinal tuberculosis? CT analysis. Eur J Radiol. 1998;28(1):55–61.
20. Chung SY, Ha HK, Kim JH, Kim KW, Cho N, Cho KS, Lee YS, Chung DJ, Jung HY, Yang SK, Min YI. Radiologic findings of Behcet syndrome involving the gastrointestinal tract. Radiographics. 2001;21(4):911–24; discussion 924–16.
21. Gore RM, Levine, MS. In: Gore RM, Levine, MS, editors. Textbook of gastrointestinal radiology. Colon. Philadelphia, PA; Saunders Elsevier: 2008.
22. Gore RM. CT of inflammatory bowel disease. Radiol Clin North Am. 1989;27(4):717–29.
23. Wiesner RH, LaRusso NF. Clinicopathologic features of the syndrome of primary sclerosing cholangitis. Gastroenterology. 1980;79(2):200–6.

9 New Endoscopic Modalities in IBD

Makoto Naganuma, Naoki Hosoe, and Haruhiko Ogata

9.1 High-Resolution Endoscopy (HRE)

High-definition white-light endoscopy or high-resolution endoscopy (HRE) has been recently developed and is expected to increase polyp detection during colonoscopy. High-definition white-light endoscopy produces images with a resolution of higher pixels (e.g., >1 million pixels) [1]. HRE enables endoscopists to observe the detailed mucosal and vascular information (Fig. 9.1). In IBD, vascular pattern can be observed in detail; thus, endoscopic remission can be strictly defined especially in patients with UC. As HRE has clinical benefits in the detection of polyps and adenomas in high-risk groups of patients with IBD, it is also shown to be useful to detect colitis-associated dysplasia/cancer in patients with IBD (Fig. 9.2). Although HRE with indigo carmine dye is useful to detect colitis-associated dysplasia/cancer, it has been still controversy whether NBI has more diagnostic accuracy of dysplasia than conventional chromoendoscopy (see NBI).

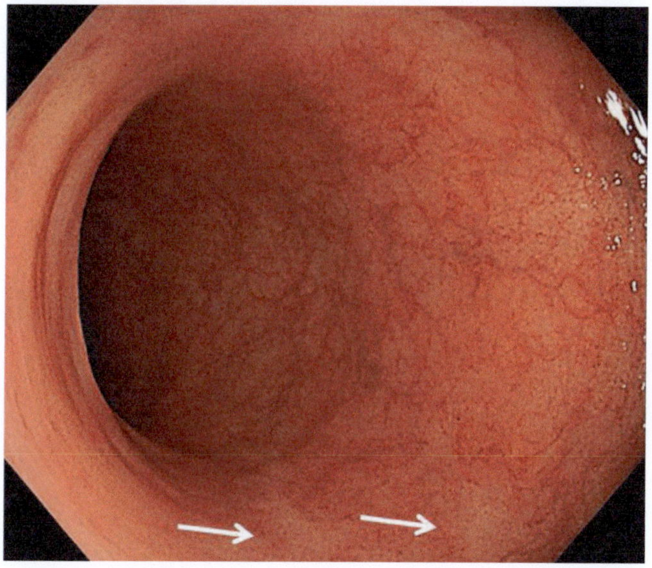

Fig. 9.1 High-resolution endoscopy can observe detailed mucosal inflammation in patients with UC. Even though endoscopic remission is obtained, vessel pattern is not completely normal, and white scars are detected (*arrow*)

M. Naganuma (✉) • N. Hosoe • H. Ogata
Center for Diagnostic and Therapeutic Endoscopy, School of Medicine, Keio University, 35 Shinanomachi, Shinjuku, Tokyo 160-8582, Japan
e-mail: hogata@z8.keio.jp

W.H. Kim, J.H. Cheon (eds.), *Atlas of Inflammatory Bowel Diseases*, DOI 10.1007/978-3-642-39423-2_9, © Springer-Verlag Berlin Heidelberg 2015

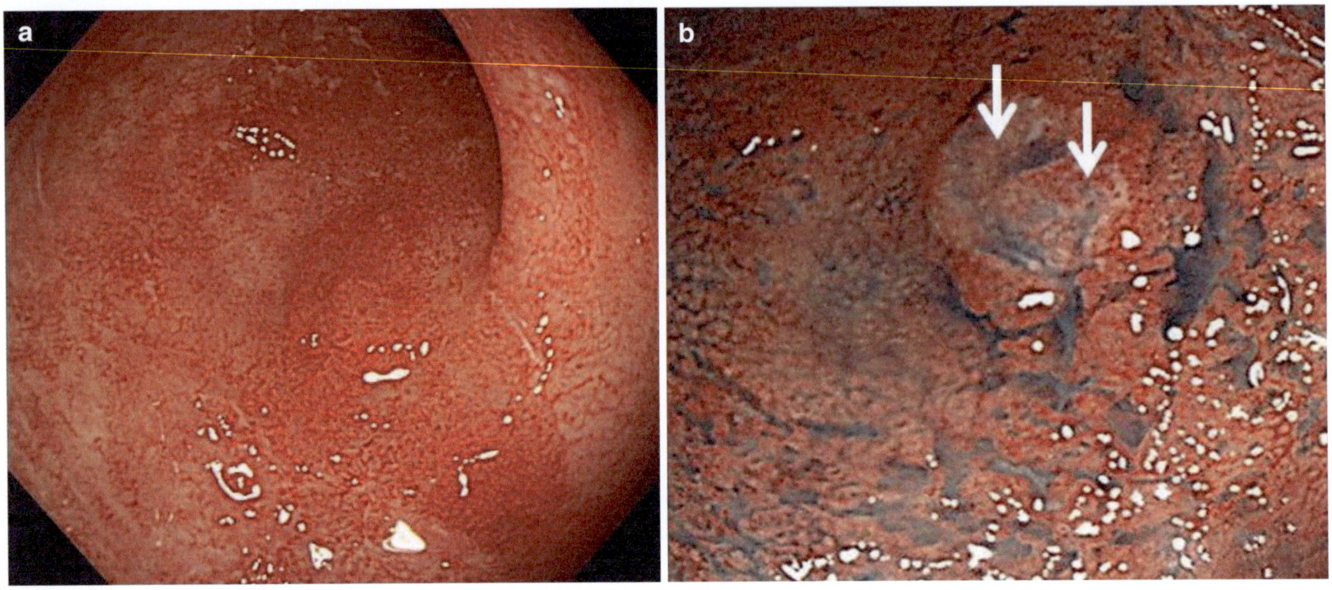

Fig. 9.2 (**a**) Five-millimeter-sized flat-elevated lesion is detected using high-resolution endoscopy. (**b**) Indigo carmine dye emphasizes the elevated lesion with slightly central depressed area (*arrow*)

9.2 Current White-Light Endoscopy for IBD Patients

To reduce patients' burden and increase the diagnostic accuracy and quality, conventional white-light endoscopy is still evolving and improving. The combination of high-definition TV image quality and high angle of view supports detailed observation and facilitates detection of lesions. Diameter of endoscopy may be critical to reduce patients' burden. Endoscopy with a relatively small diameter (e.g., Olympus PCF-PQ260, diameter 9.2 mm) is useful not only to reduce patients' pains but also to be able to pass through mild to moderate strictures in the anal area (Fig. 9.3) and anastomotic strictured site (Fig. 9.4). Endoscopy with a relatively small diameter is sometimes difficult to insert into the proximal colon and the ileum. However, the characteristics of new responsive insertion technology with passive bending and high force transmission are easier on both patients and physicians despite the smaller diameter.

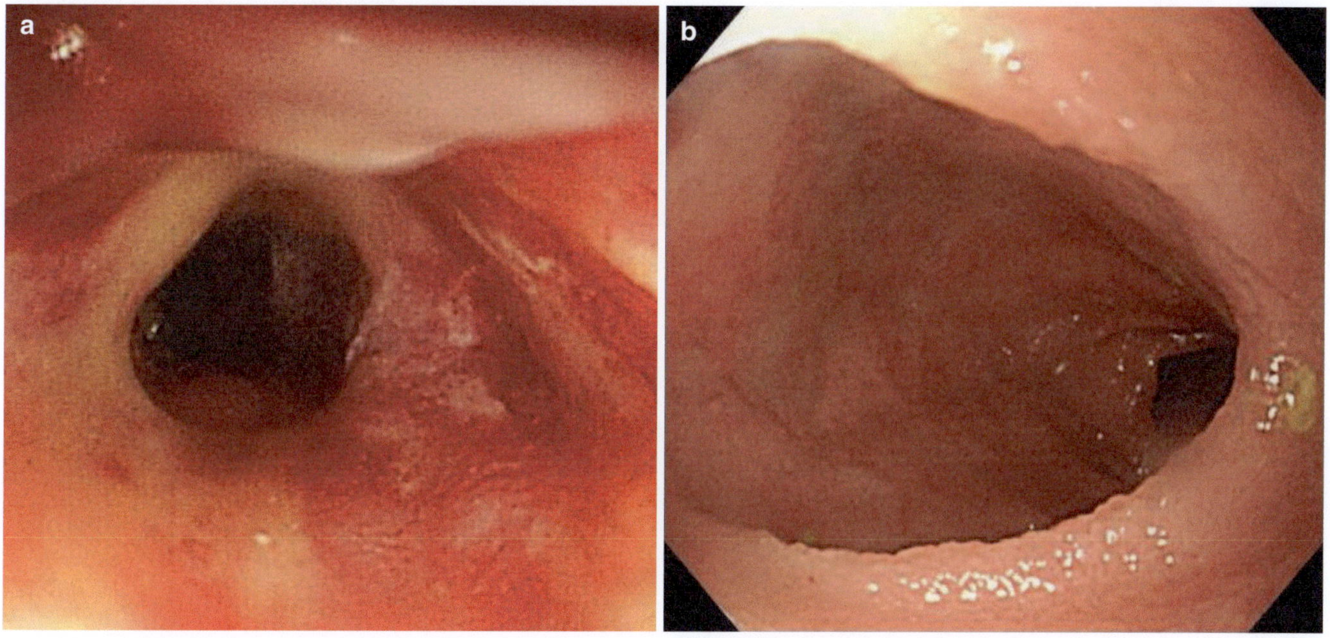

Fig. 9.3 Severe stricture with fissuring ulceration is detected. Endoscopy with 9.2 mm diameter (Olympus PCF-PQ260) can pass through the stricture (**a**), and the proximal colon is observed (**b**)

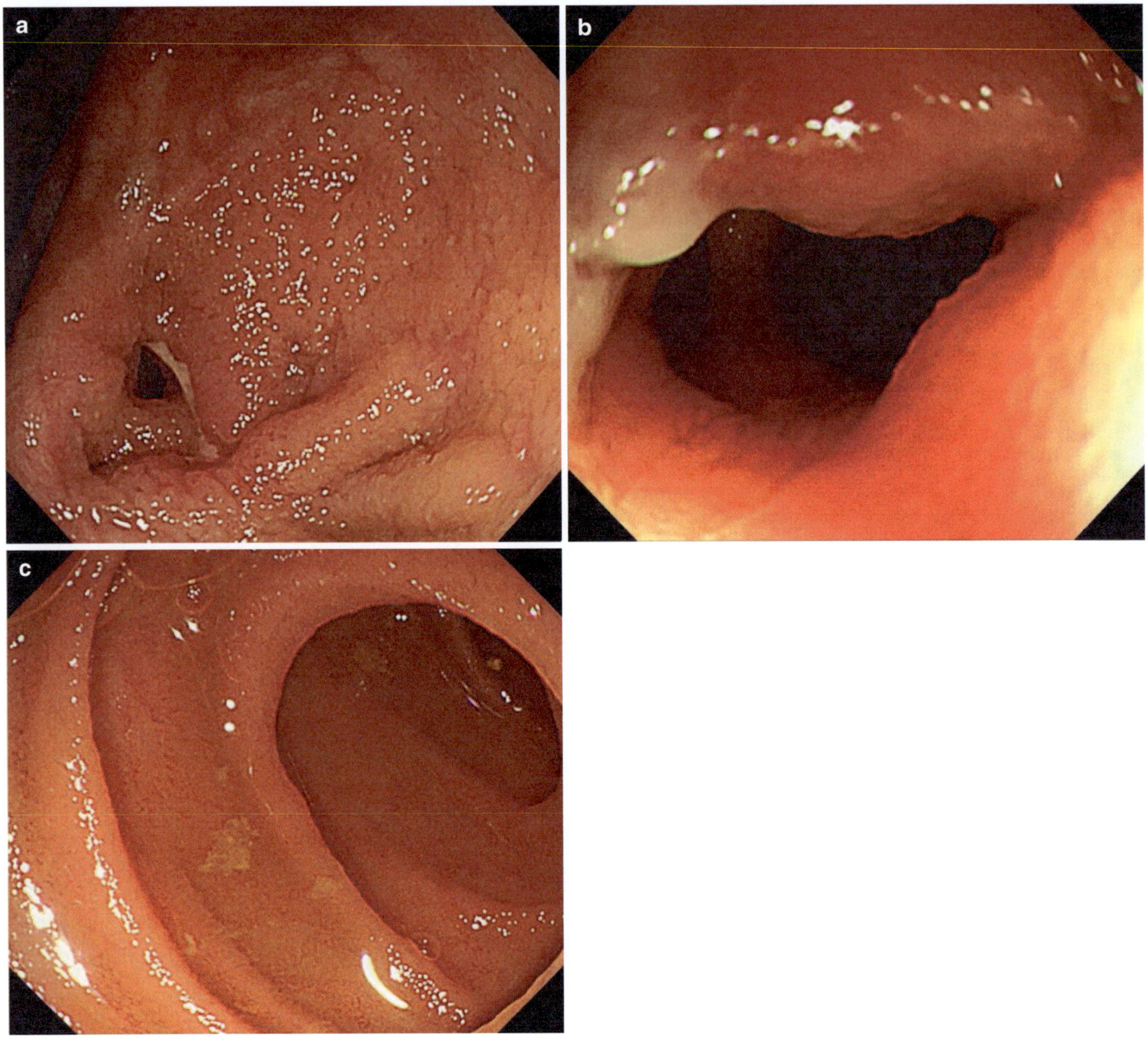

Fig. 9.4 (**a**) Conventional colonoscopy did not pass through the stricture at the anastomosis. (**b**) Endoscopy with a small diameter passes through the strictured site, and (**c**) the terminal ileum could be observed

9.3 Narrow Band Imaging

Clinical usefulness of image-enhanced endoscopy in inflammatory bowel disease in terms of determining disease severity and extent and detecting dysplasia is shown in Table 9.1. NBI has been developed to increase diagnostic accuracy of gastrointestinal adenoma/cancer by improving visual definition of the mucosal surface and by enhancing mucosal vessels. NBI enables not only to detect colon polyps easier but also to assess the possibility of endoscopic resection. Therefore, NBI is now being studied to detect colitis-associated dysplasia. Moreover, because NBI emphasizes mucosal microvessel, it is easier to detect small erosions and aphthae especially in patients with CD (Figs. 9.5 and 9.6). Indigo carmine dye is also useful to detect aphthae in the small intestinal lesions of CD (Fig. 9.6b). However, NBI may be less time-consuming and equally effective to chromoendoscopy for the detection of aphthae (Fig. 9.6c).

It is not yet clear whether NBI can be an alternative device to conventional colonoscopy or chromoendoscopy. To date, three studies have examined the usefulness of NBI to detect dysplasia in long-standing IBD [2–4]. These results suggest that NBI cannot be recommended as an alternative device to chromoendoscopy, although it is faster to perform the examination of colonoscopy. Importantly, NBI with magnification endoscopy can be used to assess extension/spread of dysplasia and to evaluate the possibility of endoscopic resection by observing visual definition of the mucosal surface and mucosal microvessels (Figs. 9.7 and 9.8).

Table 9.1 Potential clinical use of image-enhanced endoscopy in inflammatory bowel disease

	Disease severity and extent	Detection of dysplasia
Chromoendoscopy	±	+++
Magnified endoscopy	+	++
Narrow band imaging	±	+
Autofluorescence imaging	±	++
i-scan	+	++
Confocal laser endomicroscopy	++	++
Endocytoscopy	+++	+

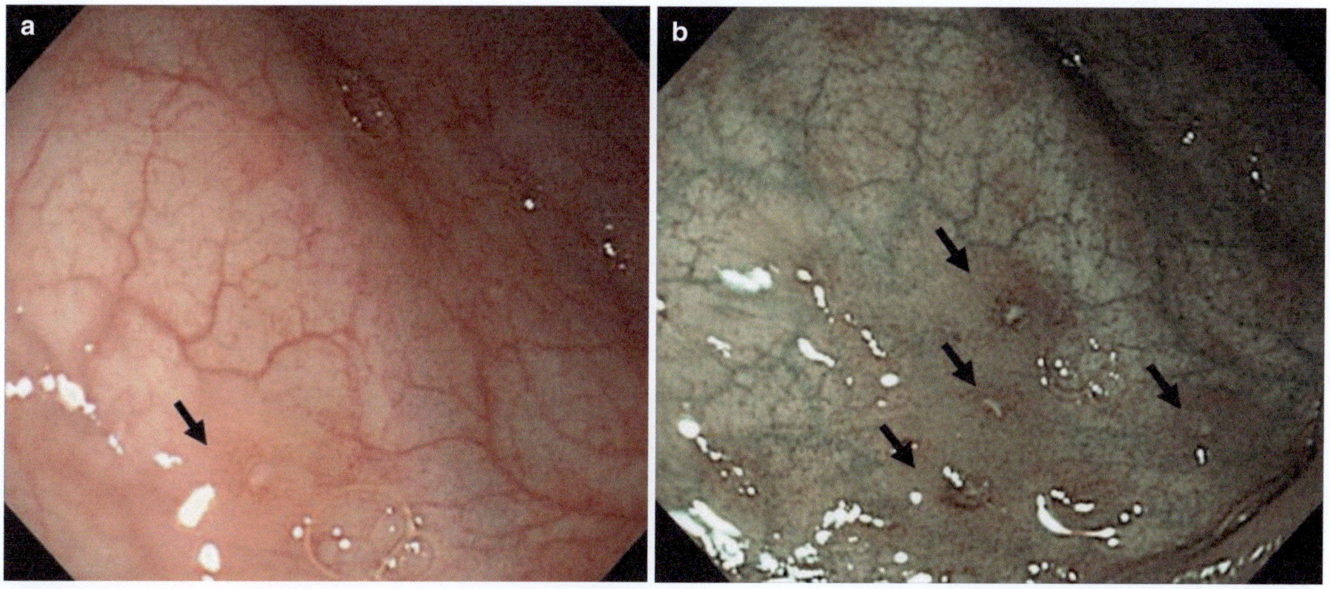

Fig. 9.5 (**a**) Colonic aphthae (*arrow*) are detected by normal white-light imaging. (**b**) NBI emphasizes microvessels, and it is easier to detect several longitudinal aphthae and several colonic lesions (*arrow*)

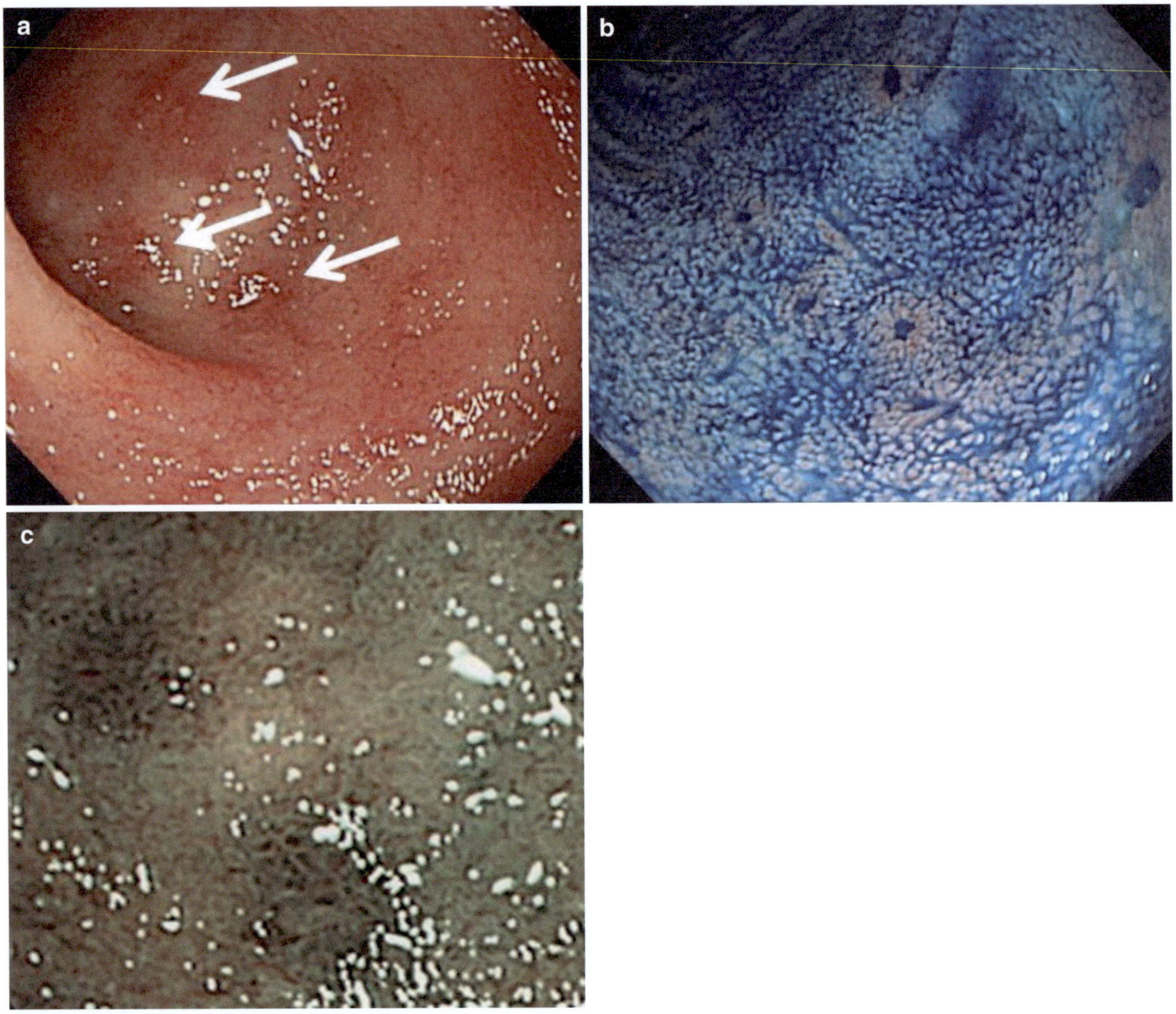

Fig. 9.6 (**a**) Small aphthoid lesions are observed using normal white-light imaging (*arrow*). Indigo carmine dye (**b**) and NBI (**c**) can easily detect these small lesions

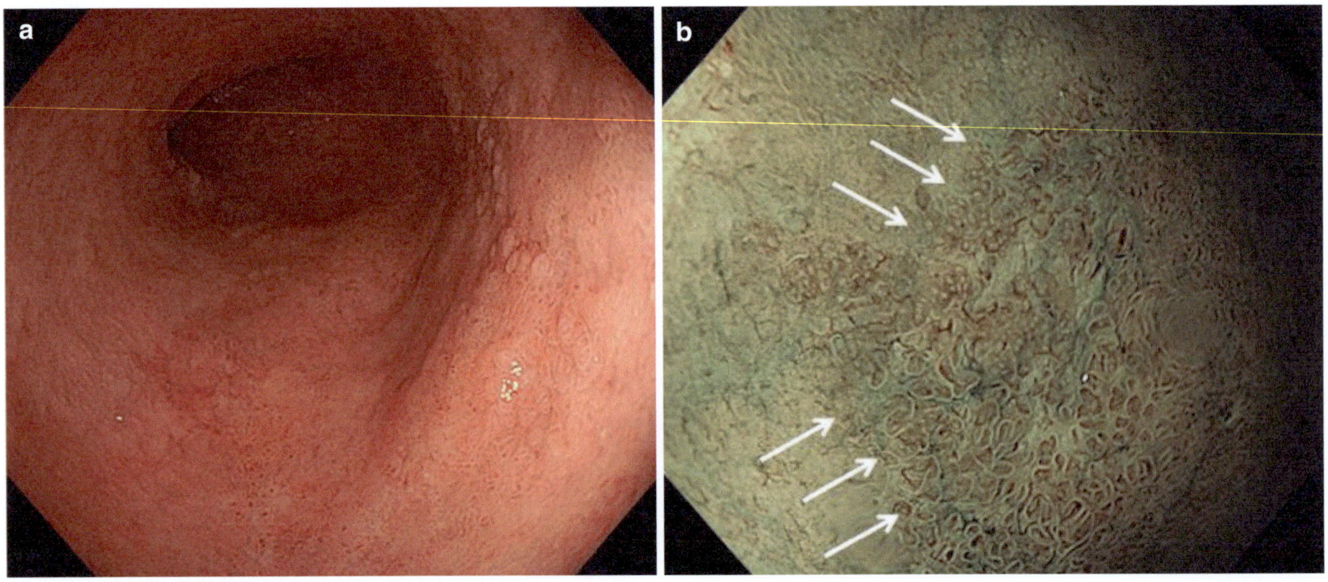

Fig. 9.7 (**a**) Irregular nodular mucosa is detected using normal white-light imaging. NBI with (**b**) normal magnification and (**c**) high magnification can distinct a dysplastic lesion from no-dysplastic area (*arrow*). (**d**) Villous-like mucosa can be detected using NBI with high magnification (*arrow*)

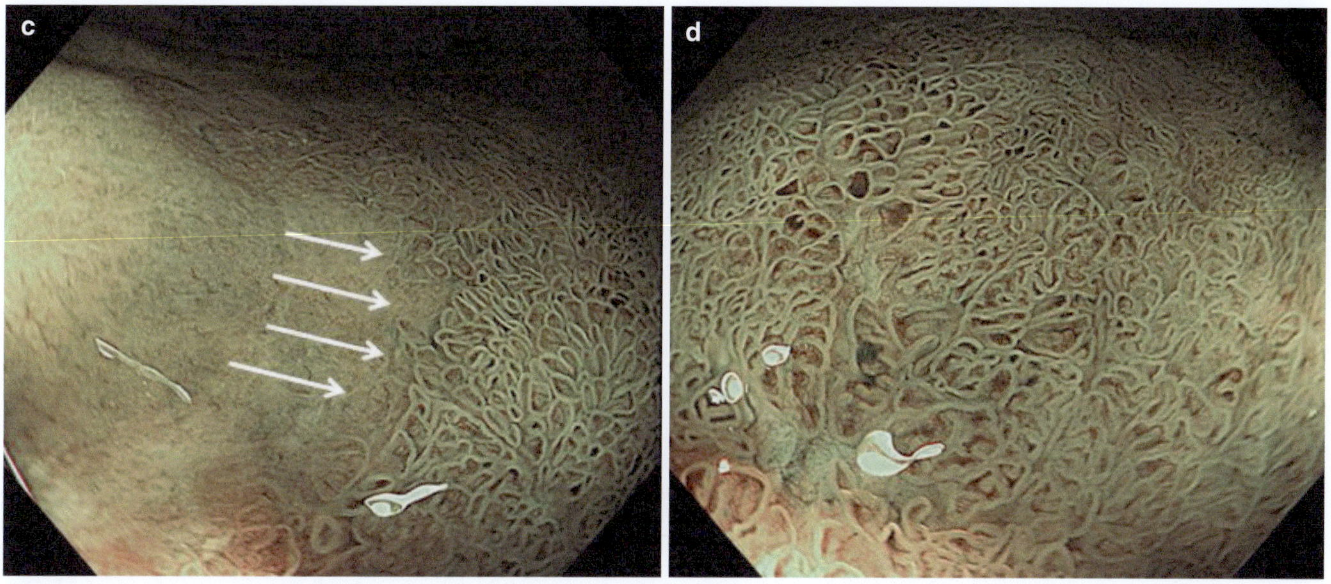

Fig. 9.7 (continued)

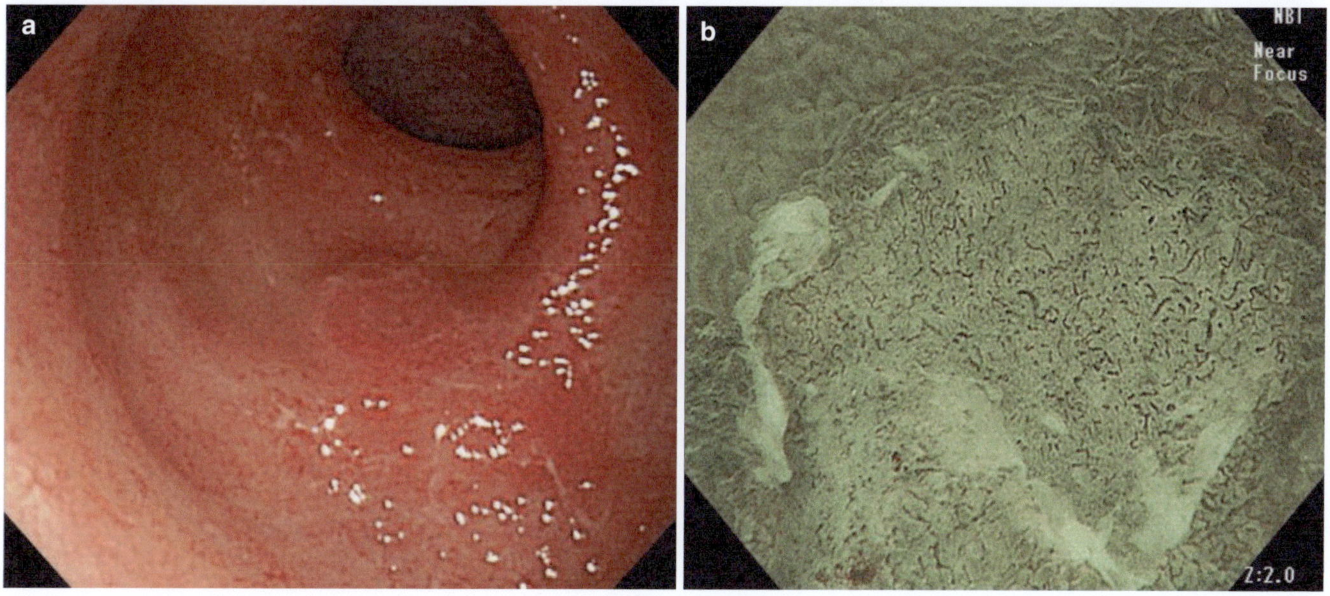

Fig. 9.8 (**a**) A flat-elevated lesion is detected in the rectum (the lesion is the same one as that in Fig. 9.7). (**b**) NBI with magnification reveals irregular vessel patterns

9.4 Magnification Colonoscopy in IBD

Magnification chromocolonoscopy has been shown to be useful in the detection of colitis-associated neoplasia in patients with chronic UC. The assessment of severity of UC using the high-magnification chromocolonoscopy correlated with the histological score to a greater degree than Matts' endoscopic classification [5]. Furthermore, magnification imaging was significantly better than conventional colonoscopy for predicting disease extent. These results suggest that magnification chromocolonoscopy may potentially be considered as an alternative to histological examination when evaluating disease severity and for the detection of colitis-associated dysplasia/cancer.

Recently, endocytoscopy and endomicroscopy have been developed. Endocytoscopy can visualize the superficial mucosal layer by allowing magnification of the mucosa up to more 1,000-fold [6]. Endocytoscopy enables the detection sharp of crypt and mucosal inflammatory cells (Figs. 9.9, 9.10, and 9.11). This new device can discriminate between histological severities of UC in patients with mucosal healing (e.g., Mayo endoscopic score 0) even if pathological examination is not performed.

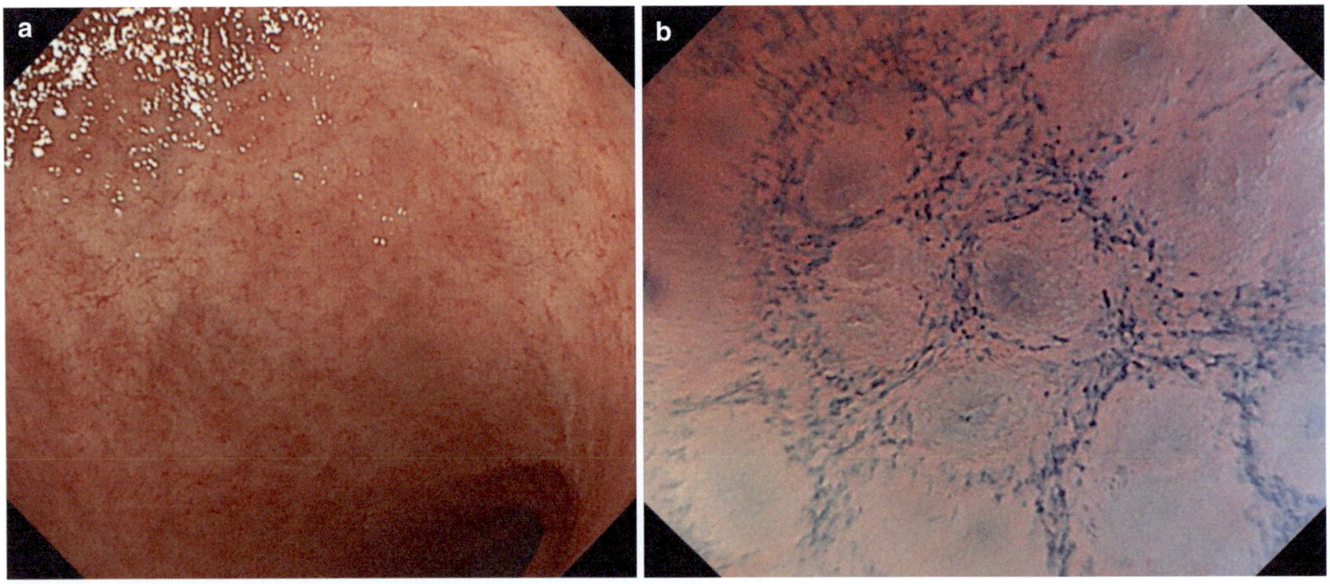

Fig. 9.9 (**a**) Endoscopic mucosal healing is observed in the rectum of patients with UC (Mayo endoscopic score 0). (**b**) Endocytoscopic findings show round crypts, and slightly inflamed cells are detected

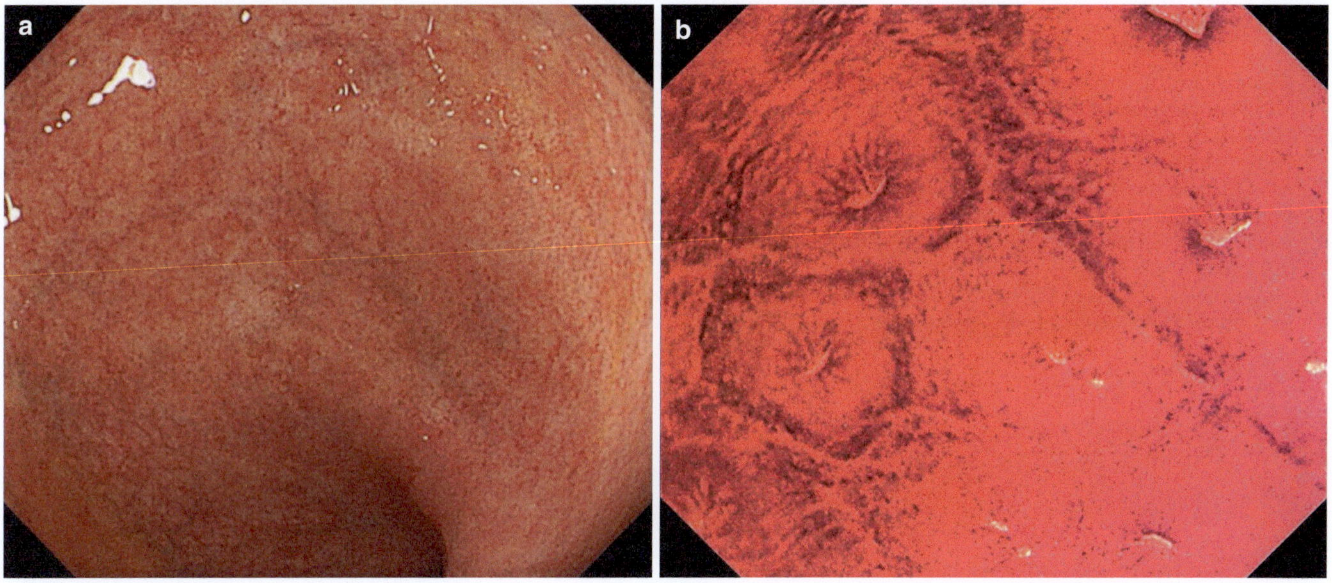

Fig. 9.10 (**a**) Endoscopic mucosal healing is observed in the rectum of patients with UC (Mayo endoscopic score 0). (**b**) Endocytoscopy reveals a few inflammatory cells with oval and round crypts

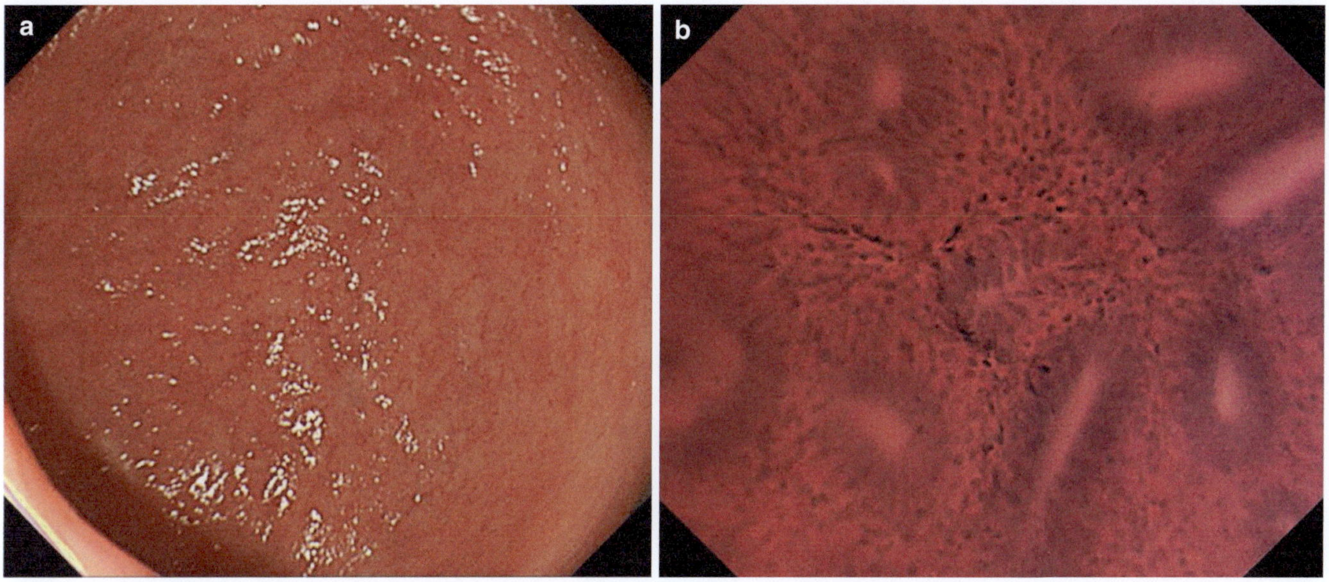

Fig. 9.11 (**a**) Mucosal vessels disappeared in the rectum of patients with UC, but there were no redness/erosions and ulcerations. (**b**) Moderate inflammation is detected, and distance between crypts was widened as revealed by endocytoscopy

References

1. Subramanian V, Ragunath K. Advanced endoscopic imaging: a review of commercially available technologies. Clin Gastroenterol Hepatol. 2014;12:368–76.e1.
2. Pellisé M, López-Cerón M, de Miguel Rodríguez C, et al. Narrow-band imaging as an alternative to chromoendoscopy for the detection of dysplasia in long-standing inflammatory bowel disease: a prospective, randomized, crossover study. Gastrointest Endosc. 2011;74:840–8.
3. Dekker E, van den Broek FJ, Reitsma JB, et al. Narrow-band imaging compared with conventional colonoscopy for the detection of dysplasia in patients with longstanding ulcerative colitis. Endoscopy. 2007;39:216–21.
4. Efthymiou M, Allen PB, Taylor AC, et al. Chromoendoscopy versus narrow band imaging for colonic surveillance in inflammatory bowel disease. Inflam Bowel Dis. 2013;19:2132–8.
5. Hurlstone DP, Sanders DS, McAlindon ME, et al. High-magnification chromoscopic colonoscopy in ulcerative colitis: a valid tool for in vivo optical biopsy and assessment of disease extent. Endoscopy. 2006;38:1213–7.
6. Neumann H, Neurath MF, Mudter J. New endoscopic approaches in IBD. World J Gastroenterol. 2011;17:63–8.

Therapeutic Endoscopy

10

Makoto Naganuma, Naoki Hosoe, and Haruhiko Ogata

10.1 Endoscopic Hemostasis

In general, blood in stool is relatively uncommon in CD patients, compared to UC patients. However, inflammation of ileocecal or small bowel lesions can cause anemia. In some cases, melena with severe anemia occurs even when they are in clinical remission.

It is not easy to detect "blood spot" using conventional colonoscopy or small bowel follow-through. Figure 10.1a, b indicates that small ulceration with massive bleeding is observed at anastomosis by colonoscopy. Endoscopic hemostasis was successfully conducted (Fig. 10.1c).

Blood in stool and melena in patients with UC are usually treated with medical treatments, such as 5-aminosalicylates, corticosteroids, or other immunosuppressive agents. Endoscopic hemostasis is very uncommon in UC patients. However, Dieulafoy's ulceration (exposed vessel on ulceration) may cause severe bleeding even when clinical and endoscopic remission is obtained (at 11 months prior to massive bleeding) as Fig. 10.2 indicates. Endoscopic hemostasis is also useful for this case.

M. Naganuma (✉) • N. Hosoe • H. Ogata
Center for Diagnostic and Therapeutic Endoscopy,
School of Medicine, Keio University,
35 Shinanomachi, Shinjuku, Tokyo 160-8582, Japan
e-mail: hogata@z8.keio.jp

W.H. Kim, J.H. Cheon (eds.), *Atlas of Inflammatory Bowel Diseases*,
DOI 10.1007/978-3-642-39423-2_10,

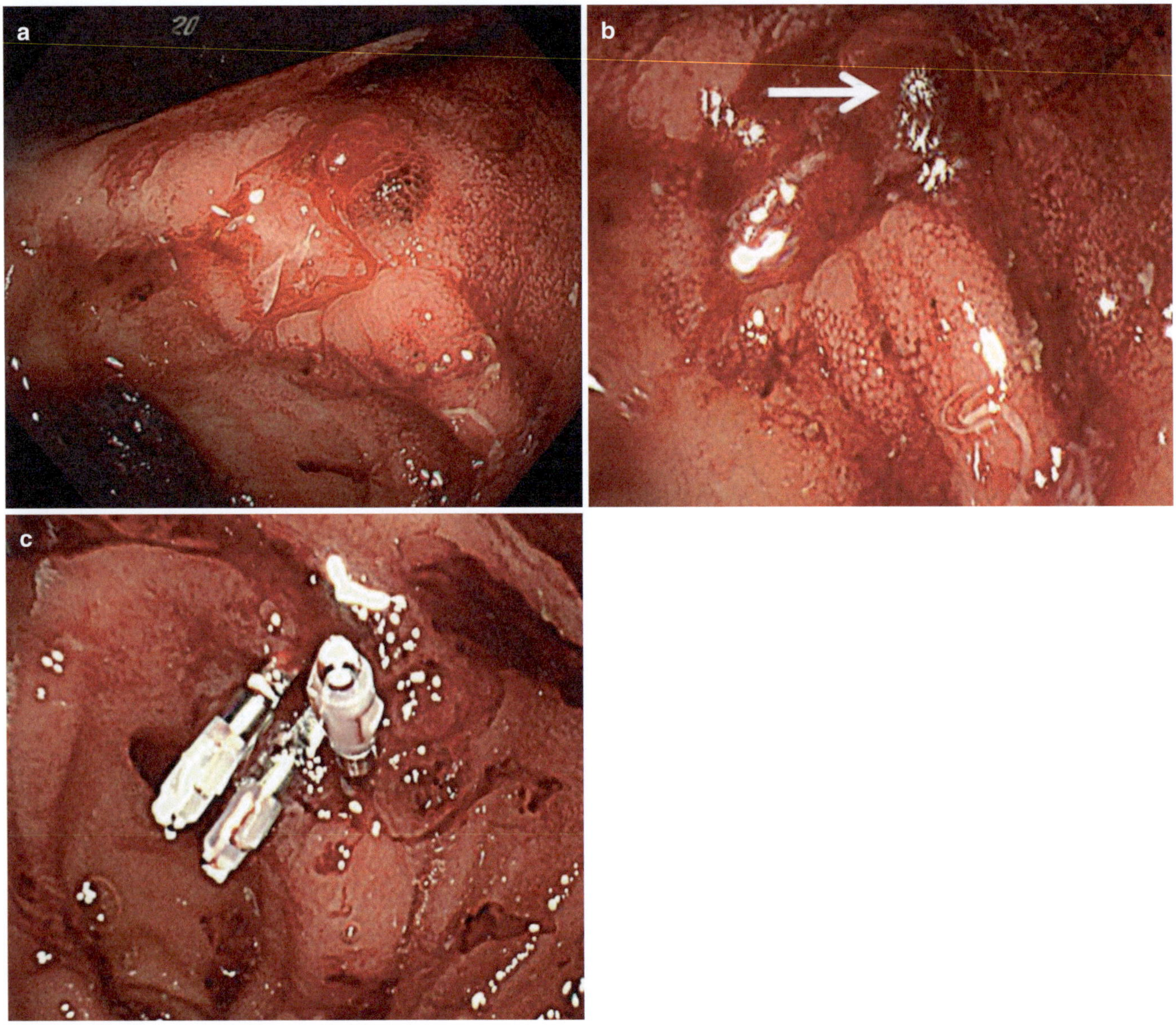

Fig. 10.1 (**a**) Massive bleeding with ulceration is observed at the ileocolonic anastomosis of patients with Crohn's disease, and (**b**) blood vessel is exposed (*white arrow*). (**c**) Endoscopic hemostasis was successfully conducted

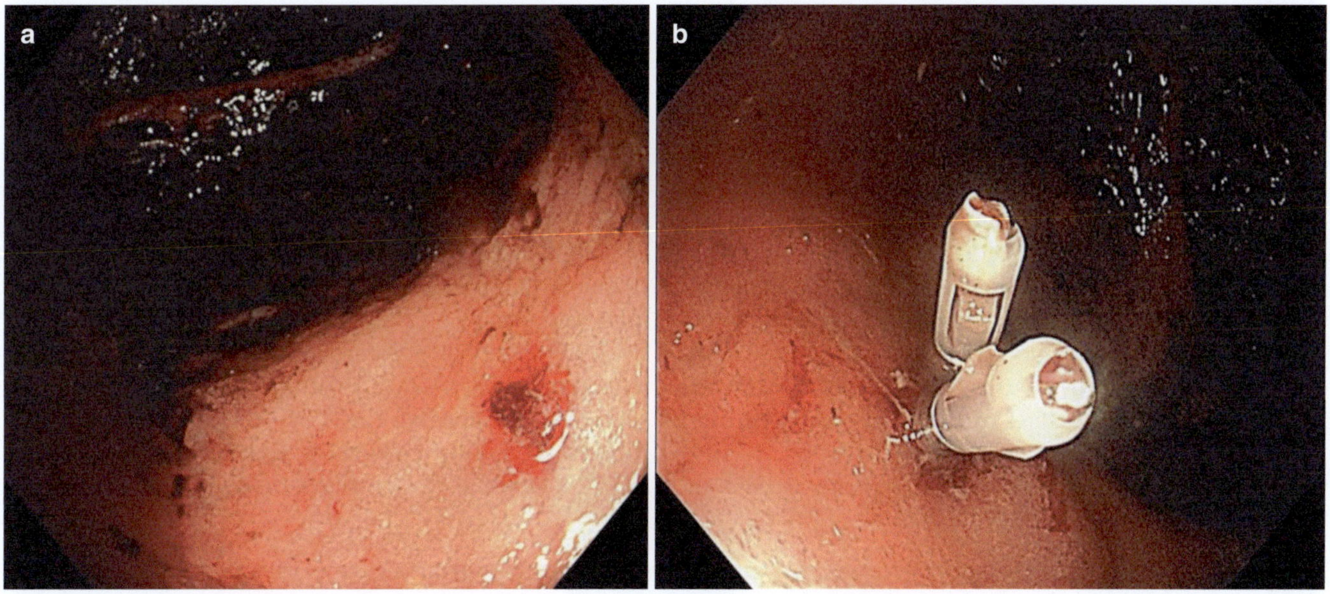

Fig. 10.2 (**a**) Dieulafoy's ulceration is detected in the rectum of patients with ulcerative colitis. Mild inflammation with friability and no-vessel pattern is observed around "bleeding spot." (**b**) Endoscopic hemostasis was successfully conducted

10.2 Endoscopic Balloon Dilatation

Strictures are observed approximately in one-third of patients with Crohn's disease, and it causes severe abdominal symptoms. More than half of patients with CD need surgery within the first 10 years after onset of disease, and strictures and obstructions were one of the common indications for surgery. To improve clinical outcome, it is critical to prevent progression of strictures as early as possible. Strictures may be categorized as fibrotic type and inflammatory types. For inflammatory strictures, medical treatments may be useful to improve the lesions, whereas these are not effective for fibrotic strictures without inflammation in most cases. Endoscopic balloon dilatation (EBD) (Figs. 10.3a–d and 10.4a–d) may relieve abdominal symptoms and prevent surgery in some cases of CD. Fibrotic, shorter length of strictures and no/mild inflammation around stenosis are indicative for EBD (Table 10.1). At the procedures of EBD, the number of strictures, length and diameter of strictures, and presence of intra-intestinal fistula should be confirmed by small bowel follow-through (Fig. 10.3e) or other diagnostic devices.

EBD is effective for patients who have small bowel strictures, and balloon-assisted enteroscopy is usually used in these patients [1]. Despott et al. showed that dilation of small bowel strictures using EBD was effective in patients with symptomatic CD [2]. Hirai et al. also reported that short-term dilation by EBD was successful in 72 % of patients [3] and the cumulative surgery-free rates were 83 and 72 % at 6 and 12 months after dilation, respectively.

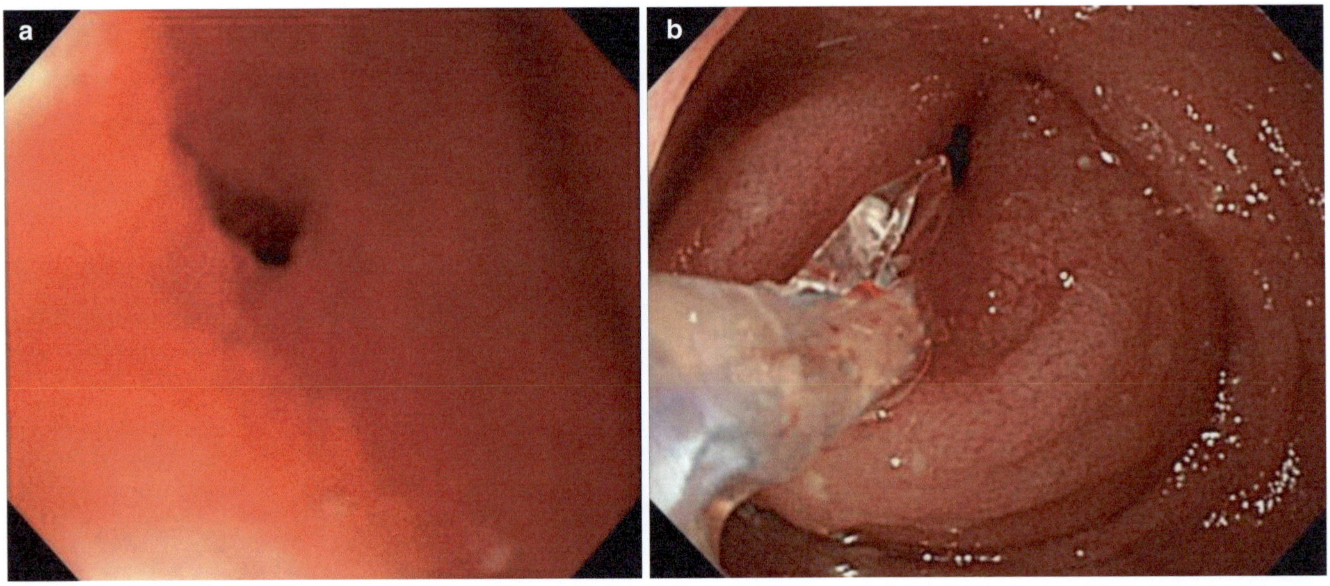

Fig. 10.3 (**a**) Severe stricture is detected in the distal ileum of patients with Crohn's disease. No ulceration is found. (**b**) Dilator is inserted into the strictures, and (**c**) endoscopic balloon dilation is performed. (**d**) Stricture was significantly improved, and colonoscopy could be passed beyond the stricture. (**e**) Before procedure of endoscopic balloon dilation, stricture without fistula was confirmed using radiological examination

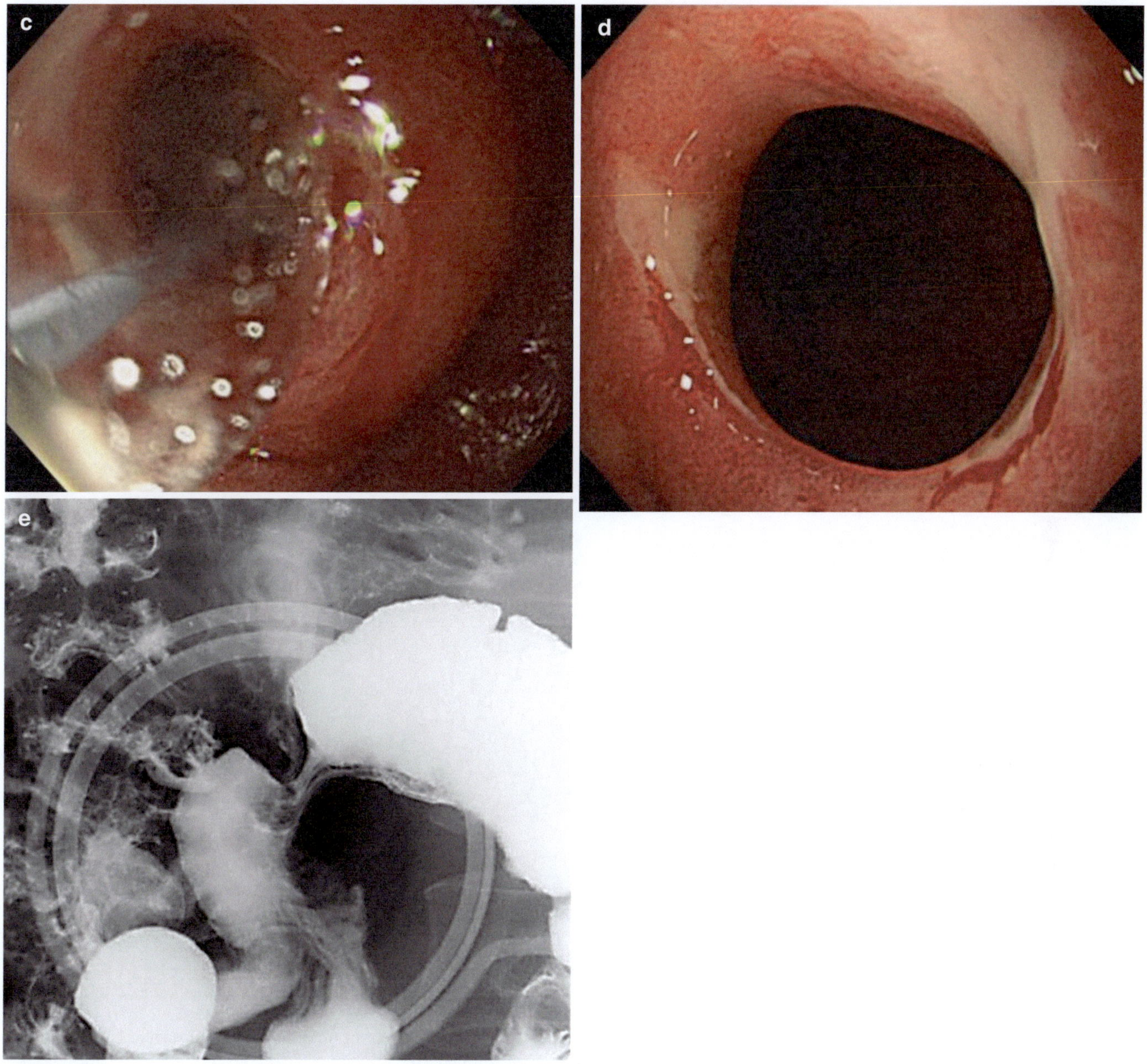

Fig. 10.3 (continued)

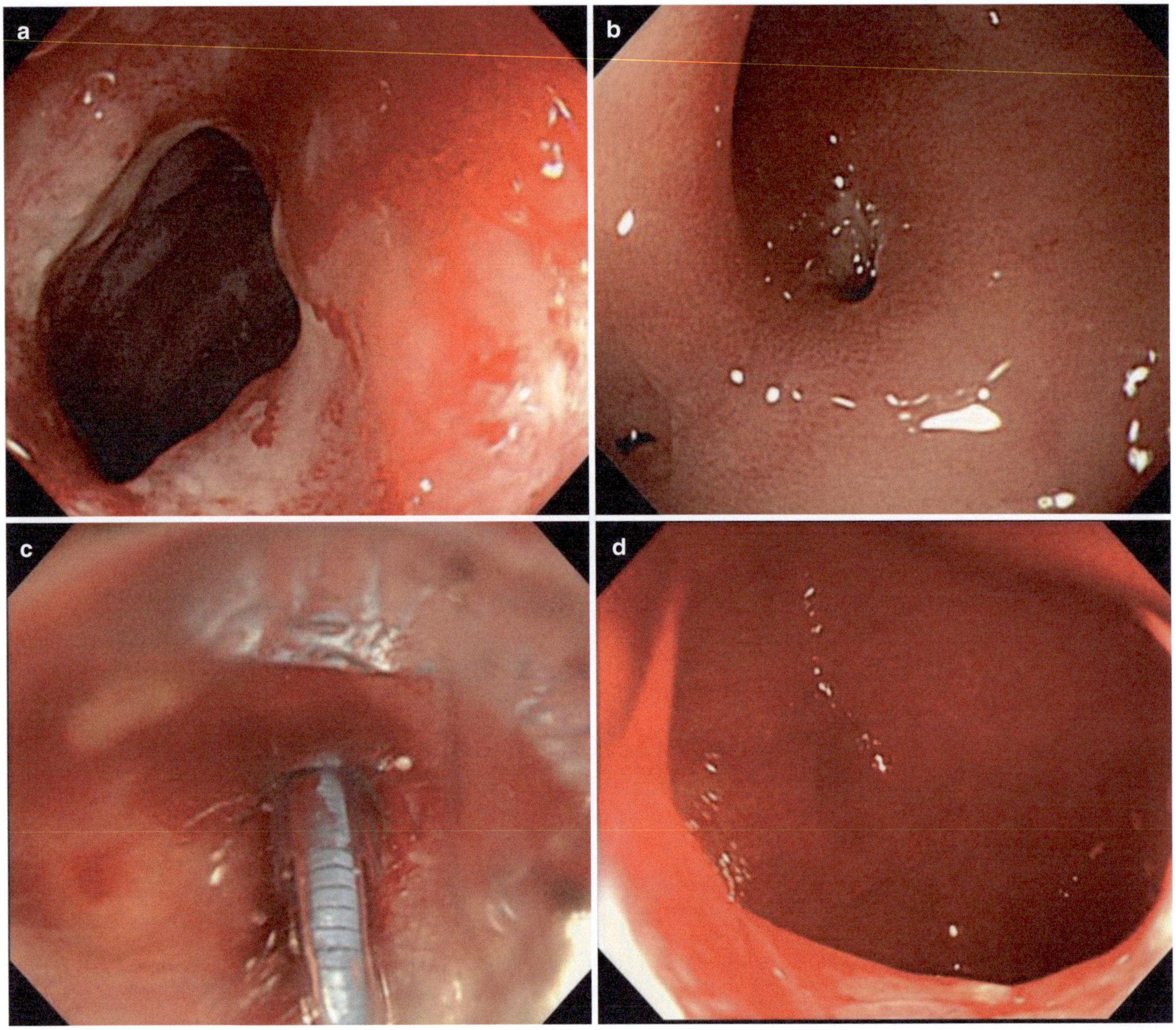

Fig. 10.4 (**a**) Patients with Crohn's disease received infliximab due to postoperative endoscopic recurrence at the anastomosis. (**b**) Endoscopic lesion on anastomosis was improved. However, severe stricture was observed after treatment of infliximab. (**c**) Endoscopic balloon dilation was performed. (**d**) Stricture was significantly improved after the procedure of dilation

Table 10.1 Indication of endoscopic balloon dilation in patients with Crohn's disease

1. No fistula and/or abscess at the stricture
2. No severe ulceration at the stricture
3. Length of stricture <5 cm
4. No severe flection at the stricture

10.3 Endoscopic Resection in Patients with IBD

Sessile polyps and adenoma are usually removed using endoscopic mucosal resection (EMR). Of note, colitis-associated dysplasia/cancer is found in patients with long-standing, chronic active UC. In case of colitis-associated dysplasia/cancer, total proctocolectomy is occasionally selected because these are typically widespread and multiple lesions and colitis-associated dysplasia may occur in any colonic mucosa where inflammations are observed. Thus, endoscopic therapeutic resection is not usually performed because other dysplasia can remain or newly develop even when endoscopic therapeutic resection is performed for "single dysplasia." However, it is difficult to distinguish colitis-associated dysplasia from sporadic dysplasia. When pathological examination is performed, diagnosis of dysplasia (colitic or sporadic) in UC patients sometimes differs even among pathologists. EMR or endoscopic submucosal dissection (ESD) can be performed and used as "therapeutic diagnosis." These endoscopic approaches are allowed in case of endoscopic remission and no dysplasia around polypoid lesions where EMR/ESD is conducted (Figs. 10.5 and 10.6). Fibrosis is moderate to severe in some cases of UC. Therefore, the technique of EMR/ESD is more difficult in UC patients than those in patients without IBD.

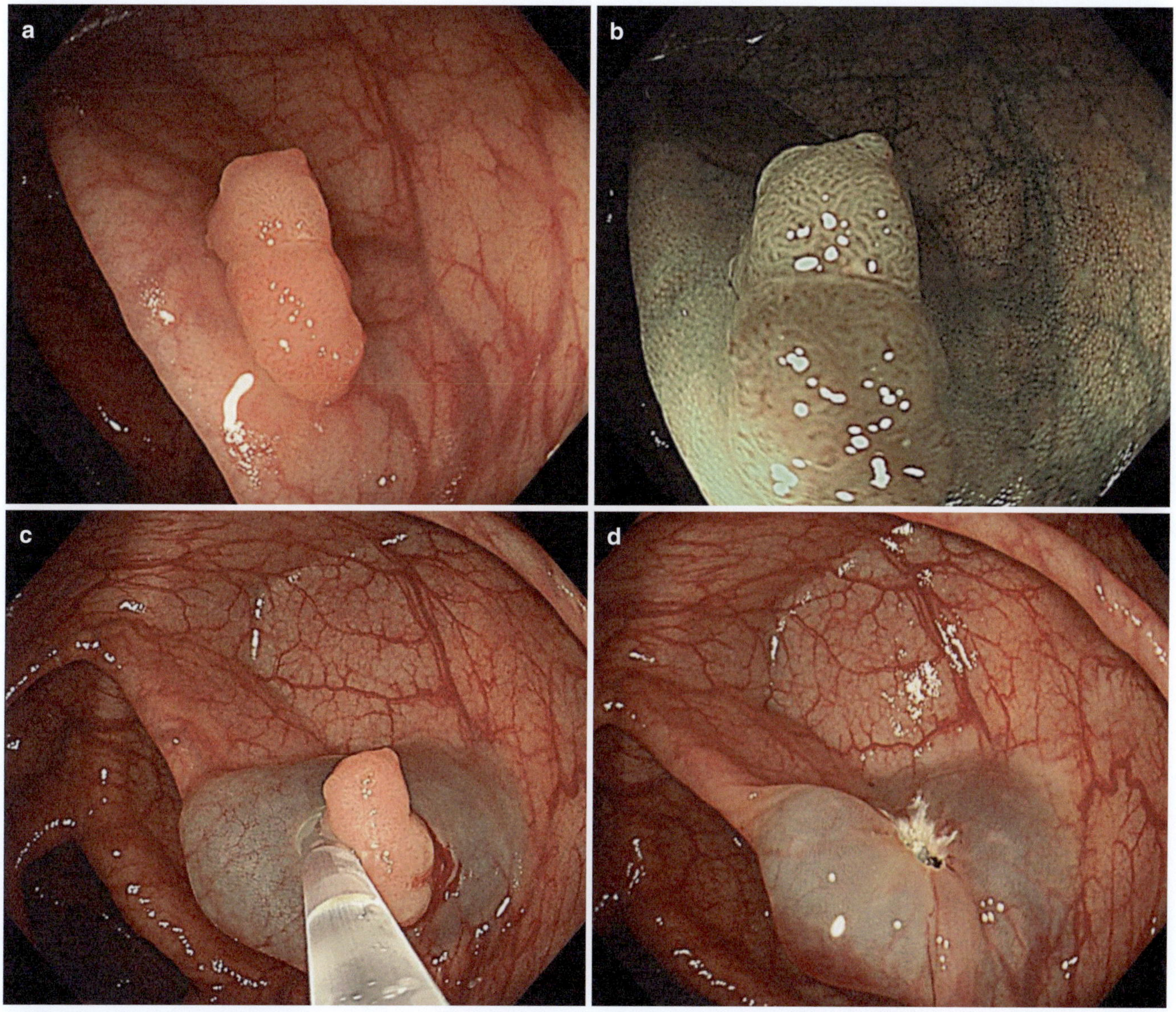

Fig. 10.5 (**a**) Ten-millimeter-sized elevated lesion (Is) is detected in the sigmoid colon of UC patients. No endoscopic inflammation with normal vessel pattern was confirmed. (**b**) Narrow band imaging revealed no abdominal vessel pattern and IIIL pit pattern. (**c**) Submucosal injection to create an undermining submucosal fluid cushion was conducted. (**d**) The lesion was completely removed

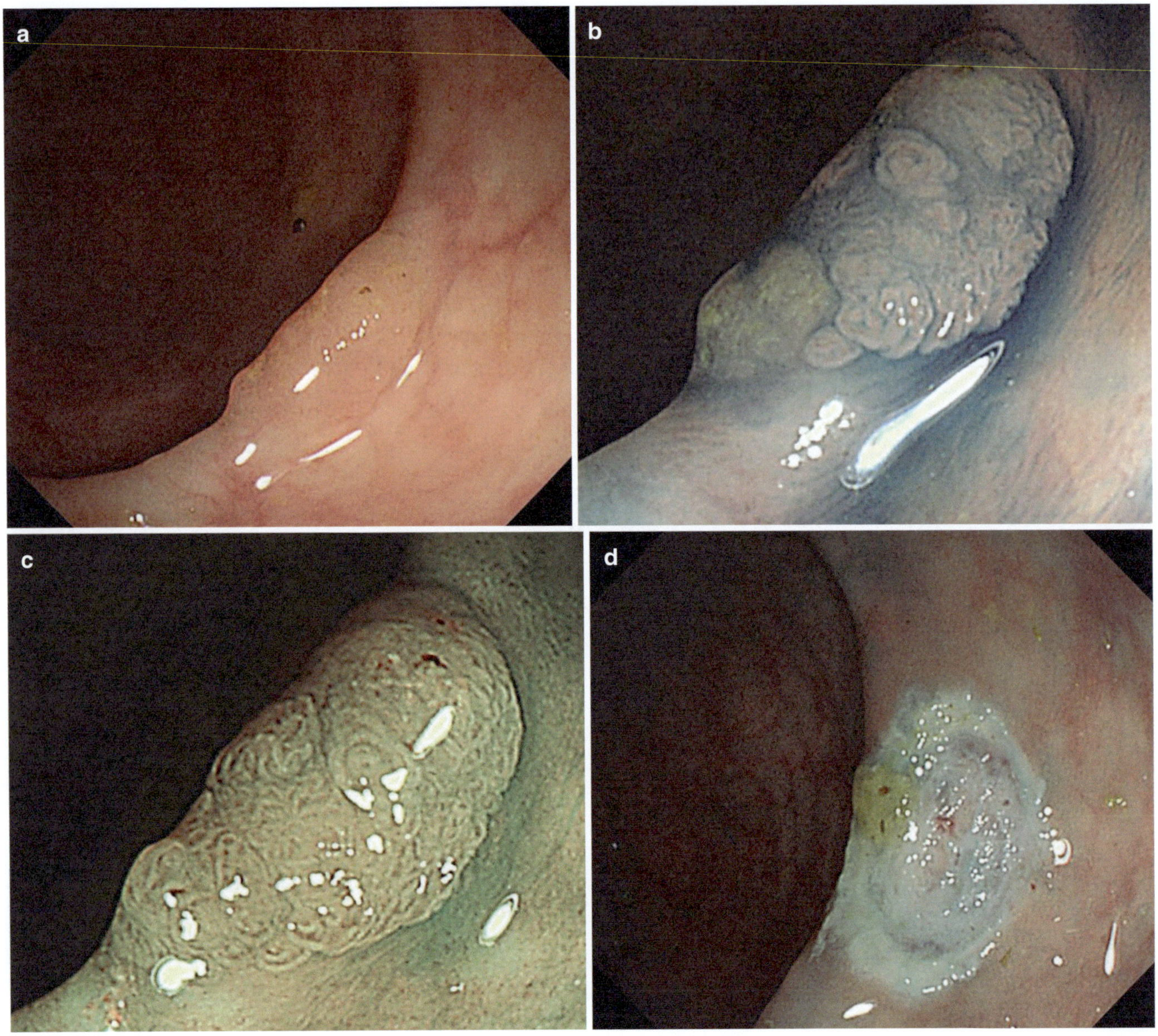

Fig. 10.6 (**a**) Ten-millimeter-sized slightly elevated lesion (IIa) was detected in the rectum of UC patients. Vessel pattern was slightly less visible, but endoscopic findings revealed no active lesion. (**b**) Indigo carmine dye could emphasize elevated lesion, and villous pattern was found on the polyp. (**c**) Narrow band imaging revealed no abdominal vessel pattern and IIIL pit pattern. (**d**) The lesion was completely removed

References

1. Naganuma M, Hosoe N, Ogata H. Inflammatory bowel disease and novel endoscopic technologies. Dig Endosc. 2014;26 Suppl 1:20–8.
2. Despott EJ, Gupta A, Burling D, et al. Effective dilation of small-bowel strictures by double-balloon enteroscopy in patients with symptomatic Crohn's disease (with video). Gastrointest Endosc. 2009;70:1030–6.
3. Hirai F, Beppu T, Sou S, et al. Endoscopic balloon dilatation using double-balloon endoscopy is a useful and safe treatment for small intestinal strictures in Crohn's disease. Dig Endosc. 2010;22: 200–4.

11 Extraintestinal Manifestations

Dongsik Bang, Do Young Kim, Suhyun Cho, and Min Ju Choi

11.1 Introduction

Extraintestinal manifestations of inflammatory bowel diseases (IBD) frequently occur, most of which are associated with Crohn's disease (CD) and ulcerative colitis (UC). However, less commonly reported manifestations of IBD include other conditions such as Behçet's disease (BD) and Hermansky-Pudlak syndrome [1–5]. In the East Asia, including Korea and Japan, where Behçet's disease is highly prevalent, gastrointestinal involvement of Behçet's disease is relatively common (5–25 % of patients with Behçet's disease) [6, 7]. However, there exist only a few reports focusing on gastrointestinal involvement of Behçet's disease.

The incidence of extraintestinal manifestations of IBD has been reported as 2–34 % [3]. Involved organs include the oral and genital mucosa, skin, eye, and joints. Extraintestinal manifestations of IBD can be classified into specific, reactive, and associated conditions in relation to gastrointestinal tract lesions [1]. The precise mechanisms underlying the pathogenic link between extraintestinal manifestations and IBD are unclear but are likely multifactorial depending upon genetics, anatomical site, microbiology, immunology, and trauma. These symptoms are highly variable and have broad spectrum regarding the underlying diseases and locations of involvement. A better understanding of characteristics of IBD extraintestinal manifestations is helpful in the early diagnosis and treatment of underlying intestinal diseases.

D. Bang, MD, PhD (✉) • D.Y. Kim • S. Cho • M.J. Choi
Department of Dermatology and Cutaneous Biology Research Institute,
Yonsei University College of Medicine,
Seoul, South Korea
e-mail: dbang@yuhs.ac

11.2 Skin and Mucosal Manifestations

11.2.1 Specific Mucocutaneous Lesions

Specific mucocutaneous lesions in IBD are relatively uncommon. Fissures and fistulas are probably the most common cutaneous manifestations and may be the presenting complaints in IBD. In a study of 569 CD patients, perianal fissures and fistulas were found in 36 % of patients [8]. Perianal fissures and fistulas associated with CD are typically multiple and involve the anus circumferentially [9]. These lesions can be associated with marked edema and chronic inflammation, abscess formation, undermined ulcers, and skin tags. In CD, direct involvement of the oral mucosa or metastatic involvements on the skin and subcutaneous tissue at sites distant from the gastrointestinal tract are considered to be disease-specific lesions. Mucosal nodularity, known as a cobblestone pattern, appears as firm plaques or confluent papules on the buccal mucosa and palate [1]. These lesions histologically show granulomas and inflammatory changes characteristic of CD.

11.2.2 Reactive Mucocutaneous Lesions

Oral and genital aphthous ulcers, erythema nodosum, pyoderma gangrenosum, papulopustular lesions, Sweet's syndrome, pathergy phenomenon, and pyodermatitis vegetans and pyostomatitis vegetans are considered to be common reactive skin manifestations of IBD. The oral mucosa is a commonly affected site in IBD. Aphtha is the most common mucous reactivity disturbance in IBD; especially in Behçet's disease, oral aphthous stomatitis may be a significant finding [10]. Nutritional deficiencies in iron, folic acid, and vitamin B12 secondary to active IBD also predispose toward aphthous ulcer formation [1]. Oral ulcers in IBD present as painful, shallow, round to oval ulcers covered with a whitish to yellowish pseudomembrane demarcated by a red hyperemic border (Fig. 11.1). Although they can occur anywhere in the

W.H. Kim, J.H. Cheon (eds.), *Atlas of Inflammatory Bowel Diseases*,
DOI 10.1007/978-3-642-39423-2_11, © Springer-Verlag Berlin Heidelberg 2015

oral cavity including the tongue, lip, gingiva, and palate, the oropharyngeal area and even the upper esophagus can also be affected in severe cases. Oral aphthae in IBD are almost indistinguishable from common ulcerations in recurrent aphthous stomatitis. However, they should be differentiated from other common conditions such as oral lichen planus or pemphigus which are frequently presenting oral ulcerations or erosions (Fig. 11.2).

Genital ulceration can occur in many patients with IBD. Importantly, genital ulcer is another cardinal manifestation of BD, and it is one of the diagnostic items in guidelines by the International Study Group for Behçet's Disease (ISGBD) [11]. They are frequently painful, round to oval lesions that are usually covered with dried crust or grayish-white exudates, which are similar findings as with oral aphthae (Fig. 11.3). Significant edema, pain, and scarring around the ulcerations are quite common. The scrotum in males and both major and minor labia in females are commonly affected sites [7].

Erythema nodosum (EN) is the most common cause of lower extremity inflammatory nodules in IBD patients (4–6 % of IBD cases), occurring more frequently in UC patients compared to CD patients [1]. More importantly, EN or EN-like lesions are cardinal cutaneous manifestations of BD [7]. EN is characterized by the sudden onset of erythematous, nonulcerating, tender nodules that are frequently located on the lower extremities (Fig. 11.4). Histopathologically, they are characterized by prominent septal and/or lobular panniculitis that is sometimes accompanied by neutrophilic vascular inflammation (Fig. 11.5).

Pyoderma gangrenosum (PG) is a severe ulcerating noninfectious neutrophilic dermatosis, which has been reported in 1–10 % of UC patients and 0.5–20 % of CD patients [12]. PG or PG-like skin ulcers are also uncommon skin manifestations in BD. Four PG variants have been described: ulcerative, pustular, bullous, and vegetative. Classically, PG begins with pain followed by pustule formation, which soon breaks down to form a rapidly enlarging ulcer. Ulcers in PG have a boggy, necrotic, nonpurulent base and are rimmed by a raised inflammatory border, which is commonly characterized by an undermined border (Fig. 11.6). Ulcerative PG most commonly occurs on the lower extremities although it can occur on any part of the body. Histologically, PG shares similar pathologic changes with other neutrophilic dermatoses including Sweet's syndrome. Tissue neutrophilia with undermining ulceration in the absence of microorganism or leukocytoclastic vasculitis favors PG when seen in the relevant clinical manifestations (Fig. 11.7).

Papulopustular lesions are frequent skin manifestation of IBD, especially in BD, with a reported prevalence ranging from 30 to 96 % among BD patients [13]. As they can be both follicular and nonfollicular papules/pustules, papulopustular lesions in BD are also referred to as pseudofolliculitis (Fig. 11.8). The most common localization in BD is the trunk followed by extremities.

The pathergy phenomenon is the hyperreactivity of the skin to a trauma. Although this phenomenon is not a pathognomic finding of BD, positivity of pathergy test is included in the diagnostic criteria by ISGBD (Fig. 11.9) [11].

In addition, pyodermatitis vegetans and pyostomatitis vegetans are rare, vegetating, pustular, eosinophilic, mucocutaneous dermatoses and have strong association with gastrointestinal diseases, being considered a marker of IBD (Fig. 11.10) [1].

11.2.3 Other Associated Conditions

There are numerous additional cutaneous lesions that are associated with IBD including psoriasis, hidradenitis suppurativa, thrombophlebitis, secondary amyloidosis, and erythema multiforme. Various autoimmune skin diseases such as vitiligo and epidermolysis bullosa are also associated with IBD [14, 15]. Rarely, there have been reports of cutaneous malignancies such as Bowen's disease and squamous cell carcinoma occurring in relation to CD or UC [15].

The most frequently associated disease is psoriasis (Fig. 11.11), and the prevalence reported in epidemiologic studies is 3–11 % in IBD patients compared to 1–2 % in the general population [16]. Psoriasis is reported to be slightly more prevalent in CD compared to UC [17]. There are also reports on concurrent psoriasis in BD [18].

The vitiligo incidence is higher in IBD patients compared to the normal population and is higher in UC than CD

(Fig. 11.12) Although the pathophysiological mechanism of vitiligo linkage to IBD is unclear, it has been proposed to be autoimmune or genetically linked [19, 20].

Epidermolysis bullosa acquisita is most frequently associated with CD [21]. Chronic inflammatory reactions in the intestine can cause patients to develop autoantibodies against type VII collagen in the bowel. These autoantibodies can in turn attack the skin dermoepidermal junction resulting in blisters and vesicle formation (Fig. 11.13) [22].

Despite that a definitive linkage of atopic diseases to IBD remains unestablished, UC patients are more likely to have atopic dermatitis (Fig. 11.14) compared to healthy controls [23].

Secondary amyloidosis, which is more common in CD compared to ulcerative colitis, is caused by a systemic response to chronic inflammation resulting in amyloid A-type skin amyloidosis. The high degree of inflammation in CD can possibly cause secondary amyloidosis, but this is a rare event [24]. There also have been rare reports of scrotal and penile lymphedema and purpura as cutaneous manifestations of CD [25, 26]. Alopecia areata, rosacea, leukocytoclastic vasculitis (Fig. 11.15), and lichen planus are also reported to be possibly associated with IBD (Fig. 11.16) [15, 27, 28].

Because inflammatory bowel lesions can lead to dietary malabsorption, skin lesions related to nutrient imbalances, such as acrodermatitis enteropathica, pellagra, scurvy, stomatitis, glossitis, angular cheilitis, xeroderma, eczema, and hair and nail abnormalities, can also be observed in these patients (Fig. 11.17) [2]. Furthermore, skin lesions caused by adverse drug reactions developing during IBD treatment can also occur. These include, for example, folliculitis, acne, acneiform eruption, drug eruption, urticaria, angioedema, and Stevens–Johnson syndrome. The skin and mucosal manifestations in IBD are summarized briefly in Table 11.1 [15, 26].

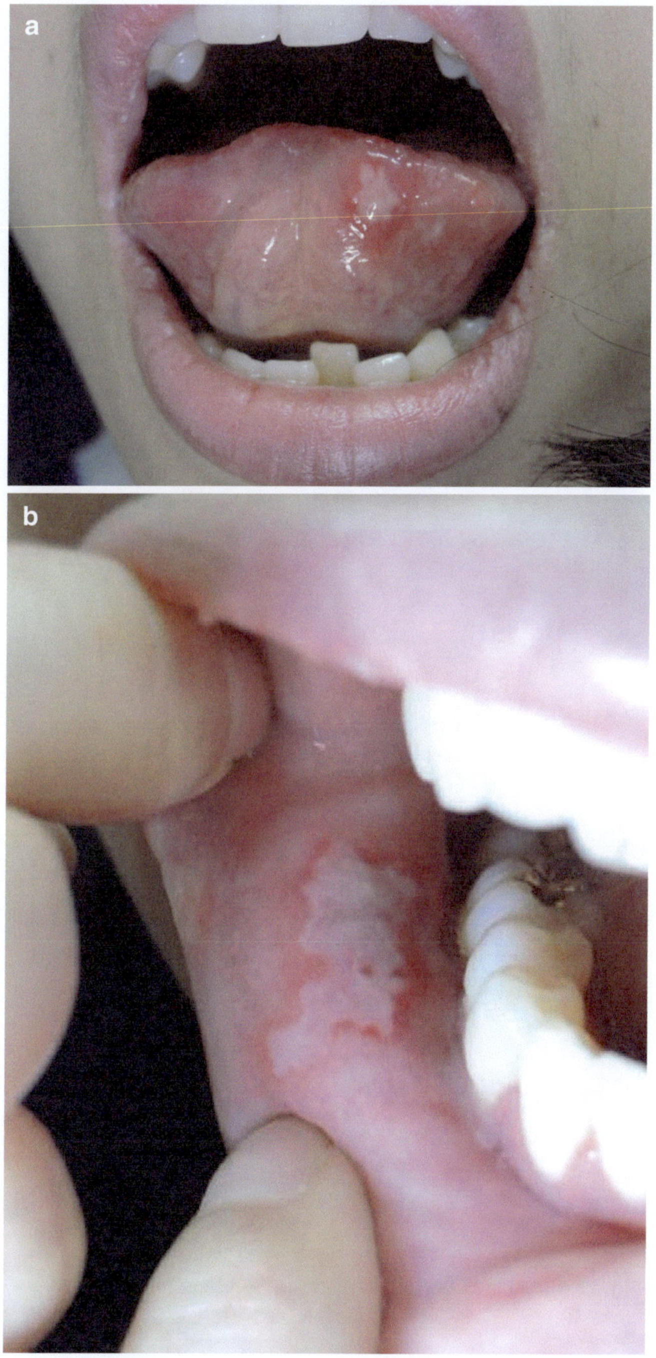

Fig. 11.1 A minor aphthous ulcer on the tongue (**a**) and a major aphthous ulcer on the lip (**b**)

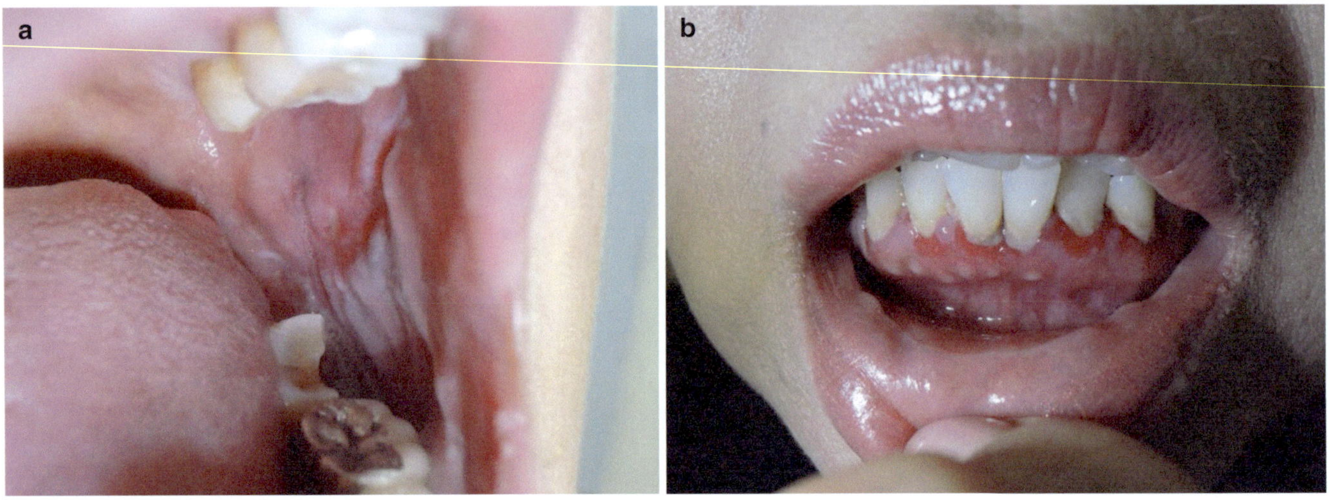

Fig. 11.2 Common mimicker of aphthous ulcer, (**a**) oral lichen planus and (**b**) pemphigus vulgaris

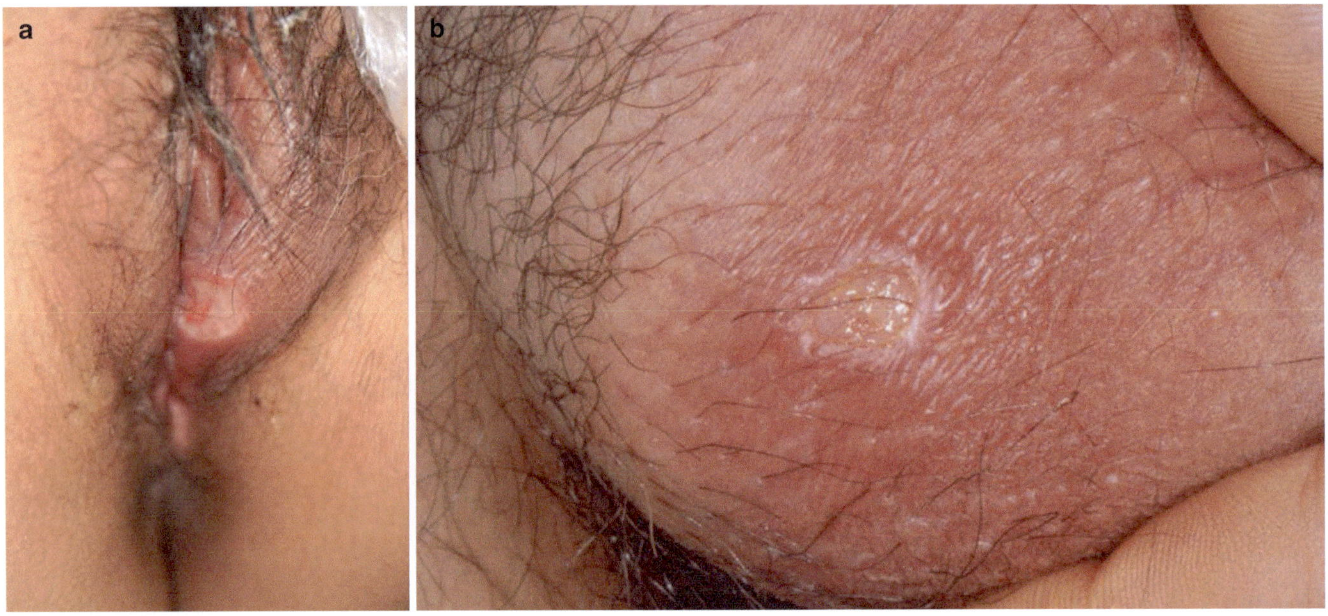

Fig. 11.3 Genital ulcers on the vulva (**a**) and scrotum (**b**)

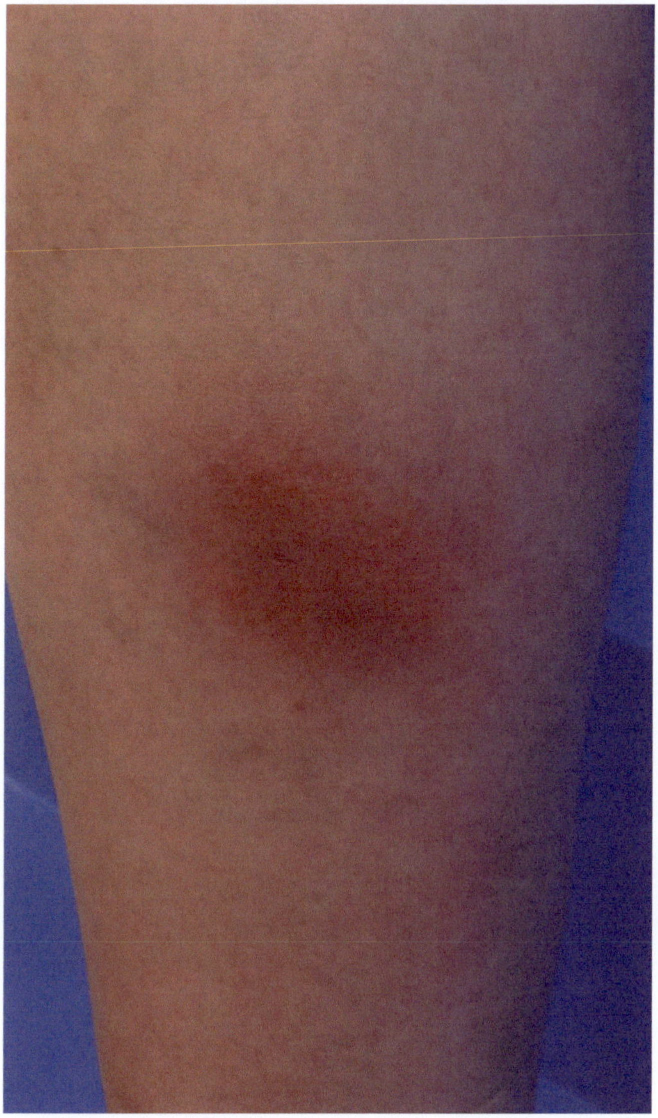

Fig. 11.4 Erythema nodosum

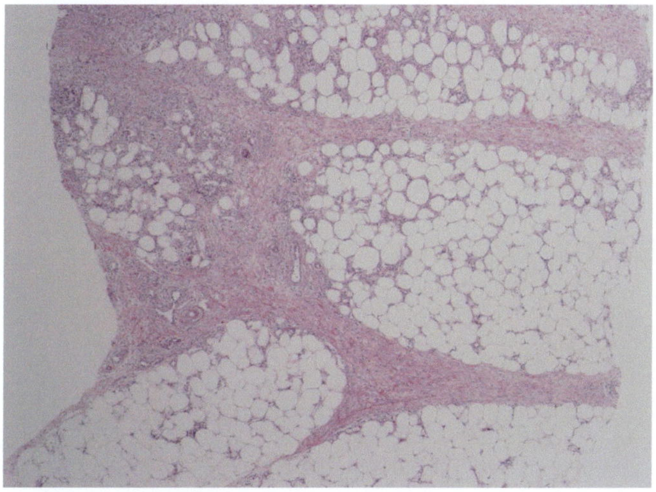

Fig. 11.5 Histopathological finding of erythema nodosum. Edema of septa with prominent lymphohistiocytic infiltrates mainly at the edge of septa and the periphery of the fat lobules, which are typical patterns of septal panniculitis

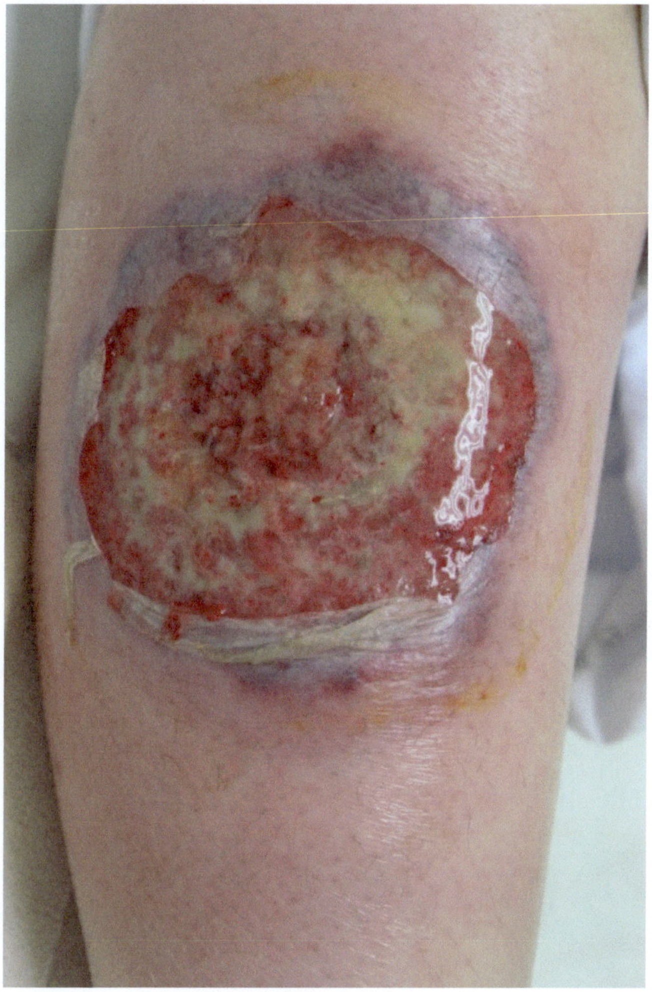

Fig. 11.6 Pyoderma gangrenosum, ulcerative variant

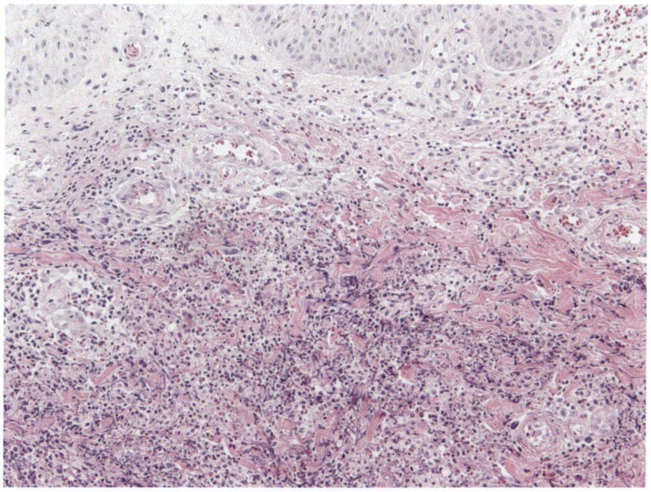

Fig. 11.7 Histopathological findings of pyoderma gangrenosum. Central necrotizing suppurative inflammation with ulceration in the absence of definite leukocytoclastic vasculitis

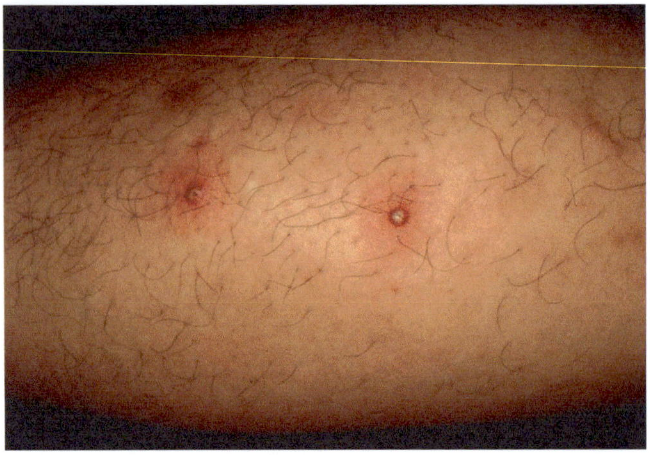

Fig. 11.8 Papulopustular lesion in Behçet's disease

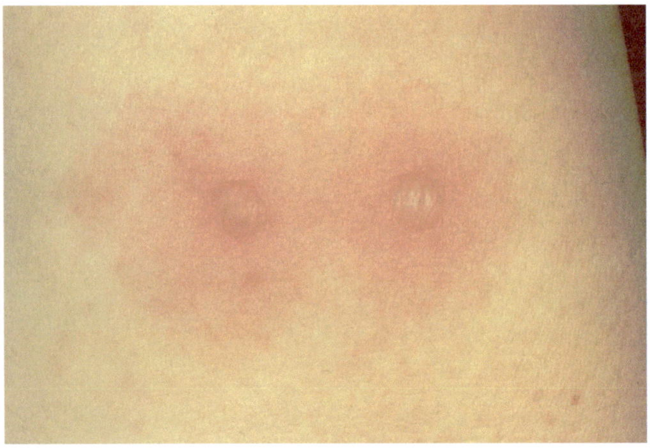

Fig. 11.9 Positive pathergy reaction on the forearm

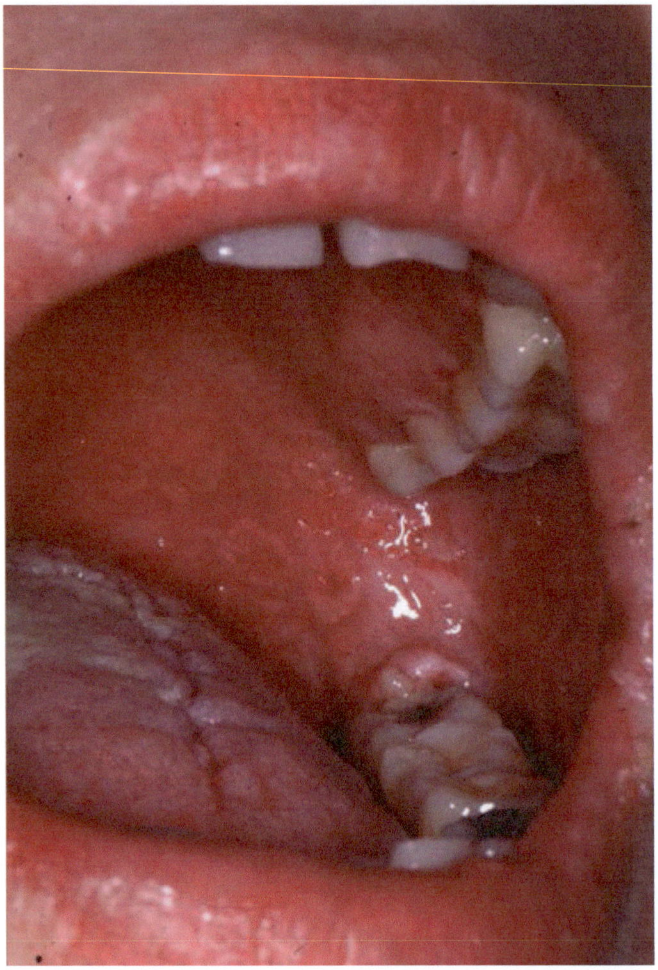

Fig. 11.10 Pyostomatitis vegetans (Courtesy of Professor Soo-Chan Kim)

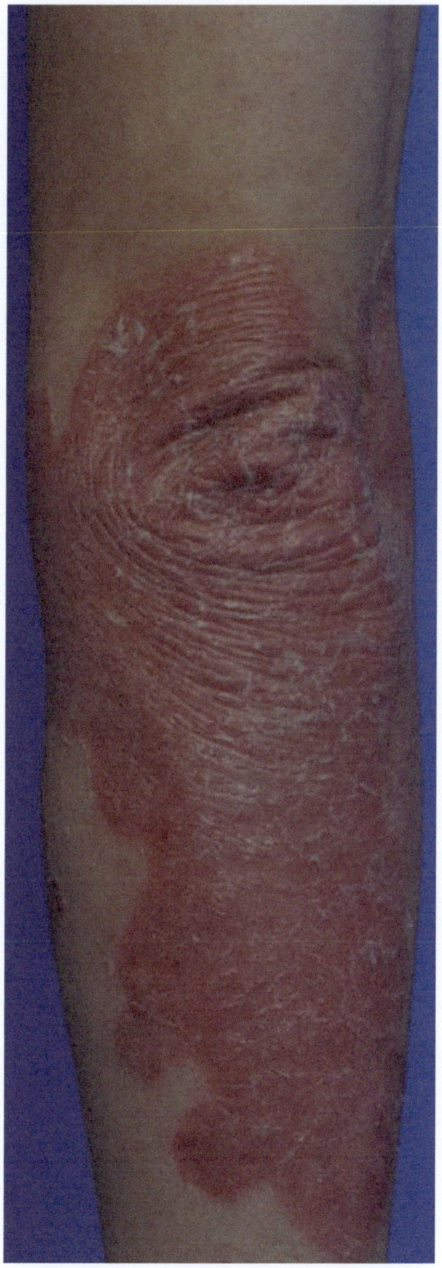

Fig. 11.11 Psoriasis

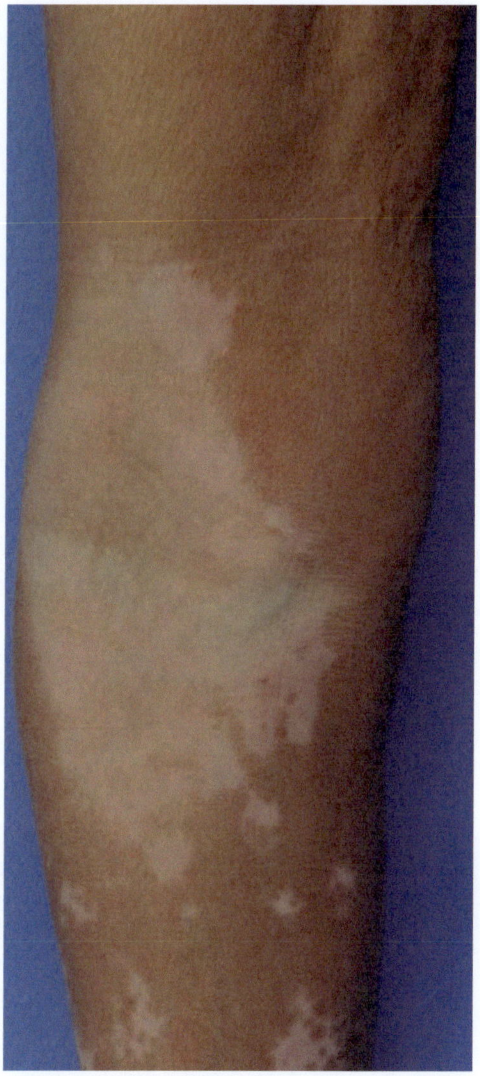

Fig. 11.12 Vitiligo

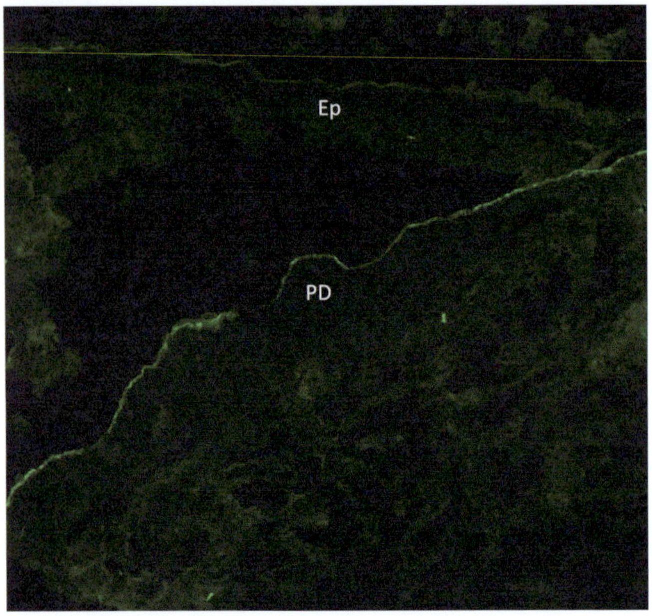

Fig. 11.13 Direct immunofluorescence staining for antihuman IgG in perilesional skin from patient with epidermolysis bullosa acquisita. Note the linear deposits of IgG along the dermal side of basement membrane zone (*Ep* epidermis, *PD* papillary dermis) (Courtesy of Professor Soo-Chan Kim)

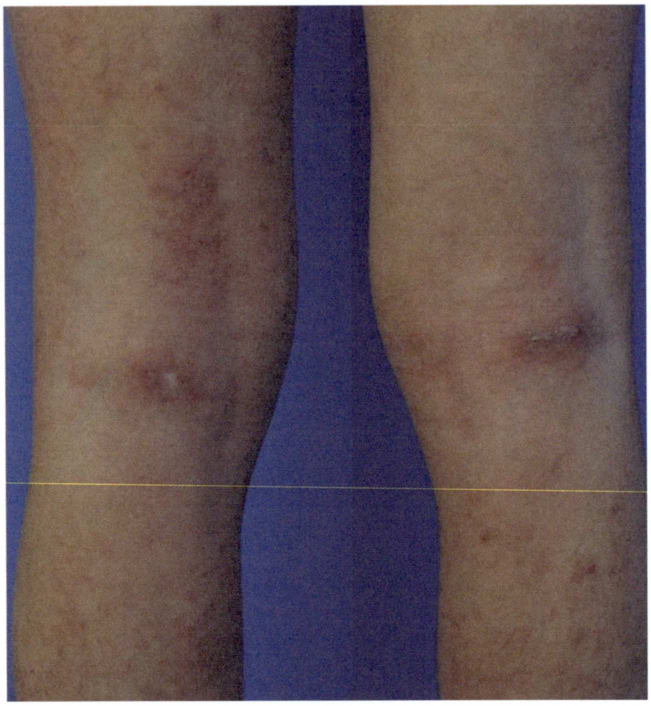

Fig. 11.14 Atopic dermatitis

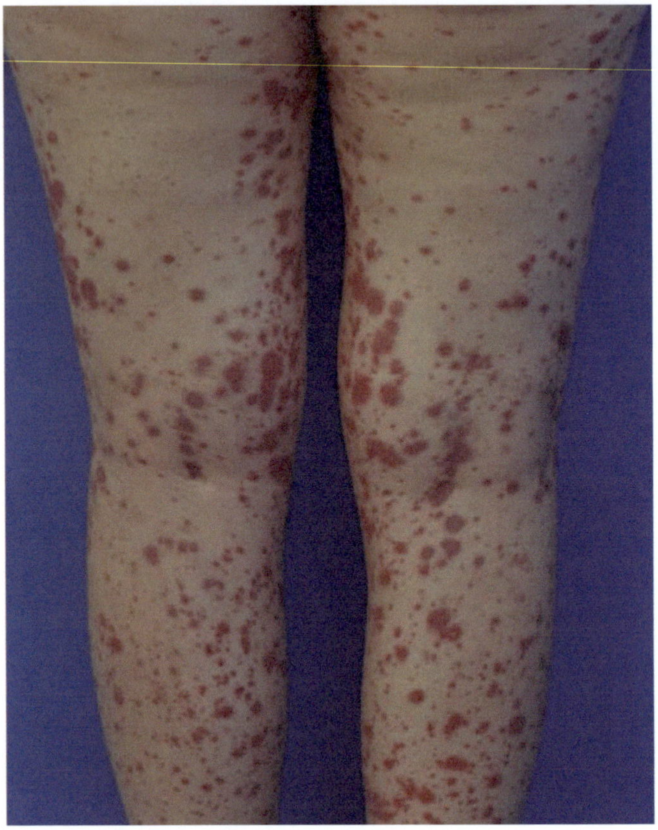

Fig. 11.15 Leukocytoclastic vasculitis

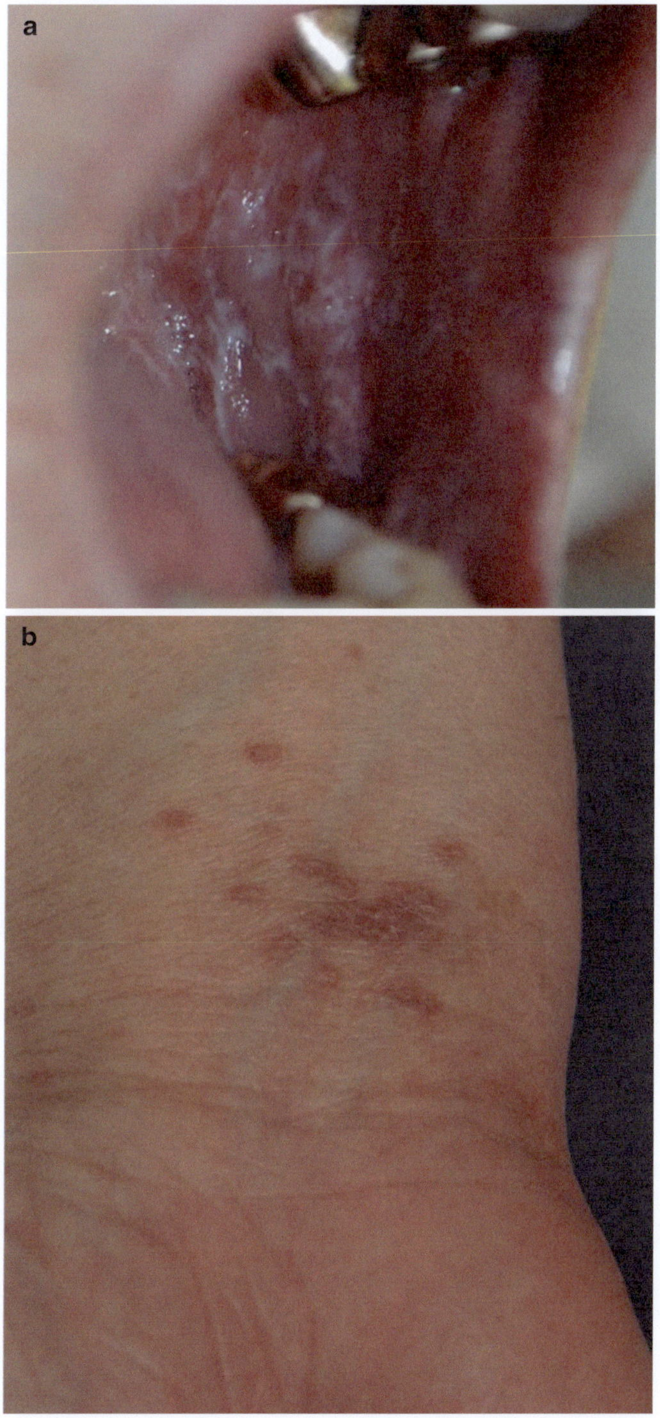

Fig. 11.16 Lichen planus on the oral mucosa (**a**) and skin (**b**)

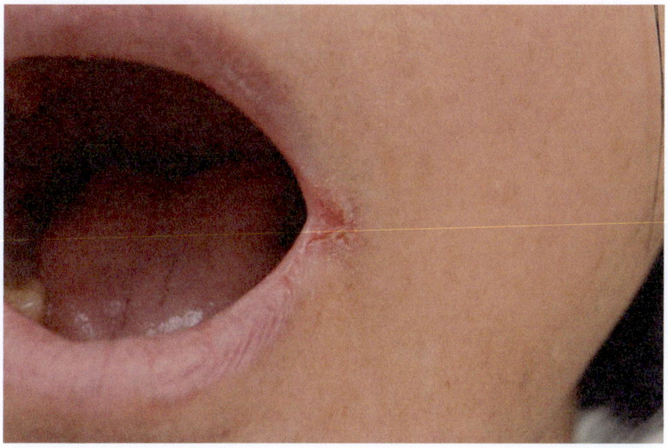

Fig. 11.17 Angular cheilitis induced by IBD-induced malabsorption

Table 11.1 Skin and mucosal manifestations in IBD

Mucocutaneous manifestations	Presentation
Specific mucocutaneous lesions	
Fissures and fistulas (perianal)	Fissures: mostly painless, located posteriorly Fistulas: It appears internally or enterocutaneously and can destroy the anal sphincter
Direct or metastatic involvements	Subcutaneous nodules or nonhealing ulcers
Reactive mucocutaneous lesions	
Oral aphthous ulcers	Painful, shallow, round to oval ulcers covered with whitish to yellowish pseudomembrane demarcated by a red hyperemic border
Genital ulcers	Painful, round to oval lesions that are usually covered with dried crust or grayish-white exudates
Erythema nodosum	Sudden onset of erythematous, non-ulcerating, tender nodules frequently located on the lower extremities
Pyoderma gangrenosum	Begins with pain followed by pustule formation, soon breaking down to form a rapidly enlarging ulcer
Papulopustular lesions	Follicular and nonfollicular papules and pustules
Sweet's syndrome	Tender nodules and papules with peripheral neutrophilia and fever
Pathergy phenomenon	Cutaneous hyperreactivity to trauma
Pyodermatitis vegetans	Vegetative papules on skin folds such as axillary or inguinal lesions
Pyostomatitis vegetans	Hyperplastic folds of the oral mucosa which progress into shallow ulcers
Other associated conditions	
Psoriasis	Scaly patches and plaques which can be associated with arthritis, nail changes
Vitiligo	Hypopigmented patches on the skin
Epidermolysis bullosa acquisita	Mucocutaneous subepidermal blisters
Atopic dermatitis	Pruritic patches with lichenification
Secondary amyloidosis	Pruritic macules, papules, patches due to amyloid deposition of the skin
Leukocytoclastic vasculitis	Ranges from palpable purpura to necrotic ulcers
Lichen planus	Mucosal lesions: lacelike whitish reticulated patches Cutaneous lesions: faintly erythematous to violaceous, polygonal papules

11.3 Eye Manifestations

The prevalence of ocular inflammation in IBD patients varies widely from 4 to 30 % [29, 30]. Ocular manifestations in IBD can be categorized according to two variables, chronicity (acute versus chronic) and location (anterior versus posterior chamber). Ocular involvement in IBD can be primary (such as uveitis, scleritis, and episcleritis) or secondary (such as iatrogenic cataracts or glaucoma from corticosteroid use or keratoconjunctivitis sicca related to 5-aminosalicylic acid medications) [29]. In a large cohort study, 32 % of IBD patients reported at least one ocular symptom [31]. Importantly, ocular involvement is one of the cardinal symptoms of Behçet's disease and is the main cause of disease-related poor prognosis causing blindness. Overall frequency of ocular lesions in BD patients varies from 50 to 70 % [7].

Most of the ocular findings in IBD involve the anterior segment and ocular surface, and conjunctivitis, episcleritis, scleritis, and uveitis are by far the most common ophthalmic complications of IBD [29]. The related symptoms are often nonspecific: tearing, burning, itching, ocular pain, photophobia, and conjunctival and scleral hyperemia. Uveitis is one of the most frequent primary ophthalmologic manifestations in IBD patients as well as the most common ocular feature in BD (Fig. 11.18a) [32]. Uveitis may include adhesion of the iris to the lens (posterior synechiae, Fig. 11.18b). Interestingly, women are at a higher risk of developing uveitis in CD and UC, whereas uveitis in BD is more frequently observed and severe in male patients [7, 29].

Episcleritis is often a common manifestation of IBD and is characterized by the injection of superficial episcleral vessels. Episcleritis may be nodular or diffuse. In scleritis, which is a less-frequent manifestation of IBD, the deep scleral vessels are dilated and injected (Fig. 11.19).

Posterior segment involvements, including posterior uveitis, retinal vasculitis, choroiditis, retinal vascular occlusion, and optic neuropathy, also may occur and lead to significant visual deterioration. Figure 11.20 shows an IBD patient with associated optic neuropathy and retinal microvascular occlusion. Panuveitis is more serious in terms of visual prognosis and occurs more frequently in BD patients than in healthy controls [33]. In conclusion, regular fundus examination of the posterior segment is important to prevent blindness in IBD patients, especially in those with BD. The ocular manifestations in IBD are summarized briefly in Table 11.2.

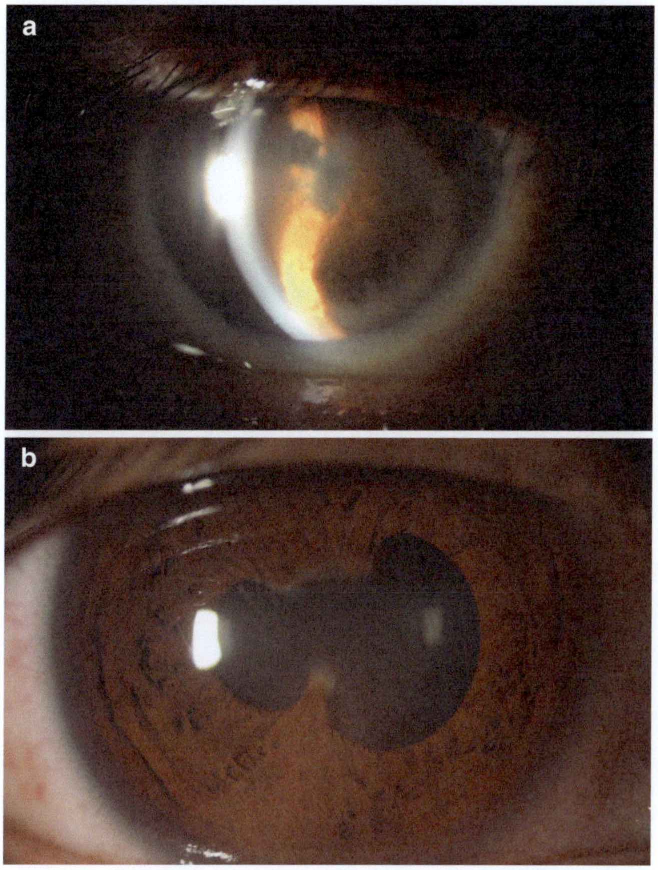

Fig. 11.18 Uveitis (**a**) with posterior synechiae (**b**) (Courtesy of Professor Sung Chul Lee)

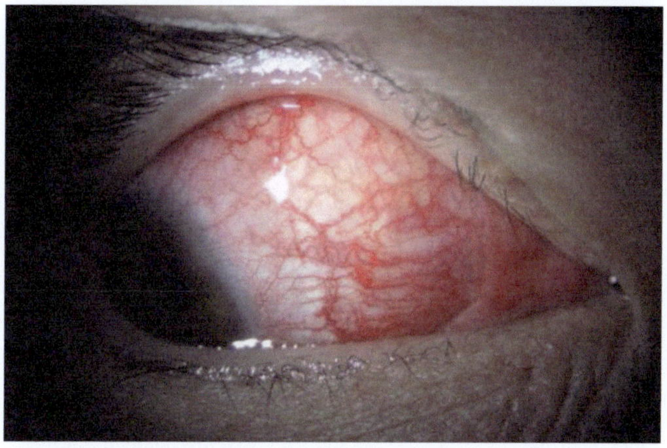

Fig. 11.19 Scleritis in a patient with Behçet's disease

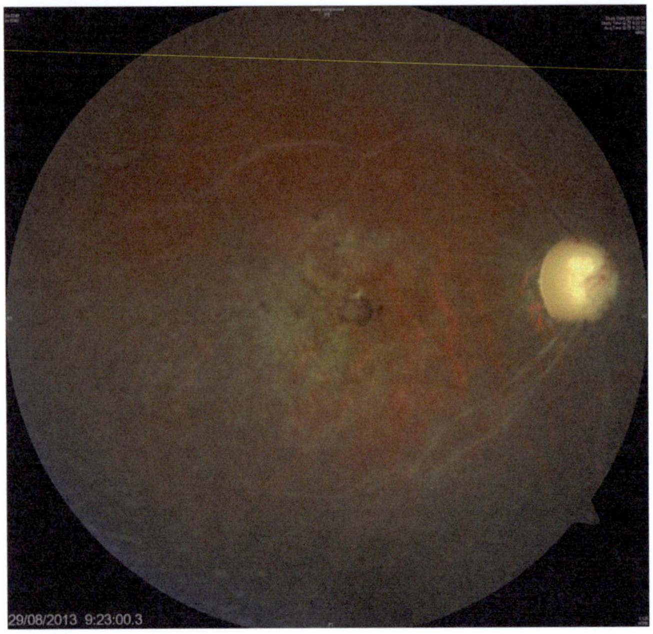

Fig. 11.20 Optic neuropathy with vessel occlusion (Courtesy of Professor Sung Chul Lee)

Table 11.2 Ocular manifestations in IBD

Eye manifestations	Presentation
Anterior segment	
Episcleritis	Injection of superficial episcleral vessels
Iridocyclitis (anterior uveitis)	Photophobia or sensitivity to light, blurred vision
Scleritis	Hyperemia, ocular pain, photophobia, tearing
Conjunctivitis	Hyperemia, chemosis, epiphora
Dry eye	Dryness, burning, irritation of the eye
Posterior segment	
Posterior uveitis	Photopsia, blurred vision, floaters
Retinal vasculitis	Painless, decrease of visual acuity, floaters, scotomas, and metamorphopsia
Optic neuritis	Sudden visual loss, sudden blurred vision, pain on movement of the affected eye
Retinal vascular occlusion	Sudden blurring or loss of vision

11.4 Joint Manifestations

Joint symptoms are common extraintestinal manifestations of IBD and occur in approximately 20–30 % of patients [34, 35]. Arthritis is more common in CD than in UC. The frequency of joint involvement in BD patients varies greatly from 9 to 70 %, depending on the study [7, 33].

Joint involvement can be classified as either peripheral or axial arthropathy. Peripheral arthritis and/or inflammatory axial involvement in IBD patients, with consistent absence of serum rheumatoid factor, is classified as a spondyloarthritis (SpA) according to the classification criteria of the European Spondyloarthropathy Study Group (ESSG) [36]. Peripheral arthritis can be divided into two groups: oligoarticular large joint arthritis and bilateral symmetrical polyarthritis [37]. Type 1 (pauci-/oligoarticular) peripheral arthritis is characterized by joint pain with evidence of swelling or effusion that affects fewer than five joints and mainly affects the large weight-bearing joints of the lower limbs such as the knee and ankle (Fig. 11.21). Type 2 (polyarticular) peripheral arthritis affects more than five joints, with a symmetrical distribution, and affects predominantly the small joints of the upper limbs including the fingers (Fig. 11.22). Although less frequently identified, enthesitis is also common in IBD. Peripheral enthesitis refers to inflammation of the site where a tendon or ligament inserts into the bone. An example of enthesitis at the Achilles tendon/calcaneus bone insertion site is shown in Fig. 11.23.

Axial arthropathies associated with IBD include isolated sacroiliitis, inflammatory back pain, and ankylosing spondylitis. The reported prevalence of sacroiliitis in IBD patients varies widely from 2 to 32 % [38]. According to the Calin criteria, inflammatory back pain is due to inflammation of the sacroiliac joints and is characterized by an insidious onset, improvement after exercise but not with rest, and is associated with morning stiffness [39]. Ankylosing spondylitis, the most typical representation of SpA, is a chronic inflammatory disease of the axial skeleton, with prevalence in IBD patients varying from 1 to 10 % [38]. However, nonspecific arthralgia, without objective arthritis signs such as swelling or effusion, is also common in IBD patients. The joint manifestations in IBD are summarized briefly in Table 11.3.

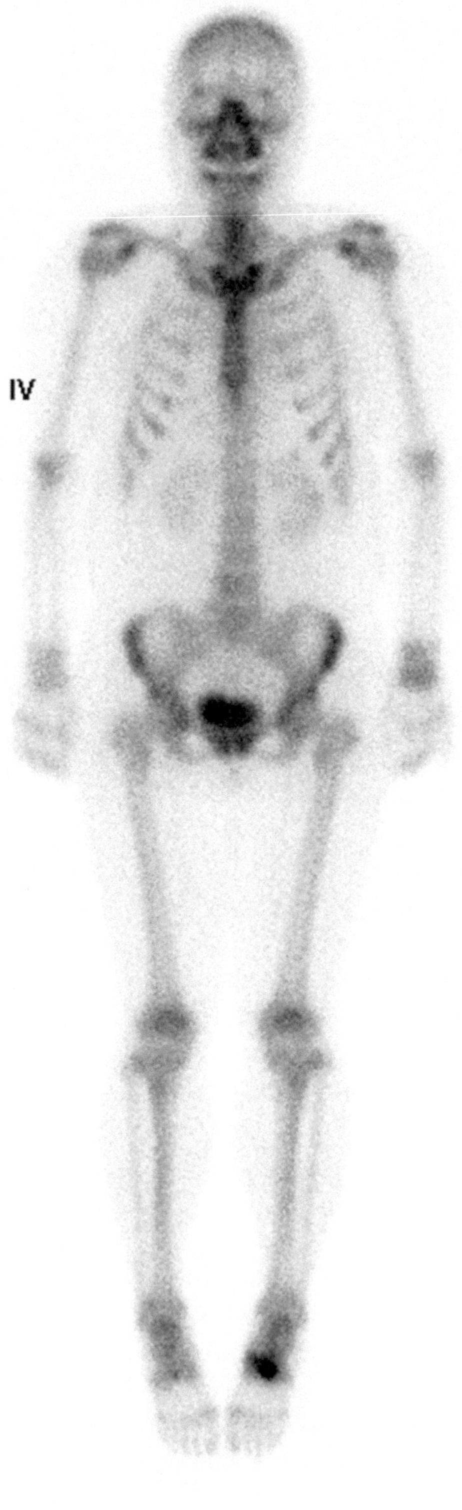

Fig. 11.21 Whole-body bone scan findings: arthritic changes in the left ankle and left wrist

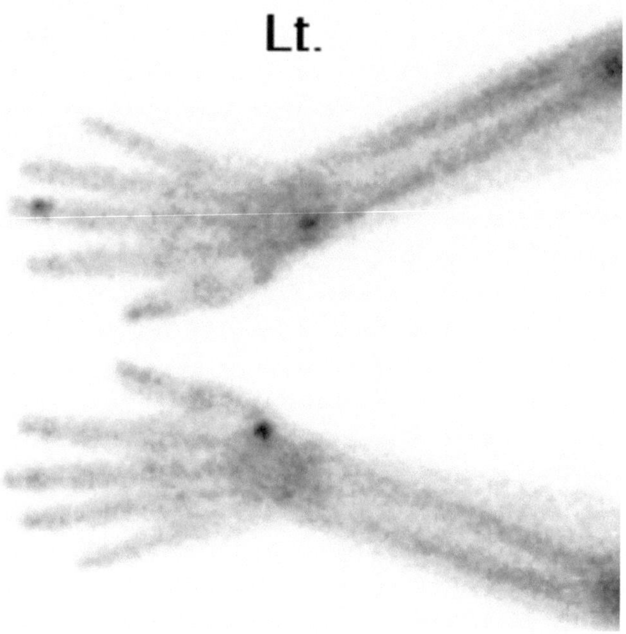

Fig. 11.22 Whole-body bone scan findings: arthritic changes in bilateral carpal bones and the left third distal interphalangeal joint

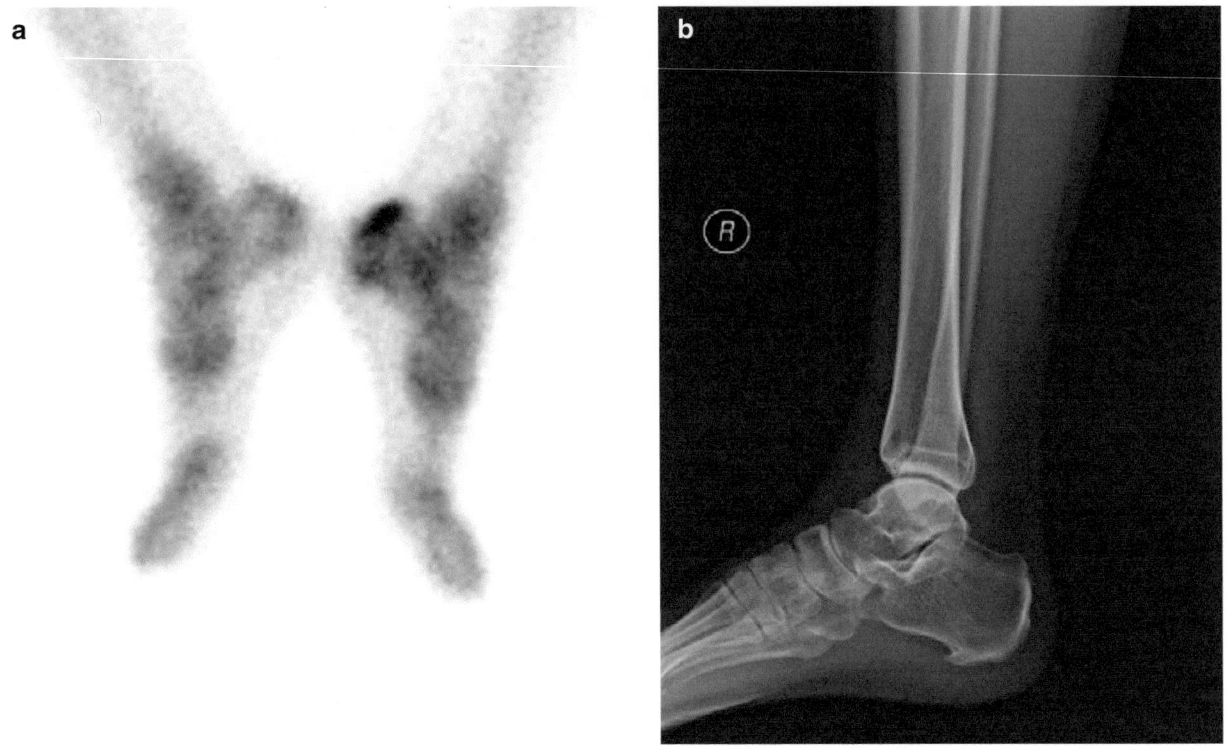

Fig. 11.23 Whole-body bone scan finding: (**a**) increased radioisotope uptake in the right calcaneal tuberosity, which is compatible with Achilles tendinitis. (**b**) Also note there is no abnormal finding on bony structures in the same heel on a plain radiograph

Table 11.3 Joint manifestations in IBD

Joint manifestations	Presentation
Peripheral arthropathy	
Type 1 peripheral arthritis (pauci-/oligoarticular)	Joint pain with evidence of swelling or effusion affecting <5 joints, mainly affects the large weight-bearing joints of the lower limbs
Type 2 peripheral arthritis (polyarticular)	Affects ≥5 joints with a symmetrical distribution, predominantly the small joints of the upper limbs
Axial arthropathy	
Sacroiliitis	Lower back pain often radiating to the buttock, groin, front of the thigh
Inflammatory back pain	Insidious onset of pain, with improvement after exercise but not with rest, associated with morning stiffness
Ankylosing spondylitis	Gradual development of back pain and stiffness

References

1. Thrash B, et al. Cutaneous manifestations of gastrointestinal disease. Part II. J Am Acad Dermatol. 2013;68(211):e1–33.
2. Gregory B, Ho VC. Cutaneous manifestations of gastrointestinal disease. Part I. J Am Acad Dermatol. 1992;26:153–66.
3. Yüksel İ, et al. Mucocutaneous manifestations in inflammatory bowel disease. Inflamm Bowel Dis. 2009;15:546–50.
4. Farhi D, et al. Significance of erythema nodosum and pyoderma gangrenosum in inflammatory bowel diseases. A cohort study of 2402 patients. Medicine. 2008;87:281–93.
5. Pozdnyakova O, et al. Nodular vasculitis – a novel cutaneous manifestation of autoimmune colitis. J Cutan Pathol. 2008;35:315–9.
6. Cheon JH, et al. Behçet's disease: gastrointestinal involvement. In: Yazici H, editor. Behçet's syndrome. 1st ed. New York: Springer; 2010.
7. Lee S, et al. Behçet's disease; a guide to its clinical understanding. Heidelberg: Springer; 2001.
8. Rankin GB, et al. National Cooperative Crohn's Disease Study: extraintestinal manifestations and perianal complications. Gastroenterology. 1979;77:914–20.
9. Lashner B. Inflammatory bowel disease. In: Carey WD, editor. Cleveland clinic: current clinical medicine. Philadelphia: Saunders; 2009.
10. Lourenço SV, et al. Oral manifestations of inflammatory bowel disease: a review based on the observation of six cases. J Eur Acad Dermatol Venereol. 2010;24:204–7.
11. International Study Group for Behçet's Disease. Criteria for diagnosis of Behçet's disease. Lancet. 1990;335:1078–80.
12. Lebwohl M, Lebwohl O. Cutaneous manifestations of inflammatory bowel disease. Inflamm Bowel Dis. 1998;4:142–8.
13. Mat C, et al. The mucocutaneous manifestations and pathergy reaction in Behçet's disease. In: Yazici Y, editor. Behçet's syndrome. 1st ed. New York: Springer; 2010.
14. Levine JS, Burakoff R. Extraintestinal manifestations of inflammatory bowel disease. Gastroenterol Hepatol. 2011;7(4):235–41.
15. Huang BL, et al. Skin manifestations of inflammatory bowel disease. Front Physiol. 2012;3:13.
16. Danese S, et al. Extraintestinal manifestations in inflammatory bowel disease. World J Gastroenterol. 2005;11(46):7227–36.
17. Yates VM, et al. Further evidence for an association between psoriasis, Crohn's disease and ulcerative colitis. Br J Dermatol. 1982;106(3):323–30.
18. Cho S, et al. Behcet's disease in concurrence with psoriasis. J Eur Acad Dermatol Venereol. 2013;27(1):e113–8.
19. Pashankar D, et al. Vitiligo and Crohn's disease in children. J Pediatr Gastroenterol Nutr. 1999;28(2):227–9.
20. Quan C, et al. Genome-wide association study for vitiligo identifies susceptibility loci at 6q27 and the MHC. Nat Genet. 2010;42(7):614–8.
21. Hoffmann RM, Kruis W. Rare extraintestinal manifestations of inflammatory bowel disease. Inflamm Bowel Dis. 2004;10(2):140–7.
22. Hundorfean G, et al. Autoimmunity against type VII collagen in inflammatory bowel disease. J Cell Mol Med. 2010;14(10):2393–403.
23. Boneberger A, et al. Atopic manifestations in patients with ulcerative colitis: a report from Chile. J Investig Allergol Clin Immunol. 2012;22(1):73–5.
24. Sattianayagam PT, et al. Systemic amyloidosis and the gastrointestinal tract. Nature reviews. Gastroenterol Hepatol. 2009;6(10):608–17.
25. Reitsma W, et al. Penile and scrotal lymphedema as an unusual presentation of Crohn's disease: case report and review of the literature. Lymphology. 2012;45(1):37–41.
26. Dudley AG, et al. Penoscrotal edema and purpura in a 12-year-old boy: a case report and review of causes. J Pediatr Urol. 2012;8(5):e47–50.
27. Mebazaa A, et al. Dermatologic manifestations in inflammatory bowel disease in Tunisia. Tunis Med. 2012;90(3):252–7.
28. Plaza Santos R, et al. Leukocytoclastic vasculitis associated with Crohn's disease. Gastroenterol Hepatol. 2010;33(6):433–5.
29. Calvo P, Pablo L. Managing IBD outside the gut: ocular manifestations. Dig Dis. 2013;31:229–32.
30. Felekis T, et al. Spectrum and frequency of ophthalmologic manifestations in patients with inflammatory bowel disease: a prospective single-center study. Inflamm Bowel Dis. 2009;15:29–34.
31. Kitaichi N, et al. Ocular features of Behçet's disease: an international collaborative study. Br J Ophthalmol. 2007;91:1579–82.
32. Kand SJ, Kim HB. Behçet's disease in Korea. J Korean Ophthalmol Soc. 1992;33:332–41.
33. Ozyazgan Y, Bodaghi B. Eye disease in Behçet's syndrome. In: Yazici Y, editor. Behçet's syndrome. 1st ed. New York: Springer; 2010.
34. Vavricka SR, et al. Frequency and risk factors for extraintestinal manifestations in the Swiss inflammatory bowel disease cohort. Am J Gastroenterol. 2011;106:110–9.
35. Bernstein CN, et al. The prevalence of extraintestinal diseases in inflammatory bowel disease: a population- based study. Am J Gastroenterol. 2001;96:1116–22.
36. Dougados M, et al. The European Spondylarthropathy Study Group preliminary criteria for the classification of spondylarthropathy. Arthritis Rheum. 1991;34(10):1218–27.
37. Orchard TR, et al. Peripheral arthropathies in inflammatory bowel disease: their articular distribution and natural history. Gut. 1998;42(3):387–91.
38. Brakenhoff LK, et al. The joint-gut axis in inflammatory bowel diseases. J Crohn's Colitis. 2010;4(3):257–68.
39. Calin A, et al. Clinical history as a screening test for ankylosing spondylitis. JAMA. 1977;237(24):2613–4.

Complications of Inflammatory Bowel Disease

12

Heyson Chi-hey Chan, Duk Hwan Kim, Phillip Fai Ching Lung, Jae Hee Cheon, and Siew Chien Ng

12.1 Introduction

Inflammatory bowel disease is a chronic, heterogenic, and lifelong illness with a high potential of individual and social disability. A general deterioration of the quality of life in patients with inflammatory bowel disease predominantly stems from localized complications regarding the natural course of the disease. Both Crohn's disease (CD) and ulcerative colitis (UC) are associated with various kinds of complications. A direct causal relationship exists between disease duration and development of complications. However, CD is frequently related with the formation of fistulae and abscess due to its transmural nature, while UC is often accompanied by the results of severe inflammations such as toxic megacolon. Despite the abundant literature discussing the pathogenesis and treatment of those complications, early detection and intervention for complication are still challenging at present. Therefore, clinical evaluation should precisely characterize the number, location, degree, and feature of the complications. In this chapter, we will review about complications of gastrointestinal tract in patients with inflammatory bowel disease.

H.C.-h. Chan • S.C. Ng, PhD (✉)
Department of Medicine and Therapeutics,
Institute of Digestive Disease,
The Chinese University of Hong Kong,
Hong Kong, The People's Republic of China
e-mail: siewchienng@cuhk.edu.hk

D.H. Kim
Digestive Disease Center, CHA Bundang Medical center,
CHA University College of Medicine,
Seongnam, South Korea

P.F.C. Lung
Department of Imaging and Interventional Radiology,
The Chinese University of Hong Kong,
Hong Kong, The People's Republic of China

J.H. Cheon, MD, PhD (✉)
Department of Internal Medicine, Institute of Gastroenterology,
Yonsei University College of Medicine,
50 Yonsei-ro, Seodaemun–gu, Seoul 120-752, South Korea
e-mail: geniushee@yuhs.ac

12.2 Fistulae

Fistula is a major complication of CD which is associated with high morbidity and mortality due to sepsis, malnutrition, and fluid and electrolyte imbalance. Around one-third of CD patients have fistulizing disease after 10 years from diagnosis [1]. Fistula is defined as pathologic connection between gastrointestinal tract and adjacent organs. Fistula can involve the small or large bowels (Fig. 12.1), skin (Fig. 12.2), bladder (Fig. 12.3), vagina (Figs. 12.4 and 12.5), and any other parts nearby in the severe inflammation of disease. The majority of fistula in CD is external or perianal lesion (Table 12.1).

Crohn's perianal fistulae may arise from inflamed or infected anal glands or penetration of fissures or ulcers. Examination under anesthesia (EUA) has an important role in the diagnosis and classification of perianal fistula. It allows immediate abscess drainage (Fig. 12.6) and/or seton placement. Pelvic magnetic resonance imaging (MRI) is a highly accurate noninvasive modality for the diagnosis and classification of perianal fistulae and is regarded as the gold standard (Fig. 12.7) [3]. To ensure diagnostic accuracy and optimal management, a combination of endoscopy and MRI/endoscopic ultrasound and EUA is required. Endoscopic assessment for proctitis is essential to determine the most appropriate management strategy.

Once fistula formation is developed, it rarely heals spontaneously or even despite medical therapy, and frequently requires surgical therapy. However, a meta-analysis showed the improvement of fistulae with immunomodulatory therapy such as azathioprine [4]. Antibiotics and thiopurines may contribute to symptom improvement but are limited by their slow onset of action, low remission rates, and high recurrence rates. Infliximab and adalimumab are effective for induction and maintenance of fistula closure (36–58 %). Moreover, antitumor necrosis factor α (TNF-α) and thiopurine combination therapy may lead to a higher fistula closure rate compared to monotherapy. However, a diverting temporary stoma remains an option for patients with severe, complicated therapy-refractory fistulizing disease [5].

W.H. Kim, J.H. Cheon (eds.), *Atlas of Inflammatory Bowel Diseases*,
DOI 10.1007/978-3-642-39423-2_12, © Springer-Verlag Berlin Heidelberg 2015

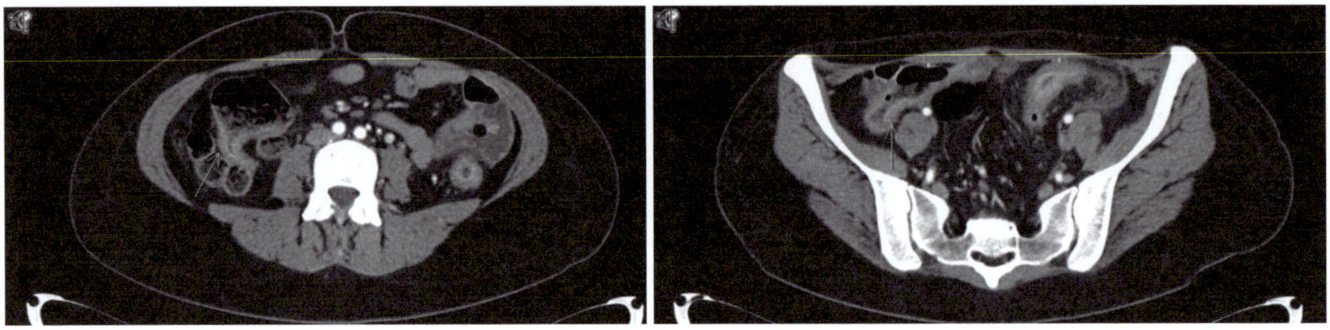

Fig. 12.1 Enterocolic fistula (*arrows*) in Crohn's disease

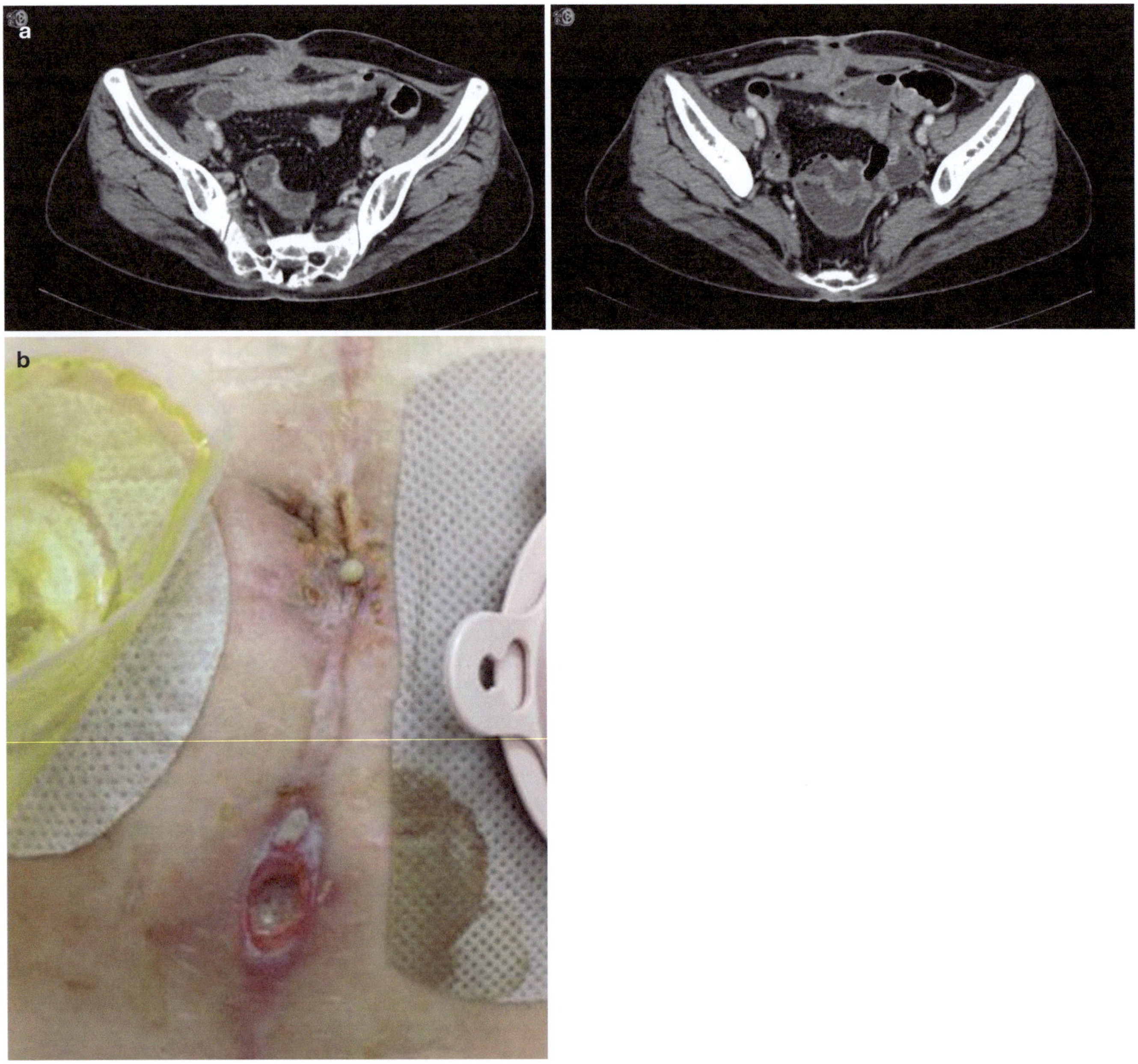

Fig. 12.2 Enterocutaneous fistula in Crohn's disease. (**a**) CT findings, (**b**) a skin photo

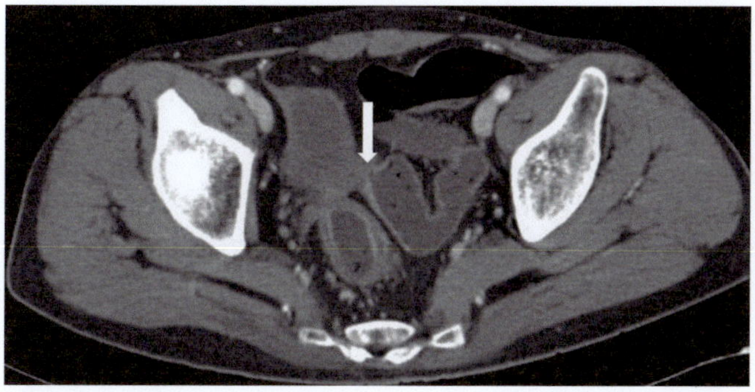

Fig. 12.3 Enterovesical fistula in Crohn's disease (*arrow*)

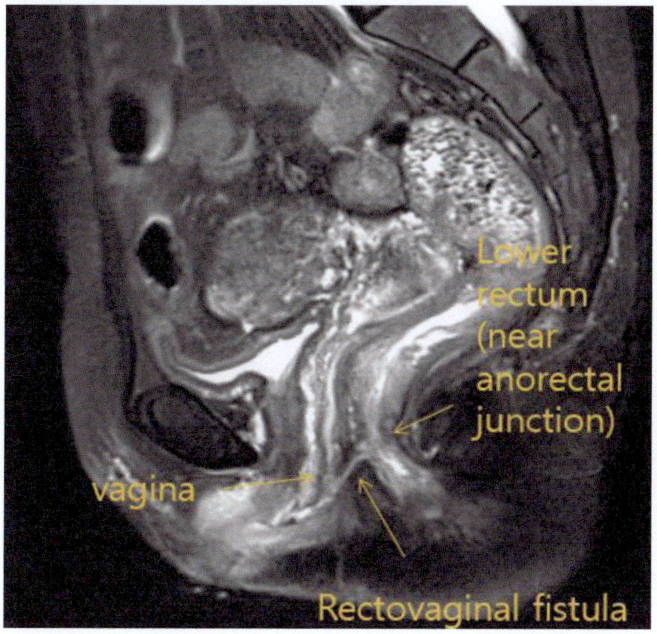

Fig. 12.4 Rectovaginal fistula

Table 12.1 Types of fistulae in patients with Crohn's disease (Modified from Table 3 of [2])

Type	Incidence (%)
External(skin)/perianal	66
Internal	34
Ileosigmoid	25
Other ileocolic	23
Ileovesical	20
Ileum/rectum to female genital tract	12
Ileoileal	11
Coloenteric	9

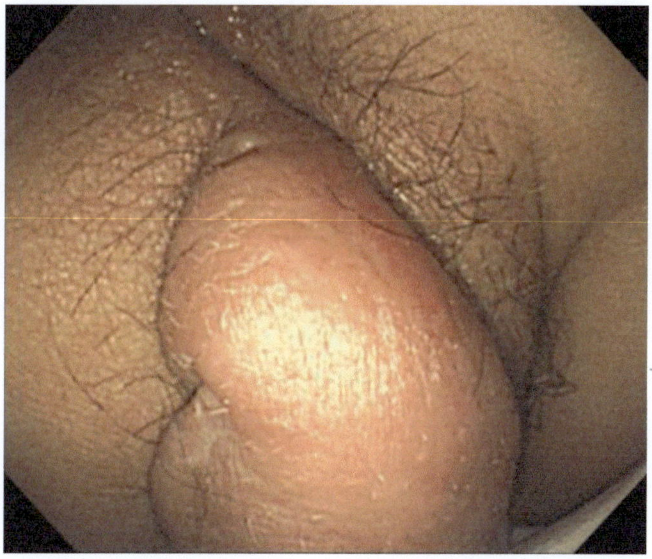

Fig. 12.5 Vulva edema due to rectovaginal fistula in Crohn's disease

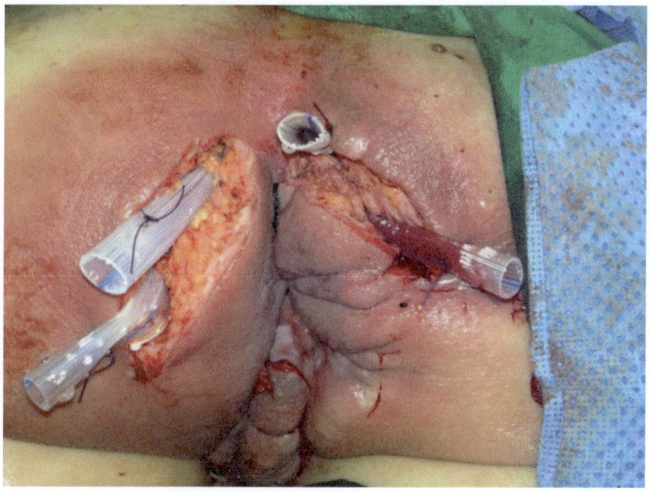

Fig. 12.6 Fistulotomy with drainage. Draining abscess and performing fistulotomy can relieve perianal fistula with abscess

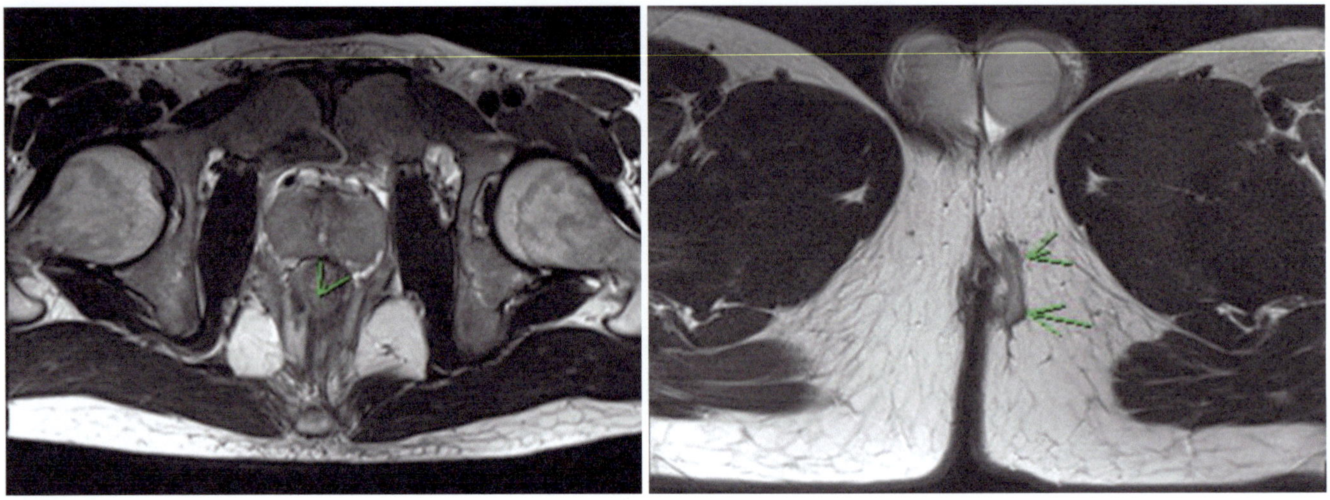

Fig. 12.7 MRI findings of perianal fistula (*arrows*)

12.3 Nonfistulizing Perianal Lesions

While various types of perianal lesions can occur in patients with CD (Table 12.2), one of the important perianal complications is anal ulceration (Fig. 12.8). Classically, anal ulcer of CD is considered as painless lesion; however, pain had been reported up to 70 % in a referral center-based study [6]. Other symptoms such as discharge, pruritus, and bleeding also can be developed. Anal ulcer in CD usually shows irregular, undermined, and detached shape with edematous border [7]. Multiple lesions can be observed, but the extension to the outside of anal canal is rare. Little is known about the long-term outcomes of anal ulceration in patients with CD; however, most of them heal spontaneously during treatment. Rarely, when the ulcer develops cavitation, it can lead to formation of abscess, stricture, or fistula with poor prognosis.

Another major anal complication is anal skin tag (Fig. 12.9). Pathogenesis of anal skin tag is explained by lymphedema secondary to lymphatic obstruction [9]. The AGA Institute classified skin tags as two types. One is large, edematous, hard, cyanotic skin tags which typically arise from a healed anal fissure or ulcer. And the other is "elephant ear" tags that are flat and broad or narrow, soft painless skin tags [10]. A report revealed that anal skin tags were found more frequently in patients with CD (75.4 %) as compared to patients with UC (24.6 %); therefore, confirming anal skin tags can aid to distinguish CD from indeterminate colitis [11]. Skin tags are usually benign; however, they can be enlarged in case with inflammatory flare-up of underlying disease. Surgical removal of anal skin tag is generally not recommended, but "elephant ear" skin tag can be treated by local excision.

Table 12.2 Types of perianal lesions in 202 consecutive patients in a Crohn's disease follow-up clinic [8]

Type of lesion	Number of patients (%)
Skin tag	75 (37)
Fissure	38 (19)
Low fistula	40 (20)
High fistula	12 (6)
Rectovaginal fistula	6 (3)
Perianal abscess	32 (16)
Ischiorectal abscess	8 (4)
Intersphincteric abscess	7 (3)
Supralevator abscess	6 (3)
Anorectal stricture	19 (9)
Hemorrhoids	15 (7)
Anal ulcer	12 (6)
Total patients with perianal lesions	110 (54)

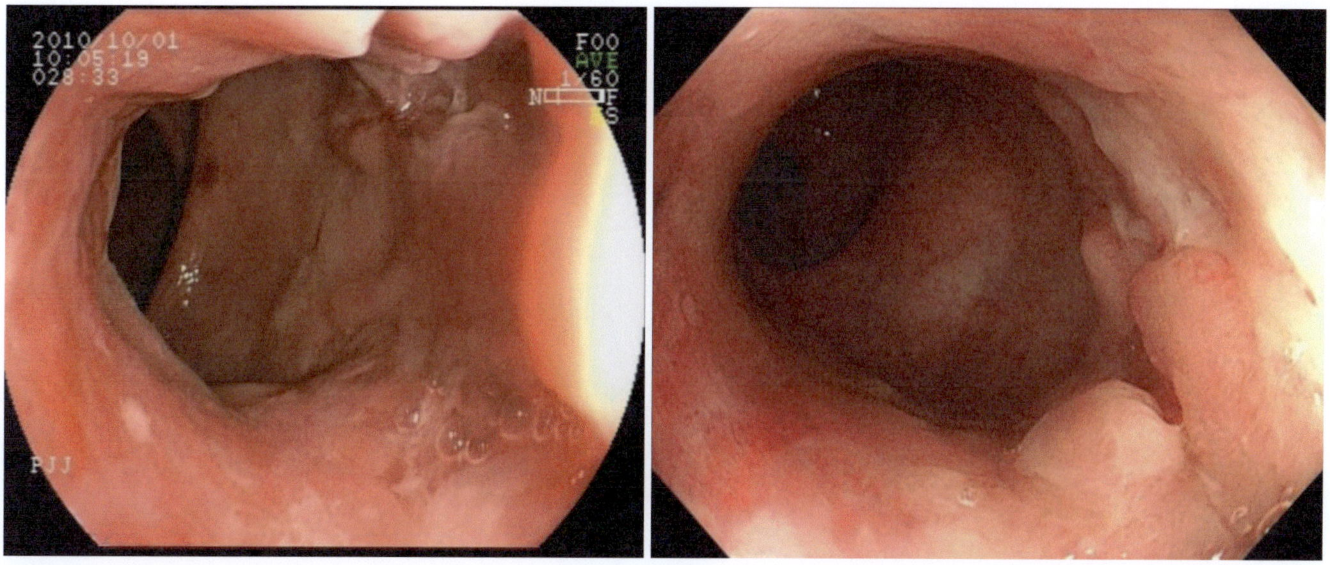

Fig. 12.8 Anal ulcers

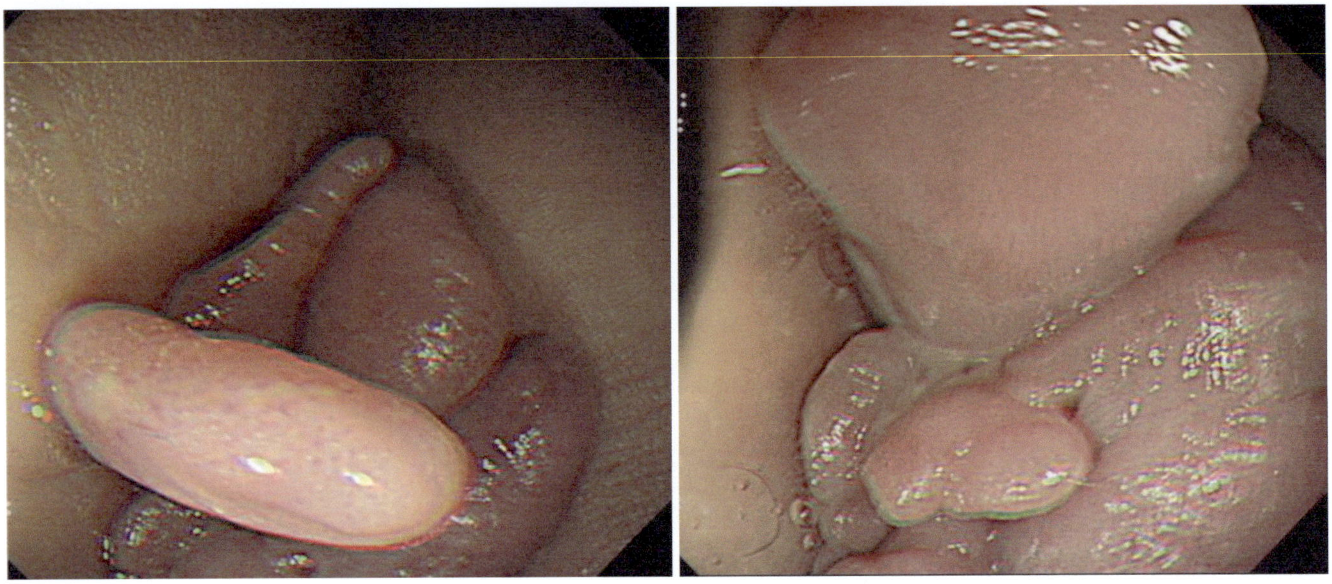

Fig. 12.9 Anal skin tags in a patient with Crohn's disease. A lobulated lump of excess skin growth near anus is seen

12.4 Abscess

Abscess formation is one of the most serious complications in patients with inflammatory bowel disease. About 7–28 % of CD patients experience this complication during lifetime [12]. Abscess in CD can be developed on any location of abdomen including peritoneal cavity, retroperitoneum, perirectum, subphrenic area, intramural space, muscle, or abdominal wall (Figs. 12.10, 12.11, and 12.12).

Abdominal abscess which is related to CD has been conventionally treated by surgical intervention, especially when the abscess is combined with other complications such as fistula or stricture [13]. Recently, however, nonsurgical treatment such as percutaneous drainage (Fig. 12.13) can be applied in accessible cases. One study revealed that the overall treatment rates and recurrence rates were not statistically different between surgical and medical treatment groups. Moreover, median hospitalization duration was significantly shorter in the medical group than in the surgical group [14].

When extramural complications are suspected, different imaging techniques of the gastrointestinal tract may be utilized to aid in the diagnosis, depending on the clinical situation. In patients presenting with an acute abdomen, contrast CT is readily available, whereas in pediatric patients, nonradiation techniques, such as ultrasound or MRI, may be more appropriate. MRI has the advantage in better tissue contrast and no radiation exposure, but may not be readily available. In addition to identifying and treating underlying sepsis using antibiotics, correcting fluid and electrolyte imbalance and assessing nutritional status with appropriate supplement (either enteral or parental nutrition) are important parts of immediate management of abdominal abscess.

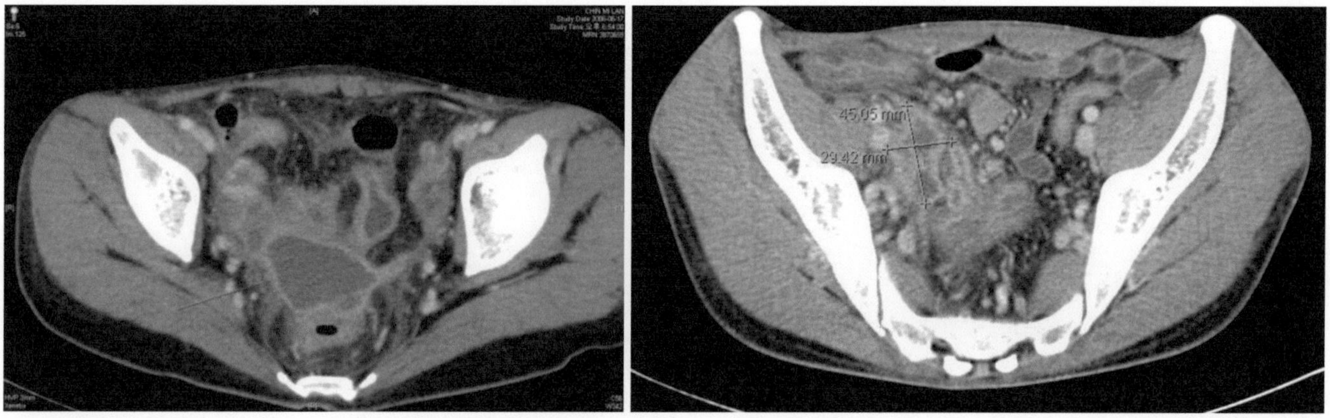

Fig. 12.10 Intra-abdominal abscess. Circumscribed round or oval water-density mass with peripheral contrast enhancement is seen in pelvic cavity (*arrow*)

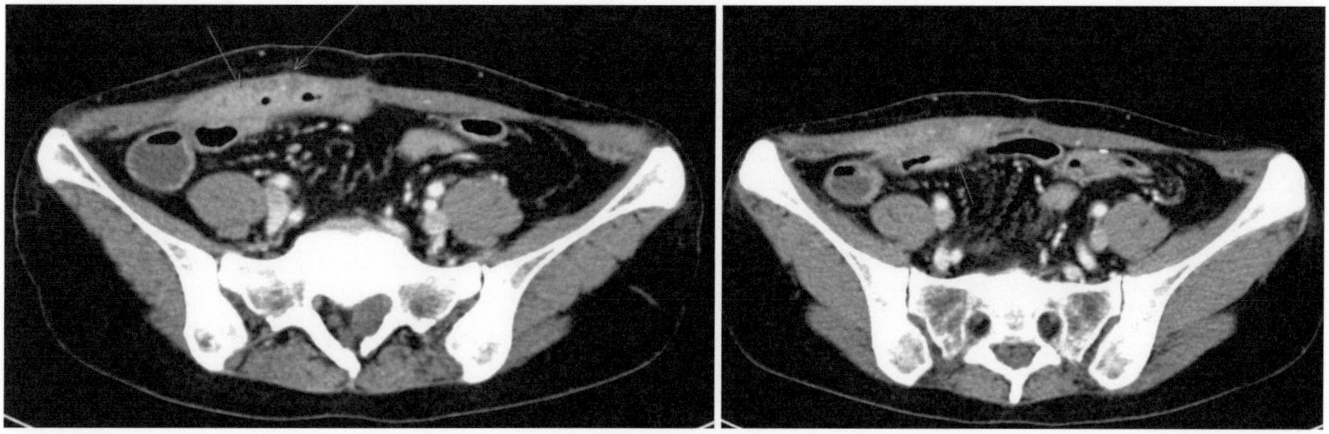

Fig. 12.11 Rectus muscle abscess. Non-enhancing fluid collection in rectus muscle with relatively well-enhanced cystic wall is seen (*arrow*). It can be single or multiple lesions. Small air bubbles in the lesion help its diagnosis

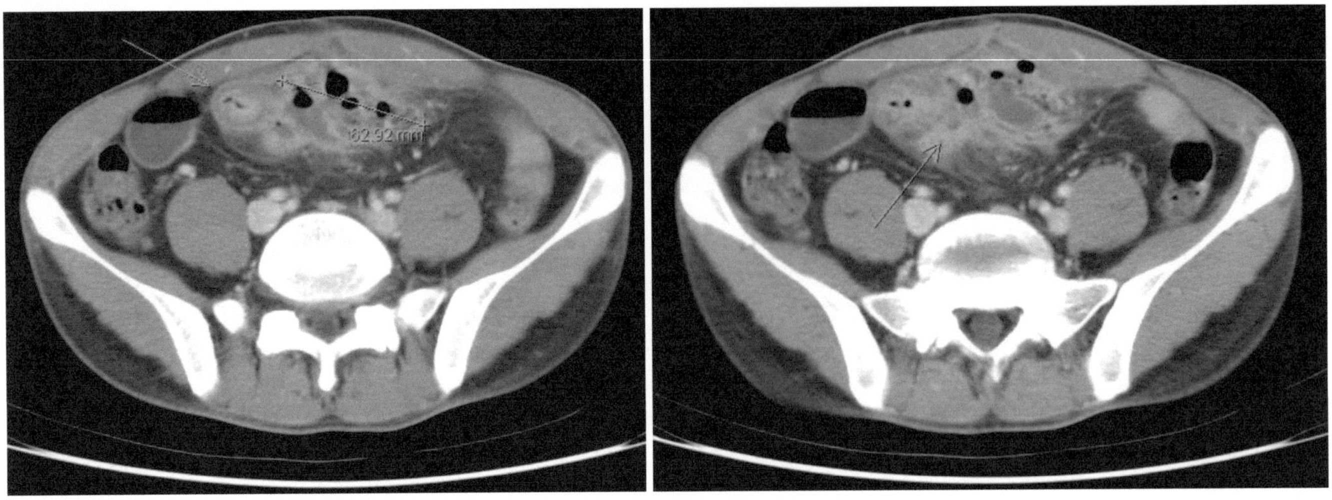

Fig. 12.12 Abscesses in the omentum in a patient with Crohn's disease. Active inflammation at the long segment of distal small bowel with abscess formation (*arrow*) due to fistula formation is seen

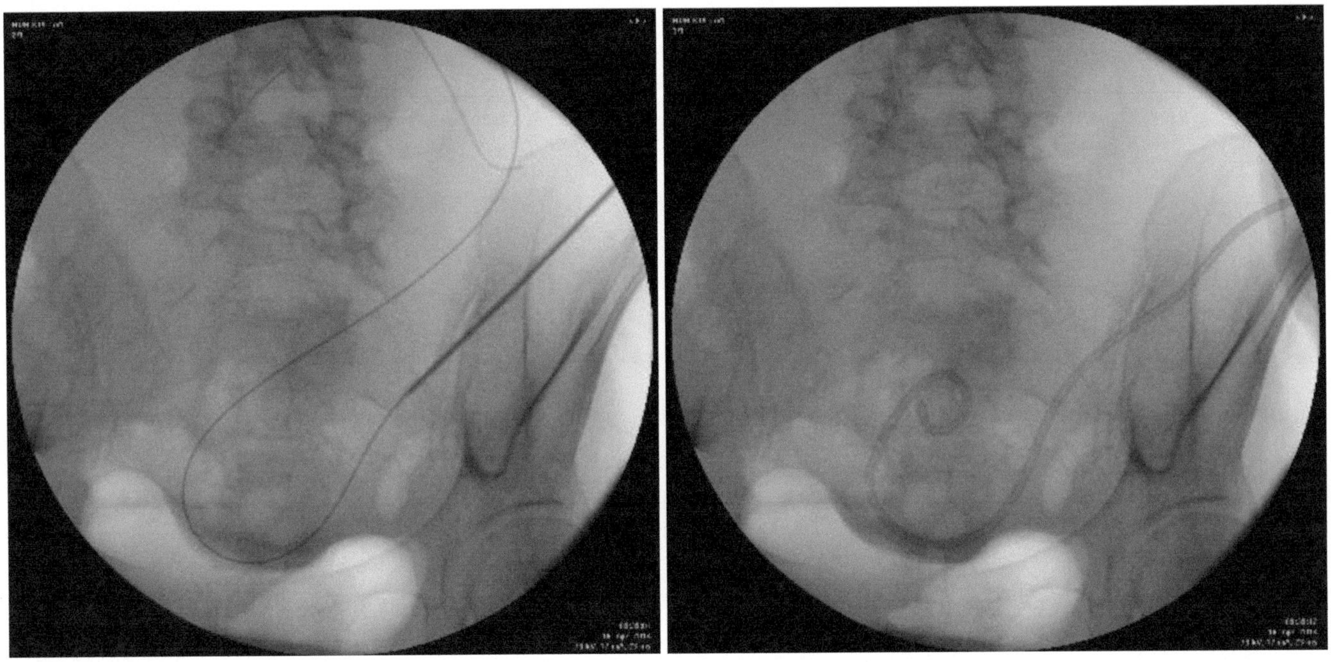

Fig. 12.13 Percutaneous drainage of intra-abdominal abscess. In selected cases, abscesses can be treated by percutaneous placement of drain catheter under imaging guidance

12.5 Stricture

Inflammatory bowel disease is frequently complicated by the formation of strictures. The majority of strictures comprise inflammatory (Fig. 12.14) and fibrotic components (Fig. 12.15), and identification of the dominant feature can help to guide therapy. In both types of strictures, severe stenosis can lead to intestinal obstruction. NOD2 carriers are more likely than non-carriers to have ileal involvement and complications related to fibrostenosis and to require intestinal resection [15]. Intestinal fibrosis is a consequence of local chronic inflammation which is much more prevalent in CD than in UC. Fibrosis is observed as abnormal deposition of extracellular matrix proteins produced by activated myofibroblasts.

Medical therapy is the first-line therapy to strictures with features mainly suggestive of active inflammation. Response to medical therapy might be reviewed, and maintenance therapy should be continued in patients with good response. In unresponsive patients, endoscopic or surgical management may be required. The treatment for strictures with features mainly suggestive of fibrotic component or anastomotic stricture depends on the length and the site of the stricture. In the patients with short and endoscopically accessible stricture, endoscopic balloon dilatation is preferred [16]. Short (<5 cm) fibrotic strictures respond well to endoscopic balloon dilatation, and in selected cases, this therapy may provide a lasting alternative to surgery (see Chap. 11, Therapeutics). While those who are not responsive to endoscopic therapy or those with long (>5 cm) strictures or not endoscopically accessible, surgical therapy by strictureplasty or resection is warranted. When surgery is required, bowel-conserving techniques such as strictureplasty should be employed if possible in order to minimize the risk of subsequent short bowel syndrome.

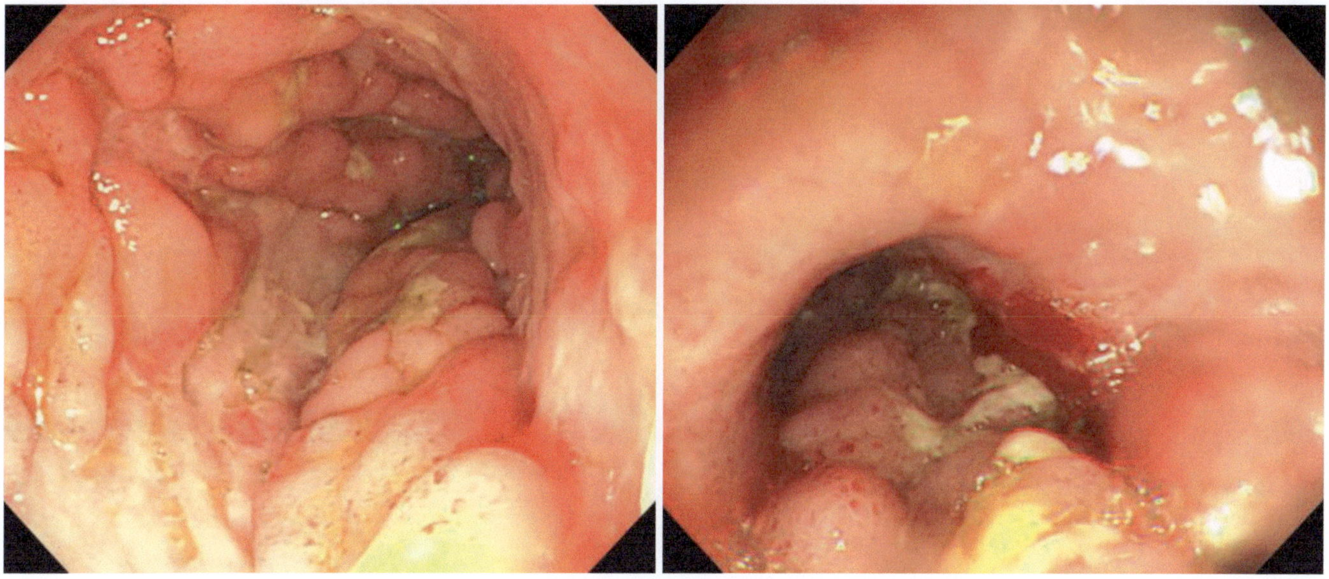

Fig. 12.14 Inflammatory stenosis with active ulcers of the colon due to Crohn's disease

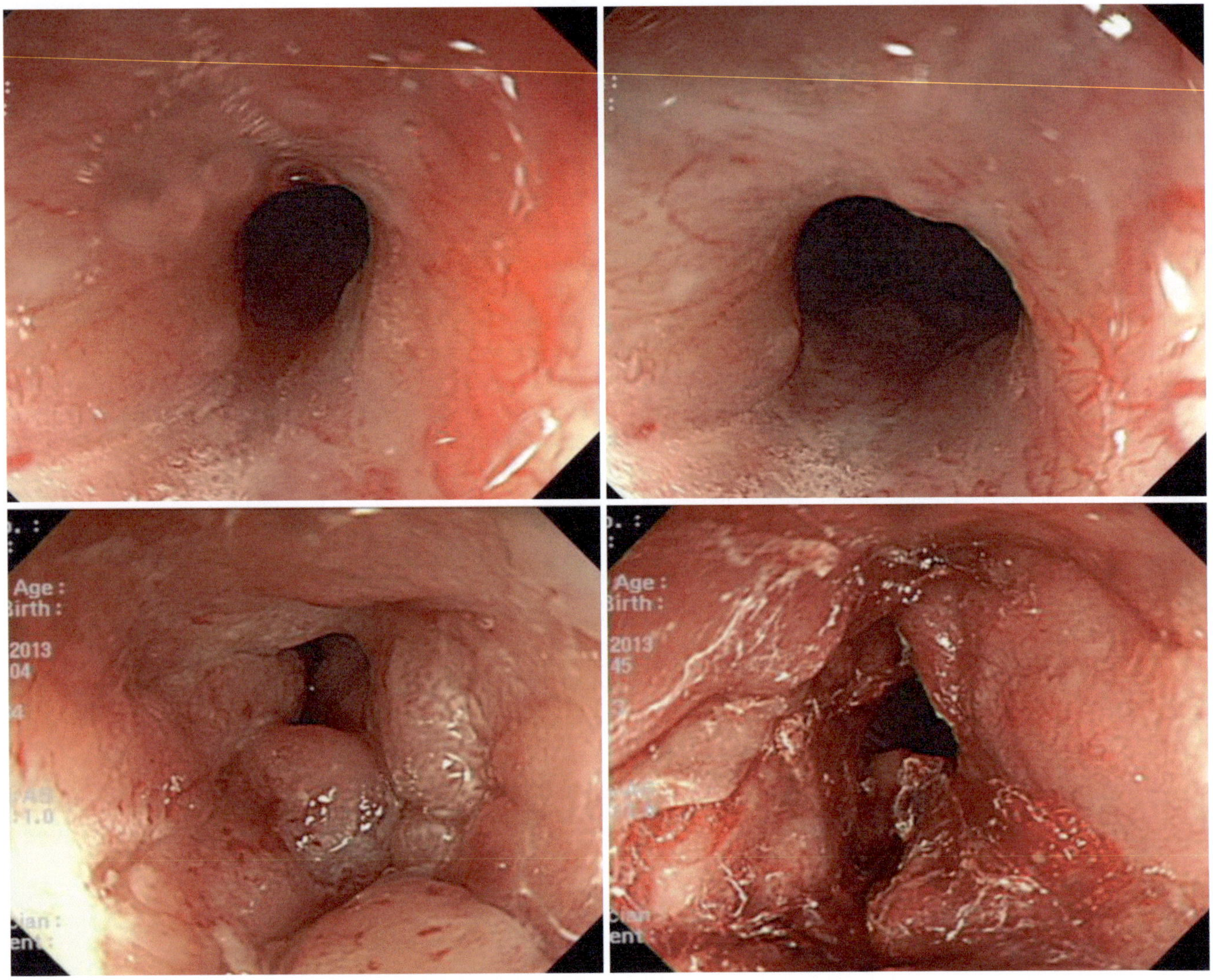

Fig. 12.15 Fibrotic stenosis of the colon in a patient with Crohn's disease

12.6 Toxic Megacolon

Traditionally, toxic megacolon was thought to be a complication of UC with a high morbidity and mortality. However, any inflammatory conditions of colon including CD can lead to this infrequent complication. It is defined as segmental or total colonic distension of more than 6 cm in diameter with signs of acute colitis and systemic toxicity [17]. Ten percent of UC and 2.3 % of CD patients with hospitalization showed toxic megacolon [18]. It is postulated that severe inflammation and damage of the colonic wall are the main causes of complication development; therefore, preceding signs such as bloody diarrhea, fevers, or abdominal cramping are typically seen before the onset of toxic megacolon. Radiological evidence is crucial for the diagnosis of this complication. And endoscopic examination may help the evaluation when the underlying disease is unclear [19]. However, endoscopy may worsen the disease course basically; therefore, extreme carefulness is essential when the physician decides the examination. General supportive care including bowel rest and decompression is necessary in this condition. There is controversy over the use of corticosteroids, but using corticosteroids in patients with inflammatory bowel disease seems reasonable regarding underlying pathogenesis. Because delay in surgical treatment may lead to colonic perforation, clinicians have to plan their treatment strategy for toxic megacolon with prudence.

References

1. Schwartz DA, Loftus Jr EV, Tremaine WJ, Panaccione R, Harmsen WS, Zinsmeister AR, et al. The natural history of fistulizing Crohn's disease in Olmsted County, Minnesota. Gastroenterology. 2002;122(4):875–80. PubMed PMID: 11910338.
2. Falconi M, Pederzoli P. The relevance of gastrointestinal fistulae in clinical practice: a review. Gut. 2001;49 Suppl 4:iv2–10. PubMed PMID: 11878790. Pubmed Central PMCID: 1766897.
3. Tozer P, Ng SC, Siddiqui MR, Plamondon S, Burling D, Gupta A, et al. Long-term MRI-guided combined anti-TNF-alpha and thiopurine therapy for Crohn's perianal fistulas. Inflamm Bowel Dis. 2012;18(10):1825–34. PubMed PMID: 22223472.
4. Pearson DC, May GR, Fick GH, Sutherland LR. Azathioprine and 6-mercaptopurine in Crohn disease. A meta-analysis. Ann Intern Med. 1995;123(2):132–42. PubMed PMID: 7778826.
5. Kamm MA, Ng SC. Perianal fistulizing Crohn's disease: a call to action. Clin Gastroenterol Hepatol. 2008;6(1):7–10. PubMed PMID: 18063415.
6. Fleshner PR, Schoetz Jr DJ, Roberts PL, Murray JJ, Coller JA, Veidenheimer MC. Anal fissure in Crohn's disease: a plea for aggressive management. Dis Colon Rectum. 1995;38(11):1137–43. PubMed PMID: 7587755.
7. Bouguen G, Siproudhis L, Bretagne JF, Bigard MA, Peyrin-Biroulet L. Nonfistulizing perianal Crohn's disease: clinical features, epidemiology, and treatment. Inflamm Bowel Dis. 2010;16(8):1431–42. PubMed PMID: 20310013.
8. Keighley MR, Allan RN. Current status and influence of operation on perianal Crohn's disease. Int J Color Dis. 1986;1(2):104–7. PubMed PMID: 3611935.
9. Hughes LE. Clinical classification of perianal Crohn's disease. Dis Colon Rectum. 1992;35(10):928–32. PubMed PMID: 1395978.
10. Sandborn WJ, Fazio VW, Feagan BG, Hanauer SB, American Gastroenterological Association Clinical Practice C. AGA technical review on perianal Crohn's disease. Gastroenterology. 2003;125(5): 1508–30. PubMed PMID: 14598268.
11. Bonheur JL, Braunstein J, Korelitz BI, Panagopoulos G. Anal skin tags in inflammatory bowel disease: new observations and a clinical review. Inflamm Bowel Dis. 2008;14(9):1236–9. PubMed PMID: 18452201.
12. Keighley MR, Eastwood D, Ambrose NS, Allan RN, Burdon DW. Incidence and microbiology of abdominal and pelvic abscess in Crohn's disease. Gastroenterology. 1982;83(6):1271–5. PubMed PMID: 7129031.
13. Ayuk P, Williams N, Scott NA, Nicholson DA, Irving MH. Management of intra-abdominal abscesses in Crohn's disease. Ann R Coll Surg Engl. 1996;78(1):5–10. PubMed PMID: 8659975. Pubmed Central PMCID: 2502682.
14. Kim DH, Cheon JH, Moon CM, Park JJ, Han SY, Kim ES, et al. Clinical efficacy of nonsurgical treatment of Crohn's disease-related intrbdominal abscess. Korean J Gastroenterol. 2009; 53(1):29–35. PubMed PMID: 19158468.
15. Lesage S, Zouali H, Cezard JP, Colombel JF, Belaiche J, Almer S, et al. CARD15/NOD2 mutational analysis and genotype-phenotype correlation in 612 patients with inflammatory bowel disease. Am J Hum Genet. 2002;70(4):845–57. PubMed PMID: 11875755. Pubmed Central PMCID: 379113.
16. Thienpont C, D'Hoore A, Vermeire S, Demedts I, Bisschops R, Coremans G, et al. Long-term outcome of endoscopic dilatation in patients with Crohn's disease is not affected by disease activity or medical therapy. Gut. 2010;59(3):320–4. PubMed PMID: 19840991.

17. Gan SI, Beck PL. A new look at toxic megacolon: an update and review of incidence, etiology, pathogenesis, and management. Am J Gastroenterol. 2003;98(11):2363–71. PubMed PMID: 14638335. Epub 2003/11/26. eng.
18. Greenstein AJ, Sachar DB, Gibas A, Schrag D, Heimann T, Janowitz HD, et al. Outcome of toxic dilatation in ulcerative and Crohn's colitis. J Clin Gastroenterol. 1985;7(2):137–43. PubMed PMID: 4008909.
19. Alemayehu G, Jarnerot G. Colonoscopy during an attack of severe ulcerative colitis is a safe procedure and of great value in clinical decision making. Am J Gastroenterol. 1991;86(2):187–90. PubMed PMID: 1992632. Epub 1991/02/01. eng.

Malignancies: Colitic Cancer and Small Bowel Cancer (Intestinal Cancer) in IBD

13

Toshiyuki Matsui

13.1 Ulcerative Colitis

13.1.1 Epidemiology

Colorectal cancer (CRC) has long been a major clinical problem in ulcerative colitis (UC), and many studies have examined its incidence and risk factors. Eaden et al. conducted a meta-analysis of CRC in UC and reported that the rate of complicating CRC was 3.7 % in all UC cases, and the cumulative cancer incidence rate was 1.6 % at 10 years after onset of UC, increasing to 8.3 % after 20 years and 18 % after 30 years [1]. As disease duration increases, so does the risk of developing CRC [2, 3]. Many recent studies have reported that this risk of acquiring CRC has decreased over recent decades. In 2004, Winther et al. reported that the risk of developing CRC at 30 years after onset of UC was 2.1 % [4], while Lakatos et al. reported a risk of 7.5 % [5]. From a surveillance study of about 600 subjects, Rutter et al. reported that the cumulative CRC onset rate was 2.5 % at 20 years, 7.6 % at 30 years, and 10.8 % at 40 years [6]. The risk of acquiring CRC has thus decreased over the decades (Table 13.1). The causes of this are thought to be advances in pharmacotherapy, increased excision of premalignant lesions, and better techniques in colon resection, as well as the spread of surveillance colonoscopy (SC).

13.1.2 Risk Factors

The clinical characteristics of UC-associated CRC are similar in Western and Eastern countries. Long-standing disease represents an important risk factor, and since the age of UC onset is young, CRC occurs at a younger age (40s) than in the general population. CRC is estimated to be the cause of death in about 20 % of UC cases [7, 8]. The incidence of multiple cancers is about 30 %. Since UC is present in the background mucosa, the morphology and histological findings vary and present different appearances from general CRC. There is a high incidence of flat and invasive types. Histologically, a characteristic of these cancers is that poorly differentiated adenocarcinoma and mucinous carcinoma account for about half of cases. A relationship with the severity of colitis has been indicated, and attention has been directed to the relationship with tissue inflammation [9, 10]. Factors raising the risk of CRC have recently been considered to be disease duration, extent of the diseased colon, family history of colon cancer, concomitant primary sclerosing cholangitis, and persistence of colitis. Conversely, factors that lower the risk are reported to be prophylactic colectomy, regular examination by a doctor, SC, chemical prevention, and adherence to treatment.

13.1.3 Purpose and Targets of SC

As mentioned above, patients with long-standing UC have a high risk of complicating CRC against a background of chronic inflammation. There is also a high rate of dysplasia, which is thought to represent a precancerous lesion. For that reason, surveillance for dysplasia as a cancer marker is recommended. Regular SC is thought to be essential for early detection of cancer or dysplasia. In fact, it has been shown that with regular SC, cancer or the related dysplastic lesions can be detected and treated at an early, curable stage [11, 12].

The main purpose of surveillance is to reduce deaths from CRC by detecting and excising precancerous lesions. A study by Choi et al. [13] looked at 41 patients who developed cancer, comprising 19 in an SC group and 22 in a non-SC group. A significant difference was seen between groups in 5-year survival, confirming the efficacy of SC [13]. In a recent study by Lutgens et al., 149 patients who developed cancer were stud-

T. Matsui
Department of Gastroenterology,
Fukuoka University Chikushi Hospital,
Chikushino, Fukuoka, Japan
e-mail: matsui@fukuoka-u.ac.jp

W.H. Kim, J.H. Cheon (eds.), *Atlas of Inflammatory Bowel Diseases*,
DOI 10.1007/978-3-642-39423-2_13, © Springer-Verlag Berlin Heidelberg 2015

ied, including an SC group of 23 patients. This SC group included many early-stage tumors than in non-SC group (52 % vs. 24 %), the mortality rate was lower (4 % vs. 24 %), and the 5-year survival rate was significantly higher than in the non-SC patients [14]. Based on the above studies, the decrease in mortality rate was concluded to be as much as 63 %. The largest study was one by Rutter et al. at St. Mark's Hospital [6]. As a result of long-term SC, cancer was detected in 5 % of patients, and their prognosis was shown to be fair. The method of SC used was not perfect but was judged to be effective.

13.1.4 Endoscopic Images

The macroscopic picture of CRC in UC is thought to be protruding cancer in many cases, but few accurate statistics are available. Matsumoto et al. classified and reported endoscopic findings of UC-associated CRC using a dye method [15] (Table 13.2).

They divided cancers into protruded lesions (Figs. 13.1 and 13.2), slightly elevated lesions (Figs. 13.3, 13.4, and 13.5), flat lesions (Figs. 13.6, 13.7, 13.8, and 13.9), depressed lesion (Fig. 13.10), and mixed-type lesions (Fig. 13.2) and presented endoscopic images of each. Appropriate endoscopic classifications like this are needed. Of course, the protruded lesion called dysplasia-associated lesion or mass (DALM) (Figs. 13.2, 13.3, 13.4, and 13.5) is the most important finding [16]. DALM presents diverse morphologies, including villiform, coarsely granular, and irregular flat-elevated shapes, with margins that are often indistinct. Changes in color tone have been confirmed in flat dysplasia, but differentiation from surrounding inflammatory regenerated mucosa is difficult (Figs. 13.5, 13.6, 13.7, 13.8, and 13.9). In endoscopy, abnormalities are seen even in non-tumor areas because of the inflammation in UC, making detection and definitive diagnosis of neoplastic lesions tricky. As mentioned above, a special care is needed in stenotic portions (Figs. 13.11 and 13.12).

Random biopsy is a method in which two to four biopsy samples are taken from the diseased colon randomly at 10-cm intervals. If sites with findings such as DALM are identified, additional biopsy is performed for pathological investigation for the presence of dysplasia. In Japan, targeted biopsy has been performed traditionally, and its effectiveness has been demonstrated [6, 17, 18]. In Western countries, concurrent use of dye methods has also been shown to be effective. The comparative studies of Matsumoto et al. and Rutter et al. using chromoendoscopy have greatly advanced the combined use of target biopsy and chromoendoscopy [7, 18].

Table 13.1 Cumulative incidence of colitis-associated cancer in UC

		Year after UC			
Author, year, area	Subject	10	15	20	30
Gilat T, 1988, Israel	Population	0.2 %	2.8 %	5.5 %	13.5 %
Lennard-Jones JE, 1990, UK	Institutional		3.0 %	5 %	
Eden JA, 2001	Meta-analysis	2 %		8 %	18 %
Winther, 2004	Population				2.1 %
Lakatos, 2006	Population	0.6 %		5.4 %	7.5 %
Rutter, 2006	Institutional			2.5 %	7.6 %
Herrinton, 2012	Institutional	60 % higher than GP			
Hata, 2003, Japan	Institutional	0.5 %		4 %	6 %

Table 13.2 Endoscopic classification for colorectal cancer associated with UC

1	Protruded lesion (DALM)	Most common, irregularity, uneven redness, surrounded by slightly elevated mucosa
2	Slightly elevated lesion	Irregular granular surface, uneven redness
3	Flat lesion	Reddish lesion with defined boundary
4	Depressed lesion	Uncommon, accompanied by slightly elevated lesion
5	Mixed-type lesion	

Matsumoto et al. [15]
DALM (dysplasia-associated lesion or mass): dysplastic polyp vs. ALM (adenoma-like mass)

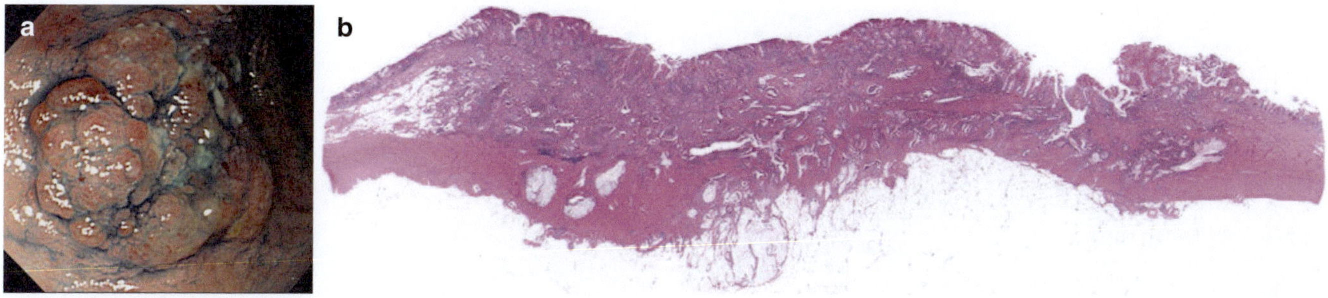

Fig. 13.1 Protruded-type cancer in long-standing UC. Endoscopic view of a protruded-type cancer showing an irregular and nodular surface (**a**). Histologic picture of a protruded-type cancer with UC (**b**). Resected specimen shows IIa-like protrusion, and histologically, this tumor was diagnosed as well-differentiated adenocarcinoma and tumor invaded down to the subserosa (Quoted from Nishimura et al. [30], under permission of publisher)

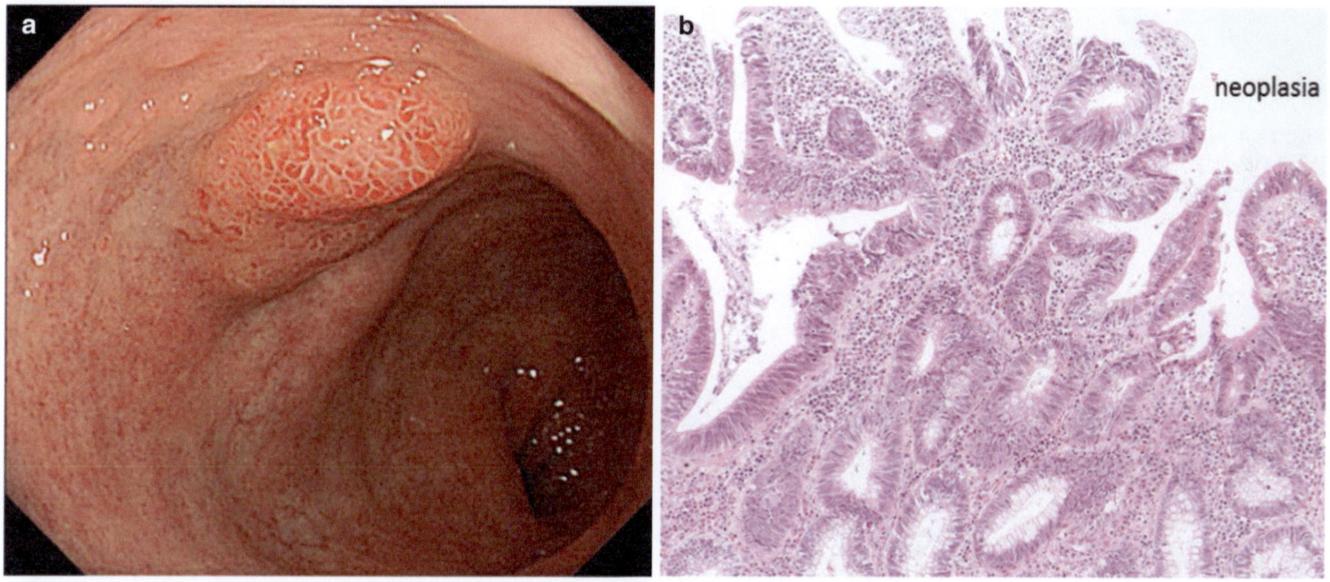

Fig. 13.2 Protruded-type cancer in UC. A 29-year-old patient with long-standing refractory UC, disease duration 11 years, total colitis. Colonoscopic view of a reddish, protruded-type cancer (Is) in the sigmoid colon (**a**). The lesion seemed to be soft, and the surface is covered by granular or papillary mucosa, but surrounding mucosa has abnormal granularity. Histological examination showed very well to poorly differentiated adenocarcinoma (**b**) with mucinous degeneration invading into the deeper portion of the submucosa and surrounding area of dysplastic epithelium

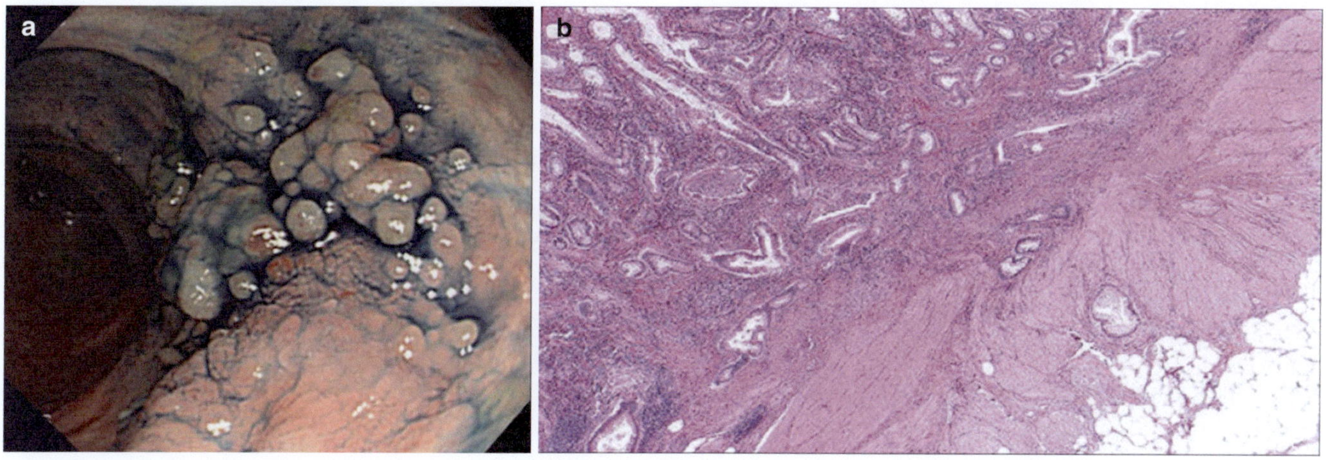

Fig. 13.3 (**a**) Endoscopic view of a slightly elevated tumor with granular surface in the transverse colon. (**b**) Histologic picture of a slightly elevated lesion. Histologically, the tumor showed IIa + Is-like advanced cancer invading down to deeper parts of the muscularis propria (Quoted from Nishimura et al. [30], under permission of publisher)

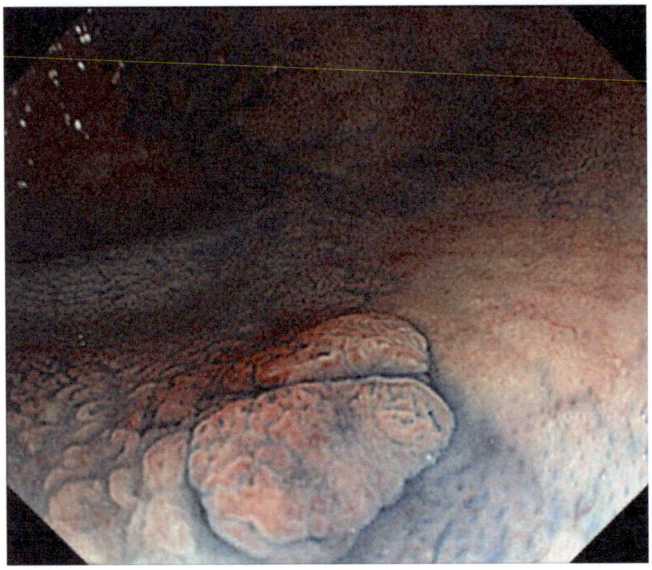

Fig. 13.4 Slightly elevated lesion in the rectum was polypectomized. A 60-year-old; disease period, 22 years; total colitis. The slightly elevated lesion of the rectum consisted of very well- to well-differentiated adenocarcinoma confined to the mucosa

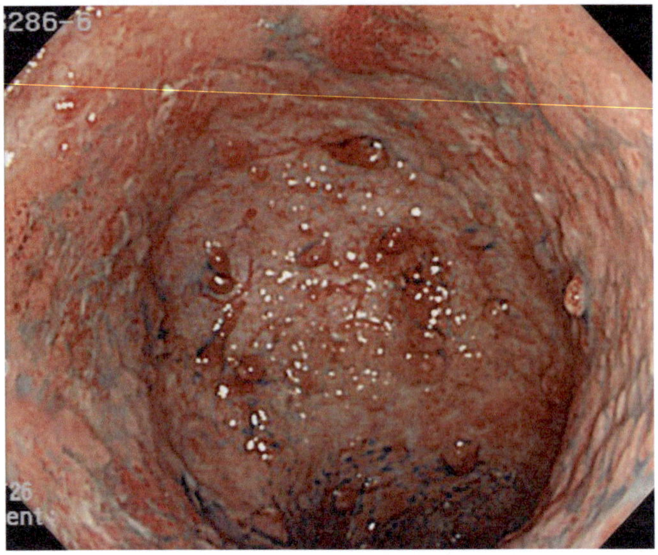

Fig. 13.6 Flat lesion. A 46-year-old patient; disease period, 18 years; total colitis. Surveillance colonoscopy detected a flat lesion with superficial irregularity. Histological diagnosis was a mucosal lesion with moderately to severely dysplastic epithelium highly suggestive of well-differentiated adenocarcinoma

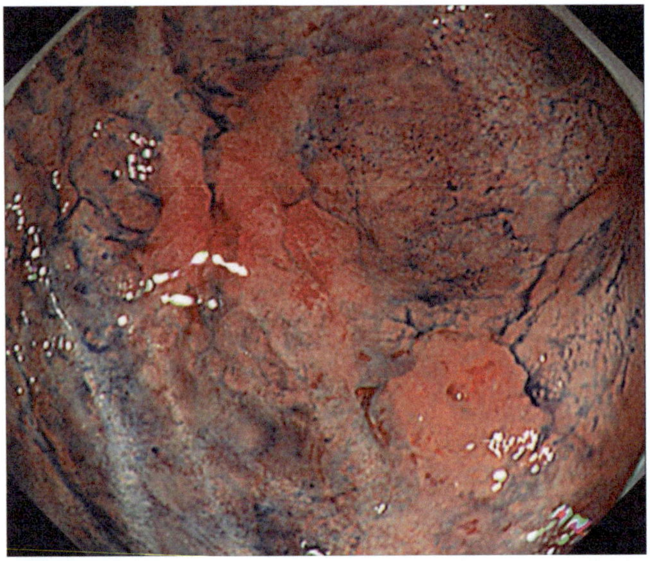

Fig. 13.5 Slightly elevated lesion. A patient in their 40s at diagnosis; disease period, 25 years; total colitis. A surveillance colonoscopy detected malignant elevations in the descending colon. The tumors comprised well- to moderately differentiated adenocarcinoma invading into the subserosa

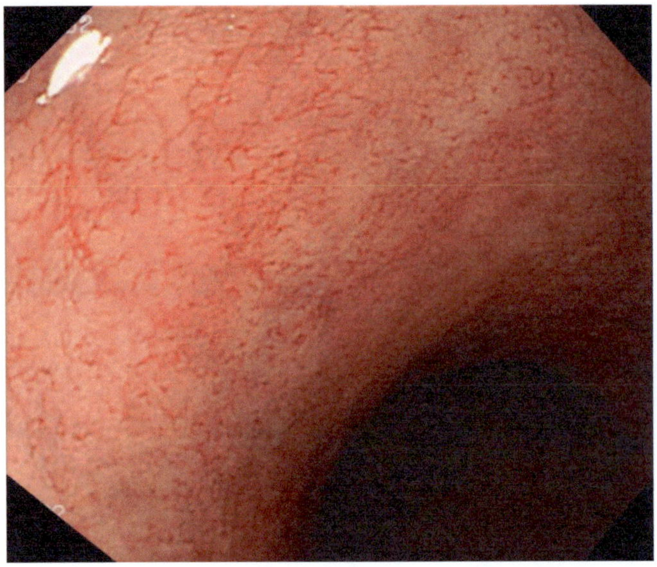

Fig. 13.7 Flat lesion. A 76-year-old patient; disease period, 4 years; left-sided type. Extremely difficult to diagnose as cancer. Endoscopic findings showed a flat lesion with low-grade inflammation and ill-defined margins. Histologically, the tumor consisted of adenocarcinoma and dysplastic epithelium in the sigmoid colon

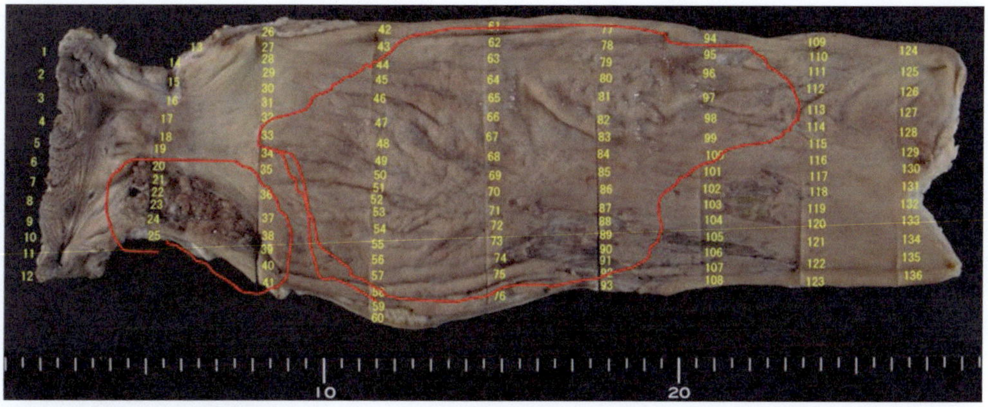

Fig. 13.8 Macroscopic picture of a flat lesion and a protrusion. A 46-year-old patient; disease period, 26 years; left-sided colitis type. Schematic illustration of the resected colon and rectum. In Rb there is a protrusion which is composed of well-differentiated adenocarcinoma with mucinous change invading into the adventitia. In Ra there showed a broad, flat lesion with well-differentiated adenocarcinoma invading into the superficial part of the submucosa

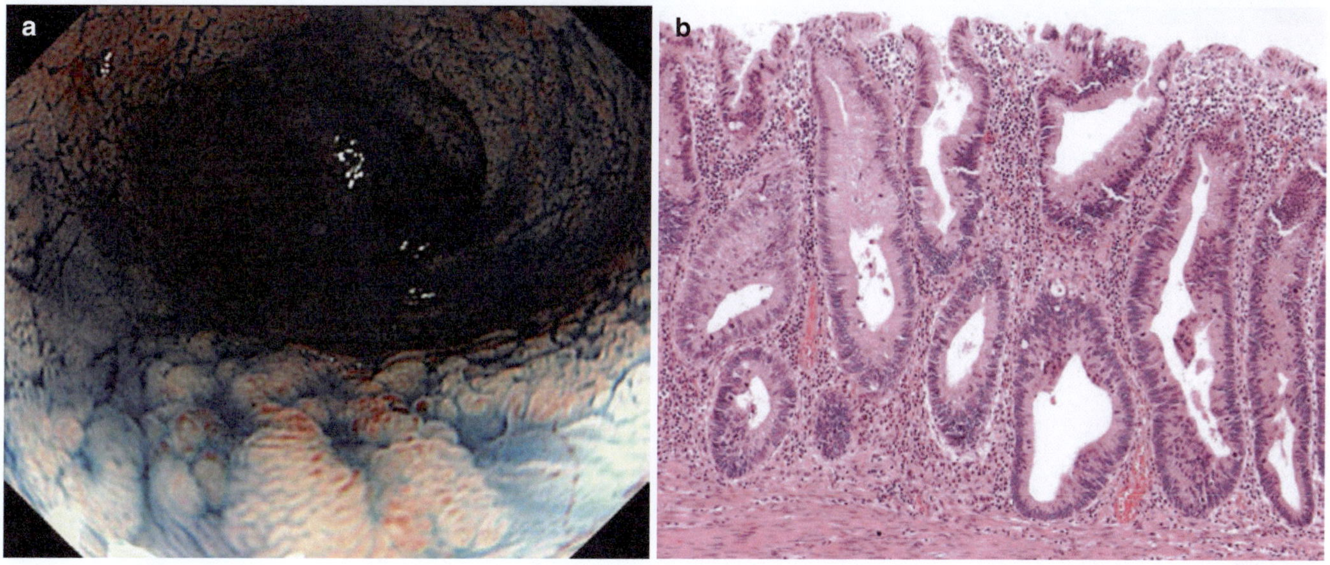

Fig. 13.9 Endoscopic view of flat lesion in the upper rectum (Ra) shown in Fig. 13.8. A flat, irregular surface lesion was detected in the upper rectum, without demarcating boundary between the mucosal cancer and inflamed area (**a**). Histologically, a flat, well-differentiated lesion is seen in Ra (**b**)

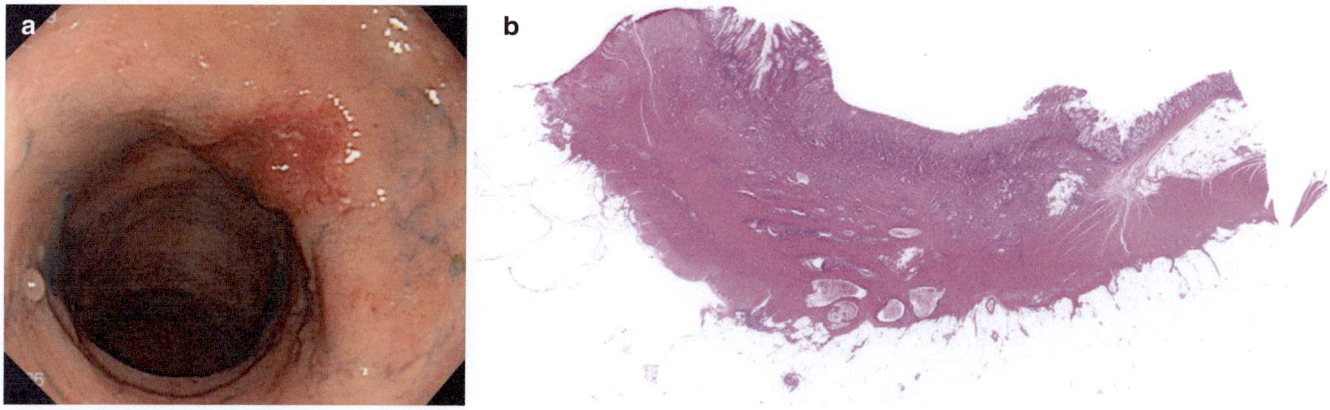

Fig. 13.10 (**a**) Endoscopic features of depressed-type cancer in UC. (**b**) Histologic picture of depressed-type cancer. In the descending colon, a depressed-type (IIc-like advanced) well-differentiated adenocarcinoma which invaded down to the subserosa was seen (Quoted from Nishimura et al. [30], under permission of publisher)

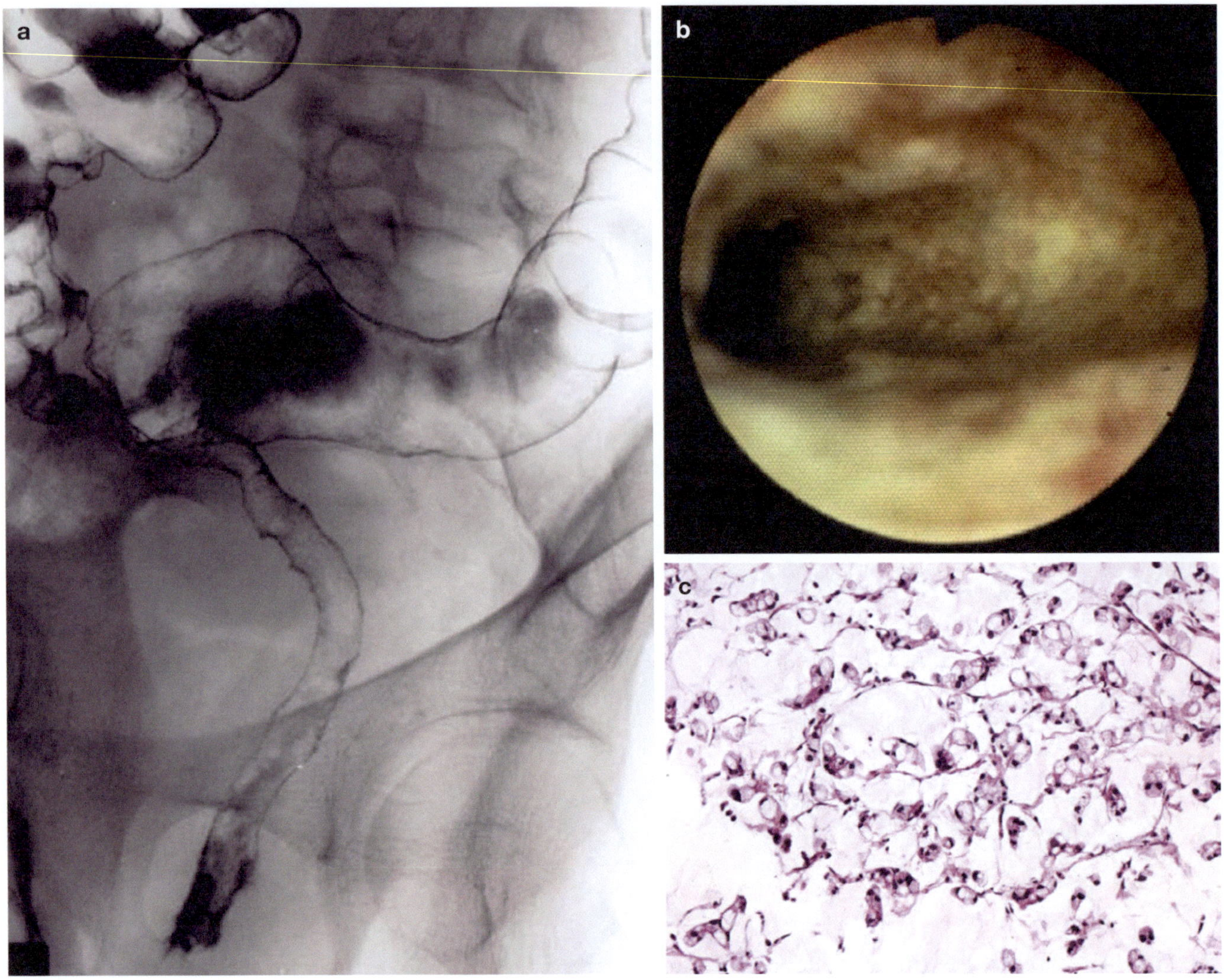

Fig. 13.11 Stenotic-type rectal cancer associated with UC. Stenosis as long as 22 cm was shown on radiography (**a**). Endoscopic picture of a CRC associated with UC, stenotic lesion (**b**). Biopsy showed mucinous adenocarcinoma with signet ring cell carcinoma (**c**) (Quoted from Nishimura et al. [30], under permission of publisher)

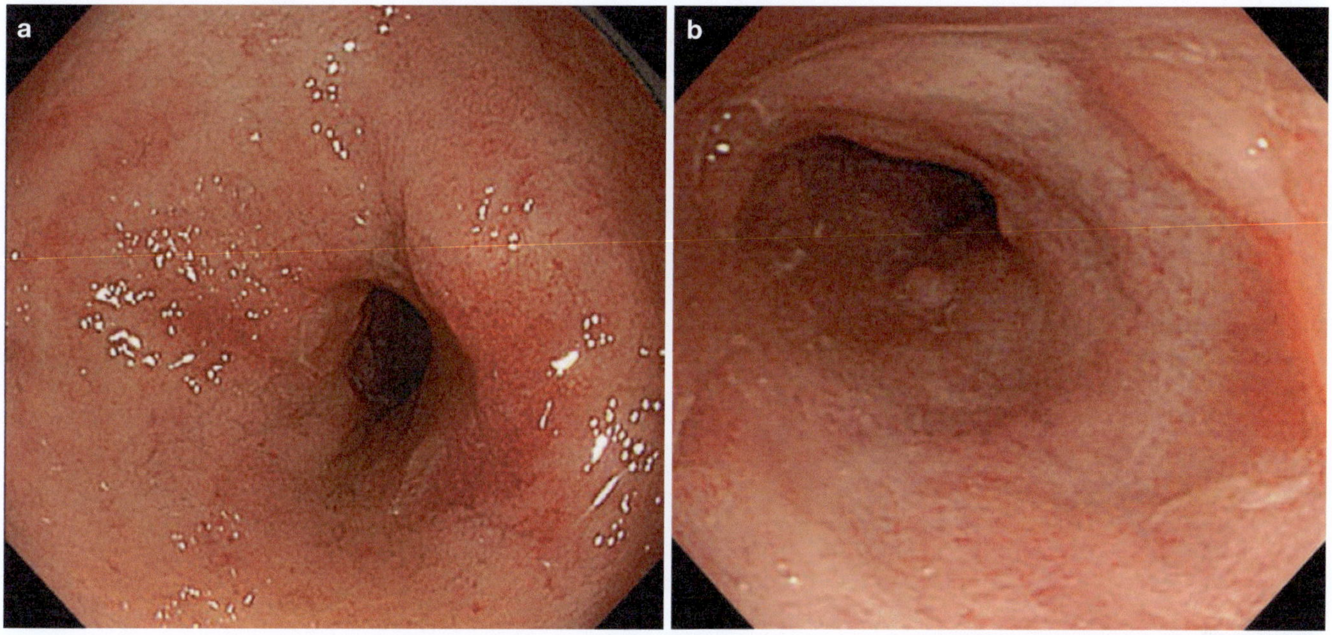

Fig. 13.12 Stenotic-type cancer in UC. A patient in their 30s; disease period, 15 years; mild persistent activity. Surveillance endoscopy revealed a tumor with severe stenosis in the descending colon (**a**). In the 4 years before final diagnosis, endoscopic findings revealed mild stenosis with mild inflammation without biopsy (**b**) (Quoted from Higashi et al. [31], under permission of publisher)

13.2 Crohn's Disease

13.2.1 Epidemiology

As in UC, CRC or small intestinal cancer also occurs in Crohn's disease (CD) patients (Figs. 13.13, 13.14, and 13.15). The relative risk (RR) of developing intestinal cancer increases with longer disease duration (Tables 13.3 and 13.4). Although this has been reported in many studies, the degree of rise in RR differs greatly depending on the population in each study [19–23]. Ekbom et al. reported an RR of 2.5 [19], whereas the regional studies of Persson et al., Munkholm et al., Fireman et al., and Jess et al. [20–23] did not find high RRs. In a study by Gillen et al. however, the RRs of CD and UC were both high, at about the same level [24]. A comparison of cancer incidence revealed rates of 7 % (20 years) in UC and 8 % (20 years) in CD, 18 and 19 times higher, respectively, than the risk in a healthy population of the same age composition. High RR was also supported in a recent meta-analysis by Canavan et al. [25]. Friedman et al. recently reported the results of continuous colon SC in 259 CD patients starting in 1980 [26, 27]. Cancer or dysplasia was diagnosed in initial (7 %) and later tests in 48 patients (adding more 14 %). SC is thus extremely important.

Our recent reports have shown a marked increase in the number of cancers detected in CD [28, 29]. The most common sites of CRC development in Japanese CD patients are from the lower rectum to anus (Figs. 13.16, 13.17, 13.18, and 13.19). A large majority of these patients have a history of anal fistula [28, 29]. Thus, in Japan, most malignant intestinal cancers associated with CD occur in the rectum or anal area, and surgical biopsy under anesthesia in the area of the anal fistula in the asymptomatic interval is thought to be effective for surveillance

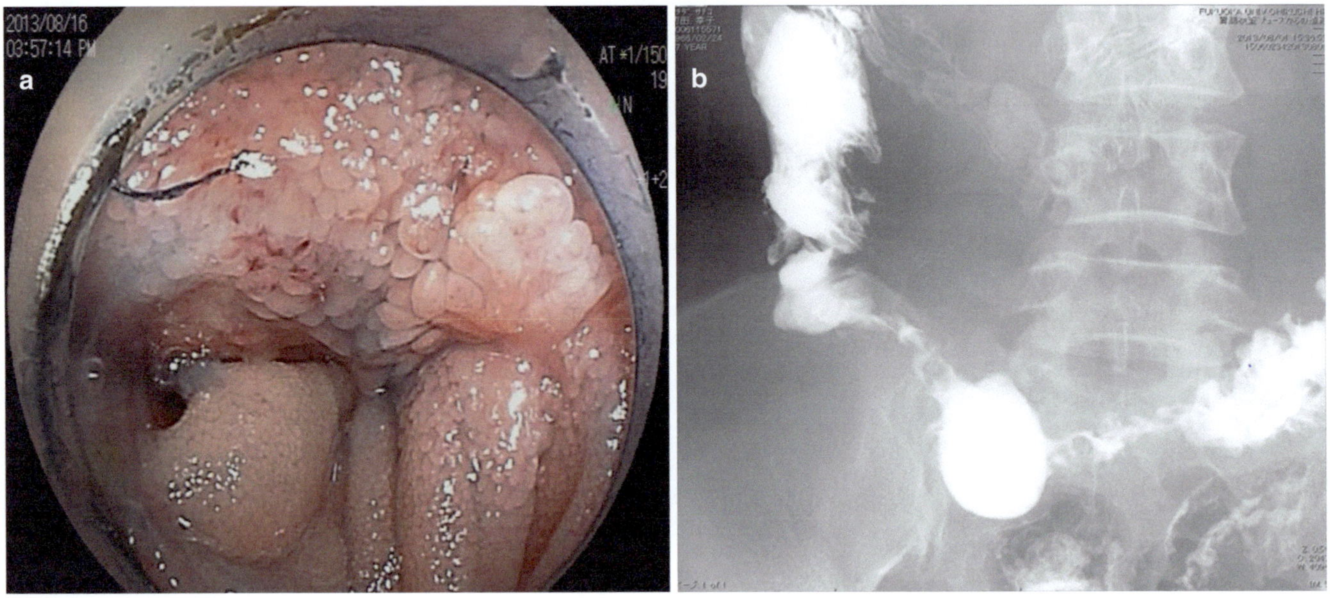

Fig. 13.13 Ileal cancer in CD. A patient in their 40s at diagnosis; disease period, 28 years. Intestinal cancer at the ileocolonic anastomosis with distant metastasis and ileus. Per-oral double-balloon endoscopy revealed segmental tumor formation at the ileocolonic anastomosis (**a**). Radiographic picture of the stenosis (**b**)

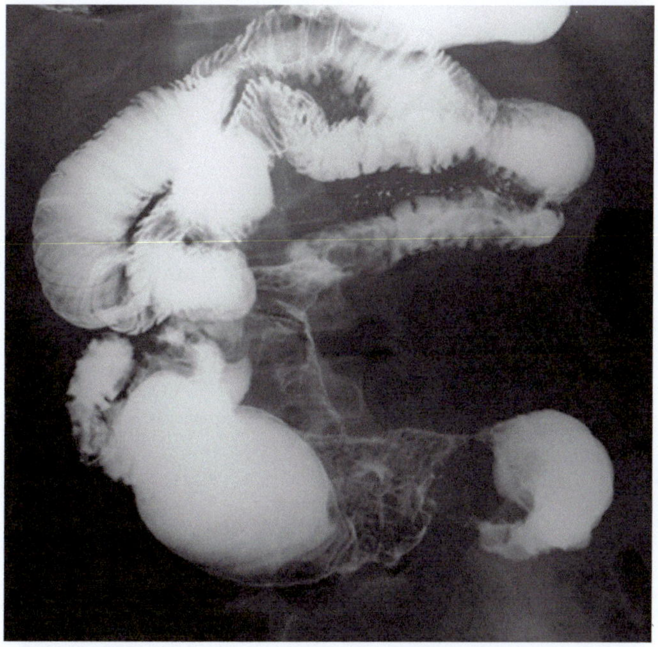

Fig. 13.14 Ileal cancer in CD. A patient in their 30s at diagnosis, with ileitis-type CD; disease duration, 23 years. A barium meal study was conducted after ileus. Multiple severe ileal stenoses were detected, but lesions seemed to be caused by Crohn's disease itself, and diagnosis of cancer was not possible preoperatively (Quoted from Higashi et al. [32], under permission of publisher)

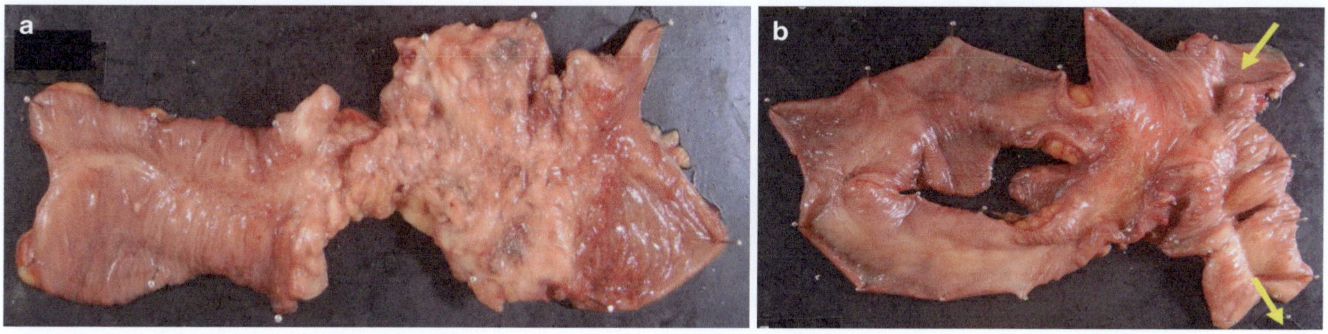

Fig. 13.15 Resected specimen of the patient as Fig. 13.14. At the stenotic site, flat cancer (**a**) with restricted shallow ulcer formation was evident. At the bypass surgery site (**b**), a cancer with ill-defined margins of shallow ulceration with mild stenosis was found. *Upper arrow* efferent loop, *lower arrow* afferent loop (Quoted from Higashi et al. [32], under permission of publisher)

Table 13.3 Relative colorectal cancer risks in CD

Author	Report year	Subjects	Relative risk	Frequency (CD onset)
Hamilton	1985	Hospital	4–20	
Fireman	1989	Field	1.0	
Ekbom	1990	Field	2.5–5.6	
Munkholm	1993	Field	1.1	
Persson	1994	Field	1.0	
Gillen	1994	Hospital	3.4–18.2	8 % (20 year)
Choi	1994	Hospital		1.3 %
Jess	2004	Field	1.1	
Yano	2008	Hospital	3.2	
Jess	2012	Field	0.85	
Canavan	2006	Meta-analysis	2.5	

Table 13.4 Relative risks of small intestinal cancer in CD

Author	Report year	Subjects	Relative risk
Fielding	1972	Hospital	100
Greenstein	1981	Hospital	85.8
Ekbom	1990	Field	3.4
Persson	1994	Field	15.6
Gillen	1994	Hospital	40.0
Mellemkjaer	2000	Field	17.9
Bernstein	2001	Field	17.4
Jess	2004	Hospital	66.7
Canavan	2006	Meta-analysis	33.2

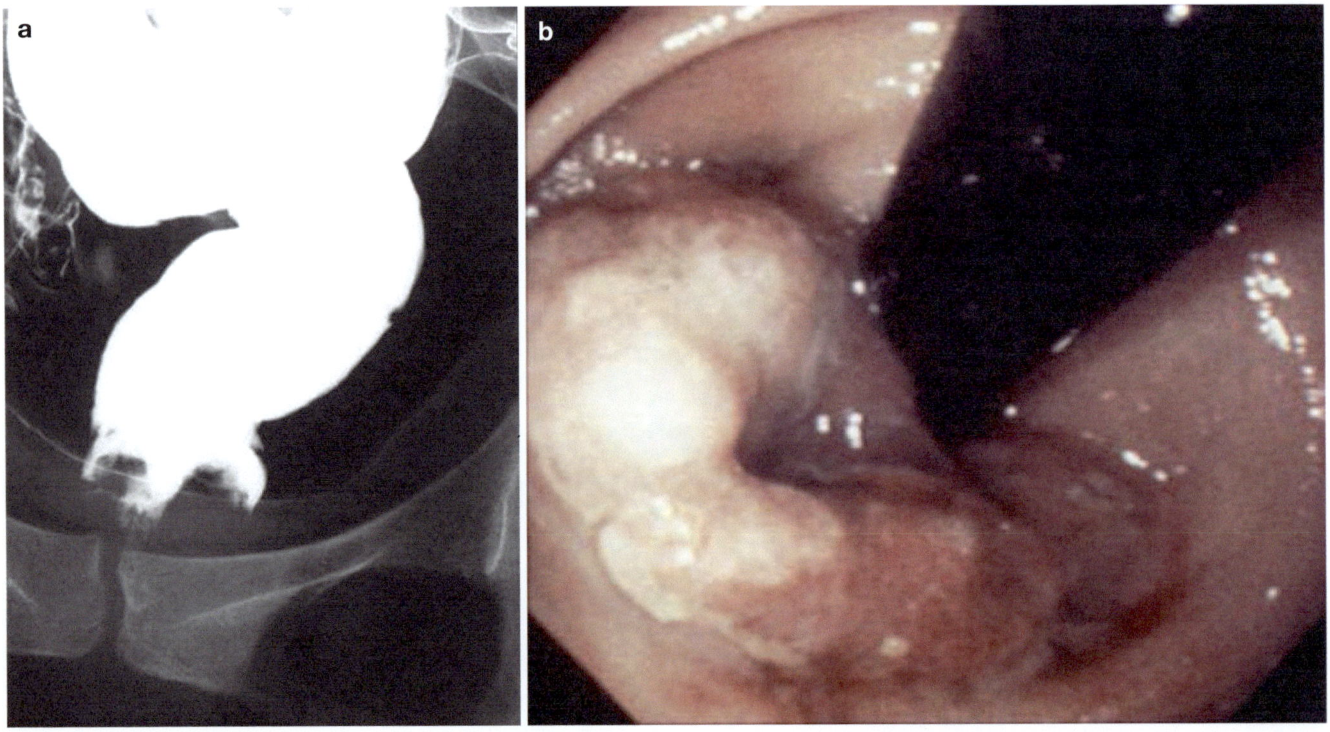

Fig. 13.16 Anal canal cancer in CD. A patient in their 40s at diagnosis. Advanced rectal cancer was detected from symptomatic change. Radiography shows advanced cancer in Rb (**a**) and endoscopic picture of the rectal tumor (**b**) (Quoted from Yao et al. [33], under permission of publisher)

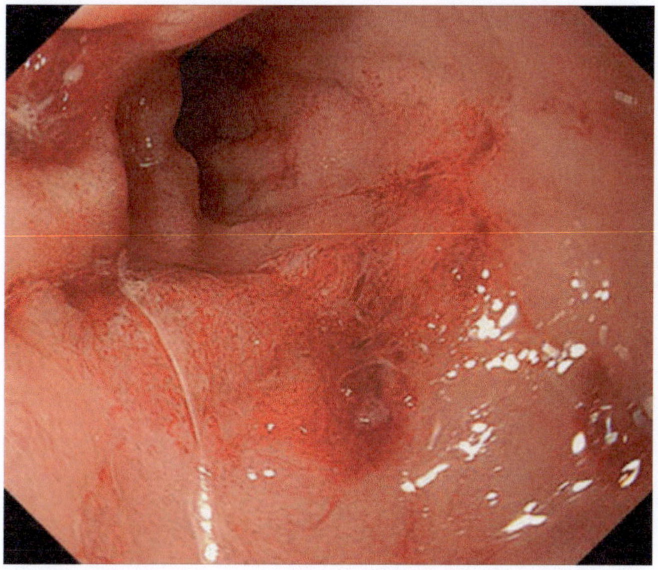

Fig. 13.17 Rectal cancer in CD diagnosed by endoscopy. Rectal stenosis and irregular mucosa were found and diagnosed as mucinous adenocarcinoma. The cancer had invaded down to the subserosa (Quoted from Futami et al. [34], under permission of publisher)

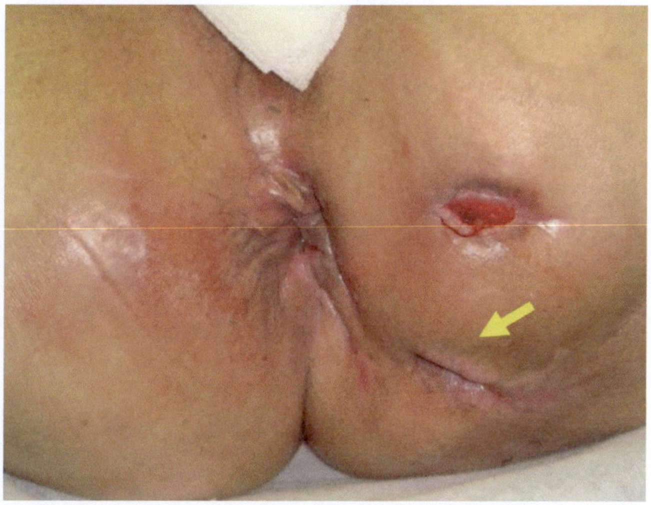

Fig. 13.18 Anal cancer in CD diagnosed by surgical biopsy in a patient with long-standing anorectal fistula. The patient had ileocolitis and a history of fistula (*arrow*). Histology showed well-differentiated adenocarcinoma with mucinous changes (Quoted from Futami et al. [34], under permission of publisher)

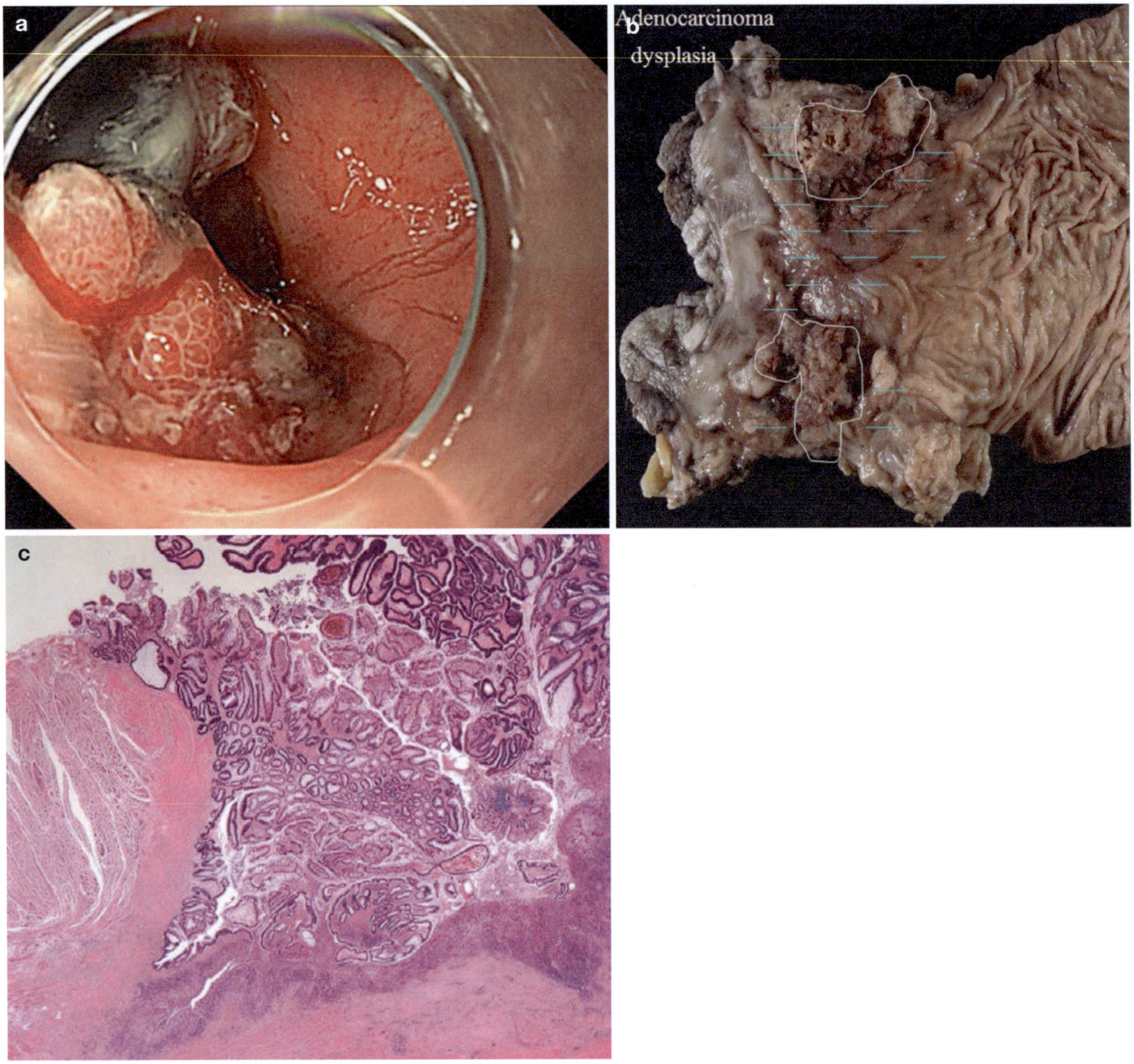

Fig. 13.19 (**a**) Protruded rectal cancer in CD. Disease period, 28 years, with long-standing ileocolitis. Endoscopic view of a protruding-type cancer with lobulation in the rectum and closeup view showing coral-like or villous appearance (**a**). Macroscopic picture of a resected specimen showing a protruded tumor with villous surface and surrounding coarse mucosa (**b**). Histologic pictures (**c**). Protruded carcinoma in the anorectal area with well-differentiated mucinous carcinoma subserosal invasion, and in the surrounding area dysplastic epithelium is seen (Quoted from Futami et al. [34], under permission of publisher)

References

1. Eaden J, Abrams KR, Mayberry JF, et al. The risk of colorectal cancer in ulcerative colitis: a meta-analysis. Gut. 2001;48:526–35.
2. Gilat T, Fireman Z, Grossman A, et al. Colorectal cancer in patients with ulcerative colitis. A population study in central Israel. Gastroenterology. 1988;94:870–7.
3. Lennard-Jones JE, Melville DM, Morson BC, et al. Precancer and cancer in extensive ulcerative colitis: findings among 401 patients over 22 years. Gut. 1990;31:800–6.
4. Winther KV, Jess T, Langholtz E, et al. Long-term risk of cancer in ulcerative colitis: a population based cohort study from Copenhagen county. Clin Gastroenterol Hepatol. 2004;2:1088–95.
5. Lakatos L, Mester G, Erdelyi Z, et al. Risk factors for ulcerative colitis-associated colorectal cancer in a Hungarian Cohort of patients with ulcerative colitis: results of a population-based study. Inflamm Bowel Dis. 2006;12:205–11.
6. Rutter M, Saunders B, Wilkinson K, et al. Thirty-year analysis of a colonoscopic surveillance program for neoplasia in ulcerative colitis. Gastroenterology. 2006;130:1030–8.
7. Gyde SN, Prior P, Allan RN, et al. Colorectal cancer in ulcerative colitis: a cohort study of primary referrals from three centres. Gut. 1988;29:206–17.
8. Higashi D, Futami K, Ishibashi Y, et al. Clinical course of colorectal cancer in patients with ulcerative colitis. Anticancer Res. 2011;31:2499–504.
9. Gupta RB, Harpaz N, Itzkowitz S, et al. Histologic inflammation is a risk factor for progression to colorectal neoplasia in ulcerative colitis: a cohort study. Gastroenterology. 2007;133:1099–105.
10. Rutter M, Saunders B, Wilkinson K, et al. Severity of inflammation is a risk factor for colorectal neoplasia in ulcerative colitis. Gastroenterology. 2004;126:451–9.
11. Rutter MD, Saunders BP, Wilkinson KH, et al. Most dysplasia in ulcerative colitis is visible at colonoscopy. Gastrointest Endosc. 2004;60:334–9.
12. Cairns SR, Scholefield JH, Steele RJ, et al. Guidelines for colorectal cancer screening and surveillance in moderate and high risk groups (updated from 2002). Gut. 2010;59:666–89.
13. Choi PM, Nugent FW, Schoetz DJ, et al. Colonoscopic surveillance reduces mortality from colorectal cancer in ulcerative colitis. Gastroenterology. 1993;105:418–24.
14. Lutgens MW, Oldenburg B, Siersema PD, et al. Colonoscopic surveillance improves survival after colorectal cancer diagnosis in inflammatory bowel disease. Br J Cancer. 2009;101:1671–5.
15. Matsumoto T, Iwao Y, Igarashi M, et al. Endoscopic and chromoendoscopic atlas featuring dysplastic lesions in surveillance colonoscopy for patients with long-standing ulcerative colitis. Inflamm Bowel Dis. 2008;14:259–64.
16. Blackstone MO, Riddell RH, Rogers BHG, et al. Dysplasia-associated lesion or mass (DALM) detected by colonoscopy in long-standing ulcerative colitis: an indication for colectomy. Gastroenterology. 1981;80:366–74.
17. Rutter M, Saunders BP, Schofield G, et al. Pancolonic indigo carmine dye spraying for the detection of dysplasia in ulcerative colitis. Gut. 2004;53:256–60.
18. Matsumoto T, Nakamura S, Jo Y, et al. Chromoscopy might improve diagnostic accuracy in cancer surveillance for ulcerative colitis. Am J Gastroenterol. 2003;98:1827–33.
19. Ekbom A, Helmick C, Zack M, Adami HO. Increased risk of large bowel cancer in Crohn's disease with colonic involvement. Lancet. 1990;336:357–9.
20. Persson PG, Karlen P, Bernell O, et al. Crohn's disease and cancer: a population based cohort study. Gastroenterology. 1994;107:1675–9.
21. Munkholm P, Langholz E, Davidsen M, Binder V. Intestinal cancer risk and mortality in patients with Crohn's disease. Gastroenterology. 1993;105:1716–23.
22. Fireman Z, Grossman A, Lilos P, et al. Intestinal cancer in patients with Crohn's disease. Scand J Gastroenterol. 1989;24:346–50.
23. Jess T, Winther KV, Munkholm P, et al. Intestinal and extra-intestinal cancer in Crohn's disease: follow-up of a population-based cohort in Copenhagen county, Denmark. Aliment Pharmacol Ther. 2004;19:287–93.
24. Gillen CD, Walmsley RS, Prior P, et al. Ulcerative colitis and Crohn's disease: a comparison of the colorectal cancer risk in extensive colitis. Gut. 1994;35:1507–8.
25. Canavan C, Abrams KR, Mayberry J. Meta-analysis: colorectal and small bowel cancer risk in patients with Crohn's disease. Aliment Pharmacol Ther. 2006;23:1097–104.
26. Friedman S, Rubin PH, Bodian C, et al. Screening and surveillance colonoscopy in chronic Crohn's colitis. Gastroenterology. 2001;120:820–6.
27. Friedman S, Rubin PH, Bodian C, et al. Screening and surveillance colonoscopy in chronic Crohn's colitis: results of a surveillance program spanning 25 years. Clin Gastroenterol Hepatol. 2008;6:993–8.
28. Yano Y, Matsui T, Uno H, et al. Risks and clinical features of colorectal cancer complicating Crohn's disease in Japanese patients. J Gastroenterol Hepatol. 2008;23:1683–8.
29. Yano Y, Matsui T, Hirai F, Okado Y, et al. Cancer risk in Japanese Crohn's disease patients: investigation of the standardized incidence ratio. J Gastroenterol Hepatol. 2013;28:1300–5.
30. Nishimura T, Matsui T, Hirai F, et al. Radiographic diagnosis of ulcerative colitis associated neoplasia. Stomach Intestine 2008;43:1281–92.
31. Higashi D, Futami K, Ishibashi Y, et al. Clinical course of colorectal cancer in patients with ulcerative colitis. Anticancer Res 2011;31:2499–504.
32. Higashi D, Futami K, Kojima D, et al. Cancer of the small intestine in patients with Crohn's disease. Anticancer Res. 2013;33:2977–80.
33. Yao S, Iwashita A, Nishimura T, et al. Colo-rectal cancer complicated with Crohn's disease. Stomach Intestine 2002;37:1047–58.
34. Futami K, Higashi D, Egawa Y et al. Intestinal cancer in patients with Crohn's disease: Diagnosis, treatment and prognosis. Anticancer Res. 2013;33:2977–80.

14 Surgery in Inflammatory Bowel Diseases

Eun Jung Park and Seung Hyuk Baik

14.1 Crohn's Disease

14.1.1 Introduction

Surgical treatment is required when medical therapy fails or complications such as free perforation, obstruction, hemorrhage, and severe inflammation or acute fulminant colitis require surgical treatments. Chronic complications such as recurrent bowel obstruction and neoplasia can also be surgical indications. Surgical treatments of Crohn's disease are divided into two main procedures: bowel-sparing surgery and resection of the involved bowel. Proper surgical indications and optimal timing for surgery are still controversial and continuously evolving.

14.1.2 Bowel-Sparing Surgery for Crohn's Disease

14.1.2.1 Strictureplasty

Strictureplasty is a bowel-sparing technique to conserve and minimize resected bowel segments. The principle is the enlargement of the narrowed bowel lumen to prevent bowel resection. A surgical technique, strictureplasty, was developed because the repeated recurrence of Crohn's disease causes frequent bowel resections, short bowel syndrome, and related nutritional deficiency.

Most strictureplasties are carried out for small bowel diseases. Jejunoileal stricture is known as the most frequent site to perform a strictureplasty [29]. Although colonic disease has lower risks for malabsorption than small bowel disease, the length of remaining viable bowel is still important to perform a strictureplasty.

The types of strictureplasty are decided by the number of strictures, the length of each stricture, the degree of inflammation of involved bowel segments, and the relationship among bowel strictures.

Surgical Indications for Strictureplasty

Surgical indications for strictureplasty are multiple strictures of the small bowel, previous significant bowel resection more than 100 cm, patients with short bowel syndrome, strictures without inflammatory lesions with a forming fistula or phlegmon, strictures at prior anastomotic sites, and growth retardation [8, 28, 39].

The contraindications are related to the nutritional status of patients, active disease progression, and complicated symptoms. The symptoms include perforation of the small bowel with or without peritonitis, malnutrition (serum albumin level <2.0 g/dl), fistula or phlegmon at the operative site, short distance of stricture near the segment requiring bowel resection, likelihood of anastomotic tension after strictureplasty, hemorrhage of stricture site, and malignant transformation of stricture site.

Surgical Techniques

The types are decided by the number of strictures, the length of each stricture, the degree of inflammation of involved bowel segments, and the relationship among bowel strictures. The strictureplasty can be categorized from the length of strictures and can be summarized as follows (Table 14.1).

The Heineke-Mikulicz (HM) strictureplasty is a conventional technique, which is most commonly used for short-segment strictures less than 10 cm [3, 19, 21] (Fig. 14.1).

E.J. Park, MD • S.H. Baik, MD, PhD (✉)
Section of Colon and Rectal Surgery, Department of Surgery, Yonsei University College of Medicine, Seoul, South Korea
e-mail: whitenoja@yuhs.ac

W.H. Kim, J.H. Cheon (eds.), *Atlas of Inflammatory Bowel Diseases*,
DOI 10.1007/978-3-642-39423-2_14, © Springer-Verlag Berlin Heidelberg 2015

The Judd strictureplasty is a useful technique for a short-segment stricture with a fistulous opening (Fig. 14.2).

The Moskel-Walske-Neumayer strictureplasty can adjust the narrow distal bowel lumen into the enlarged proximal lumen throughout the "Y"-shaped enterotomy (Fig. 14.3).

The Finney strictureplasty is a procedure for an intermediate stricture from 10 to 25 cm in length by a side-to-side approach. The "U"-shaped enterotomy and anastomosis creates a blind pouch, which can resolve the stricture (Fig. 14.4).

The Jaboulay strictureplasty is a procedure for intermediate bowel stricture like the Finney strictureplasty. However, the difference of the Jaboulay strictureplasty is the anastomotic site, which is performed with relatively healthy bowels and not including stricture sites. After facing the antimesenteric border of the bowel including the stricture site, an enterotomy is performed by a longitudinal incision of a separated healthy bowel (Fig. 14.5).

Side-to-side isoperistaltic strictureplasty is a procedure for long segments of strictures more than 20–25 cm [25] (Fig. 14.6). The Poggioli strictureplasty is a modified procedure of Michelassi's side-to-side isoperistaltic strictureplasty [27] (Fig. 14.7). The Sasaki strictureplasty is a modified side-to-side isoperistaltic anastomosis with double HM strictureplasty [32] (Fig. 14.8). The Hotokezaka strictureplasty is for a long strictured segment, which needs a bowel resection simultaneously due to severe adhesion, abscess, or intestinal fistula [12] (Fig. 14.9).

Postoperative Outcomes

The rates of recurrence requiring a reoperation were estimated at 11–32 % at 5 years, 20–44 % at 10 years, and 46–55 % at 20 years ([22, 38], [42], [98]). According to the meta-analysis of outcomes after a strictureplasty for Crohn's disease, the rate of symptomatic recurrence after a jejunoileal strictureplasty was 39 % of the patients, and the cumulative reoperation rate was 41 % at 5 years and 51 % at 10 years [43].

Septic complications such as anastomotic leakage, enteroenteric fistula, and abscess after a jejunoileal strictureplasty can occur [7, 13, 35, 37, 40]. However, the rate of septic conditions after a strictureplasty was reported in 3–50 % of the patients, which was similar with that after a bowel resection [5, 30, 41]. Hemorrhage, wound infection, or bowel obstruction can also occur after a strictureplasty. Concerns of malignant transformation of the strictureplasty sites also matter because patients with Crohn's disease are at a high risk of malignancy and are exposed to immunomodulators for a long time. However, the incidence of carcinoma after strictureplasty is extremely rare since only two cases were reported where adenocarcinoma occurred at the site of strictureplasty [17, 24].

14.1.2.2 Bypass or Exclusion

A bypass or exclusion surgery was used for ileocecal Crohn's disease in the past. However, at present, bypass surgery is not recommended any longer because of the higher incidence of septic conditions after surgery and the risk of malignant transformation in the bypassed segment [1, 9, 11]. It is performed very limitedly in gastroduodenal Crohn's disease because of the immobilization of the second and third portion.

Table 14.1 Strictureplasty compared by the length of strictures

Short segments: <10 cm	Heineke-Mikulicz (HM) strictureplasty Judd strictureplasty Moskel-Walske-Neumayer strictureplasty
Intermediate segments: 10–25 cm	Finney strictureplasty Jaboulay strictureplasty
Long segments: >25 cm (side-to-side isoperistaltic strictureplasty)	Michelassi's strictureplasty Poggioli strictureplasty Sasaki strictureplasty Hotokezaka strictureplasty

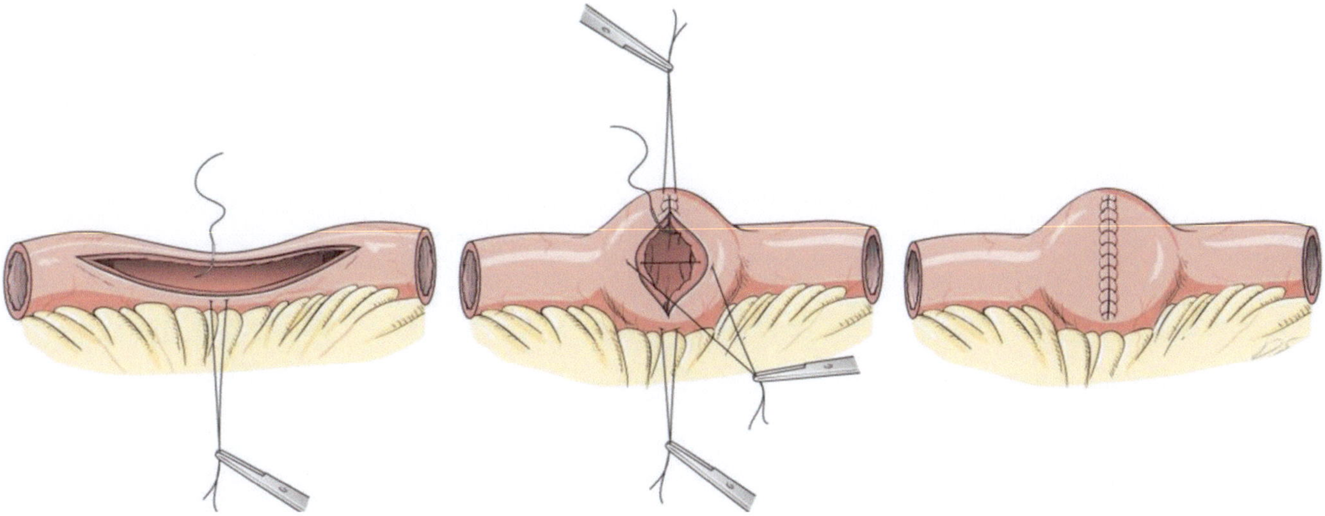

Fig. 14.1 Heineke-Mikulicz strictureplasty

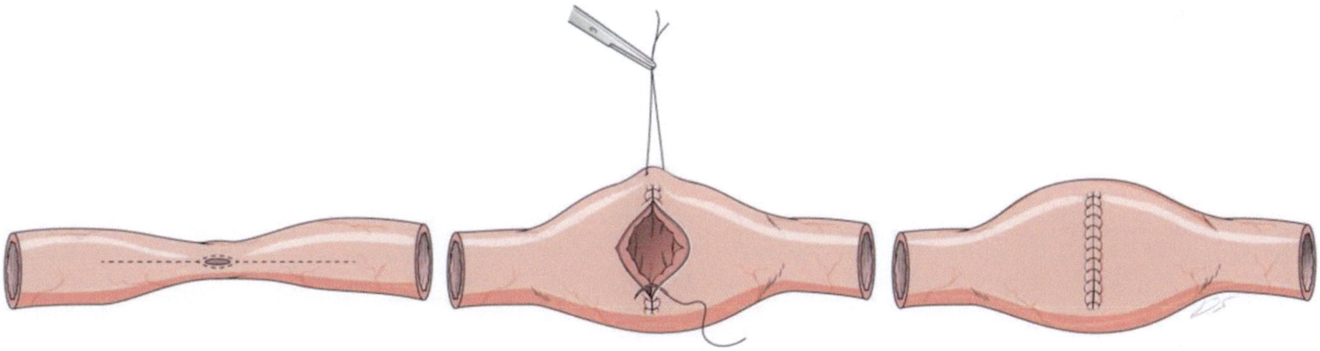

Fig. 14.2 Judd strictureplasty

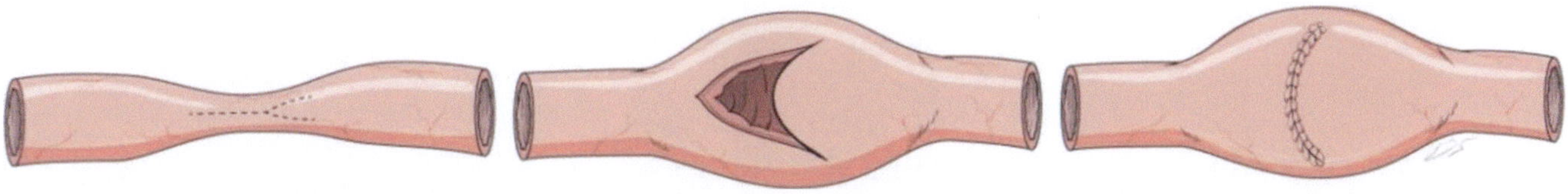

Fig. 14.3 Moskel-Walske-Neumayer strictureplasty

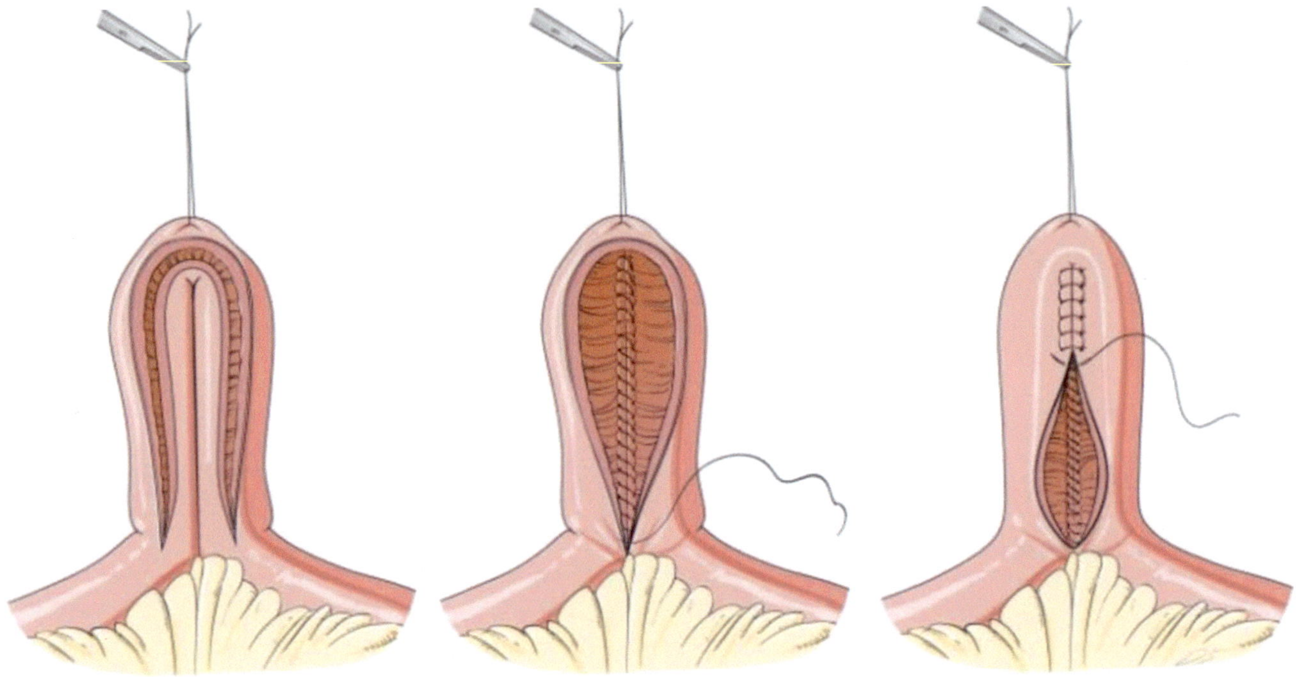

Fig. 14.4 Finney strictureplasty

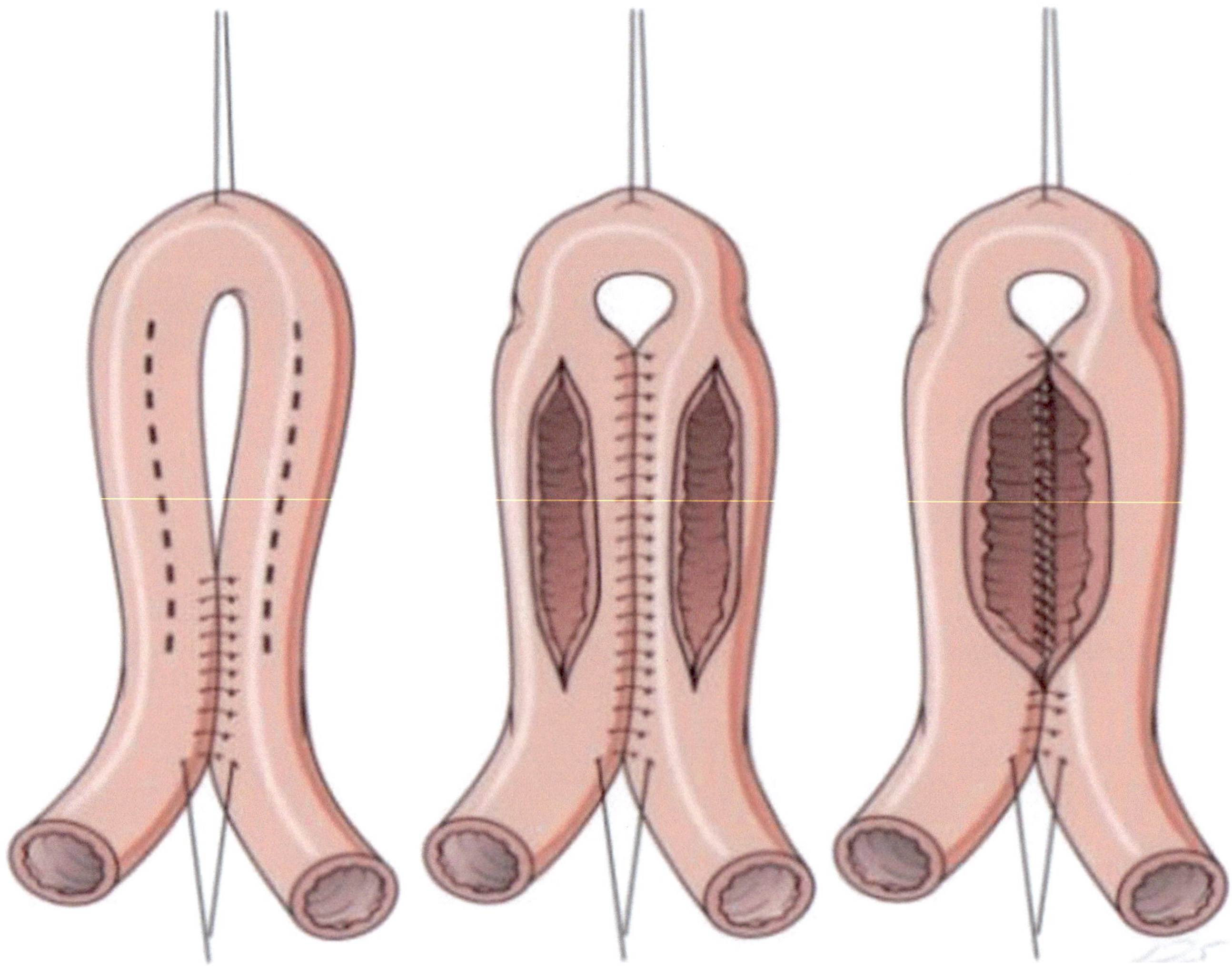

Fig. 14.5 Jaboulay strictureplasty

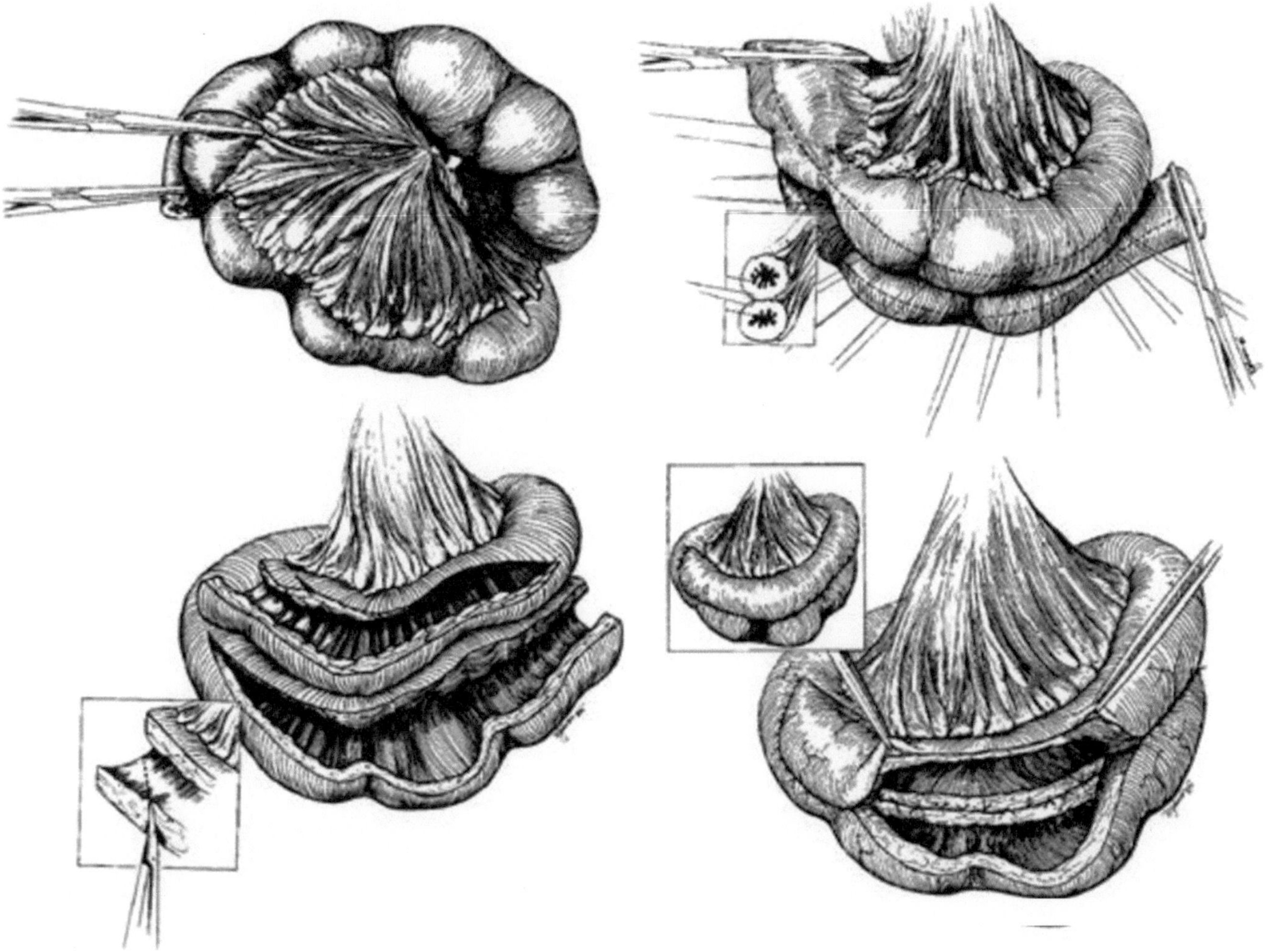

Fig. 14.6 Michelassi's strictureplasty (side-to-side isoperistaltic strictureplasty) (Printed with permission from Fabrizio Michelassi, MD)

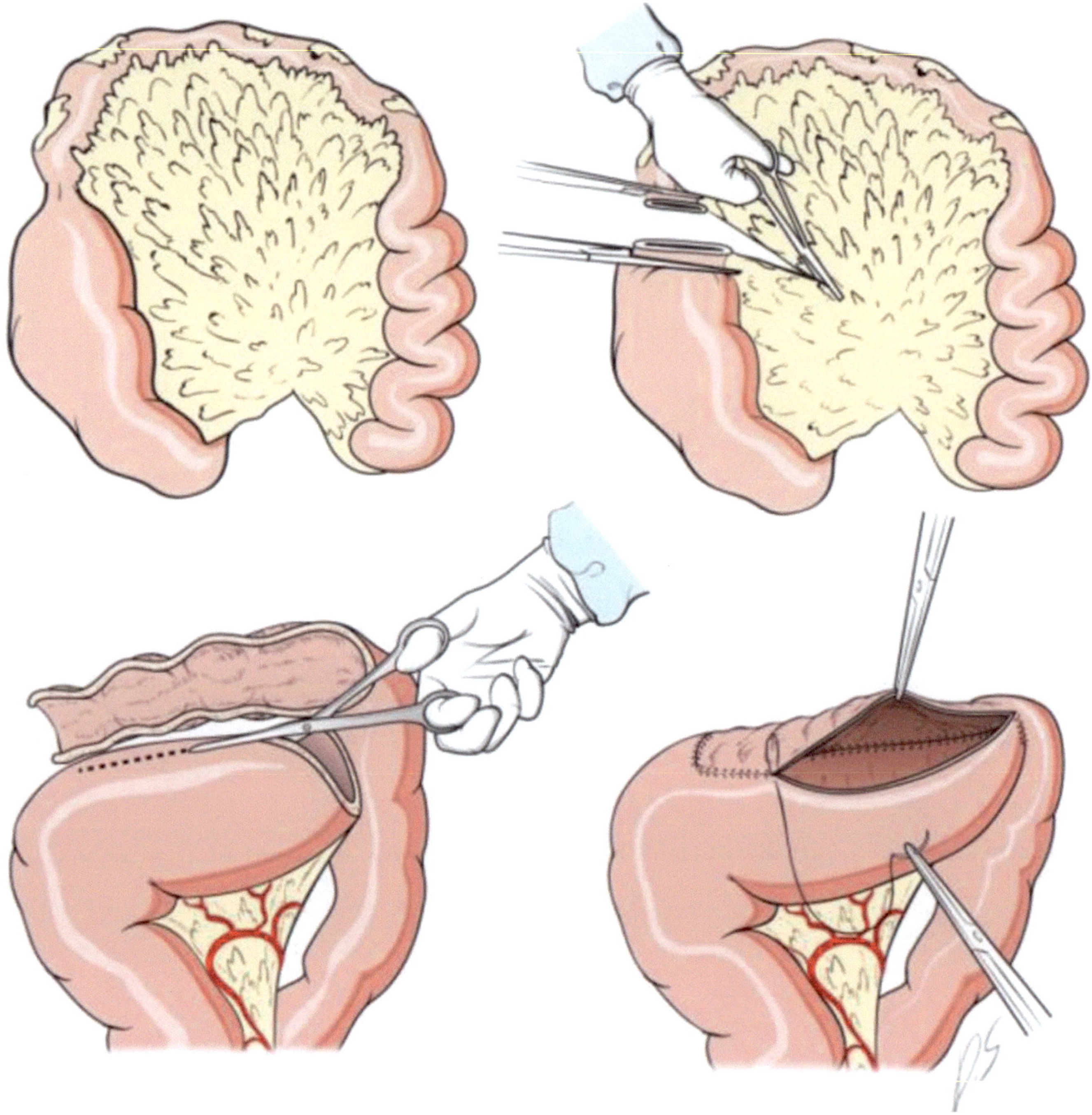

Fig. 14.7 Poggioli strictureplasty (side-to-side diseased to disease-free anastomosis)

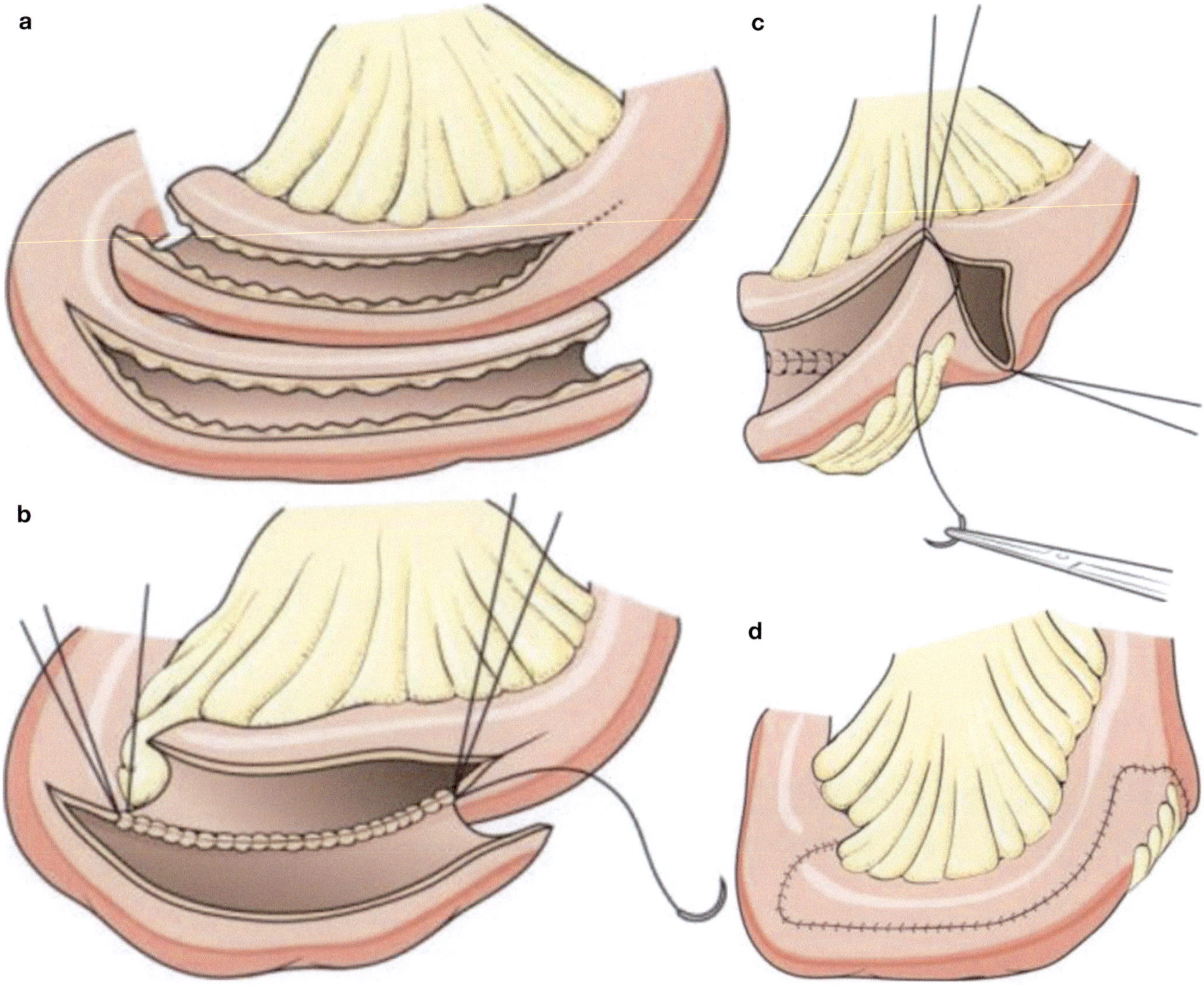

Fig. 14.8 Sasaki strictureplasty (side-to-side isoperistaltic strictureplasty with double HM strictureplasty). (**a**) The two intestinal loops are placed in a side-to-side isoperistaltic direction. (**b**) Approximated at the posterior wall of the adjacent bowels. (**c**) The end of the anastomotic site is closed transversely in the way of an HM strictureplasty. (**d**) The circumferences of both bowel ends become nonspatulated and lengthened

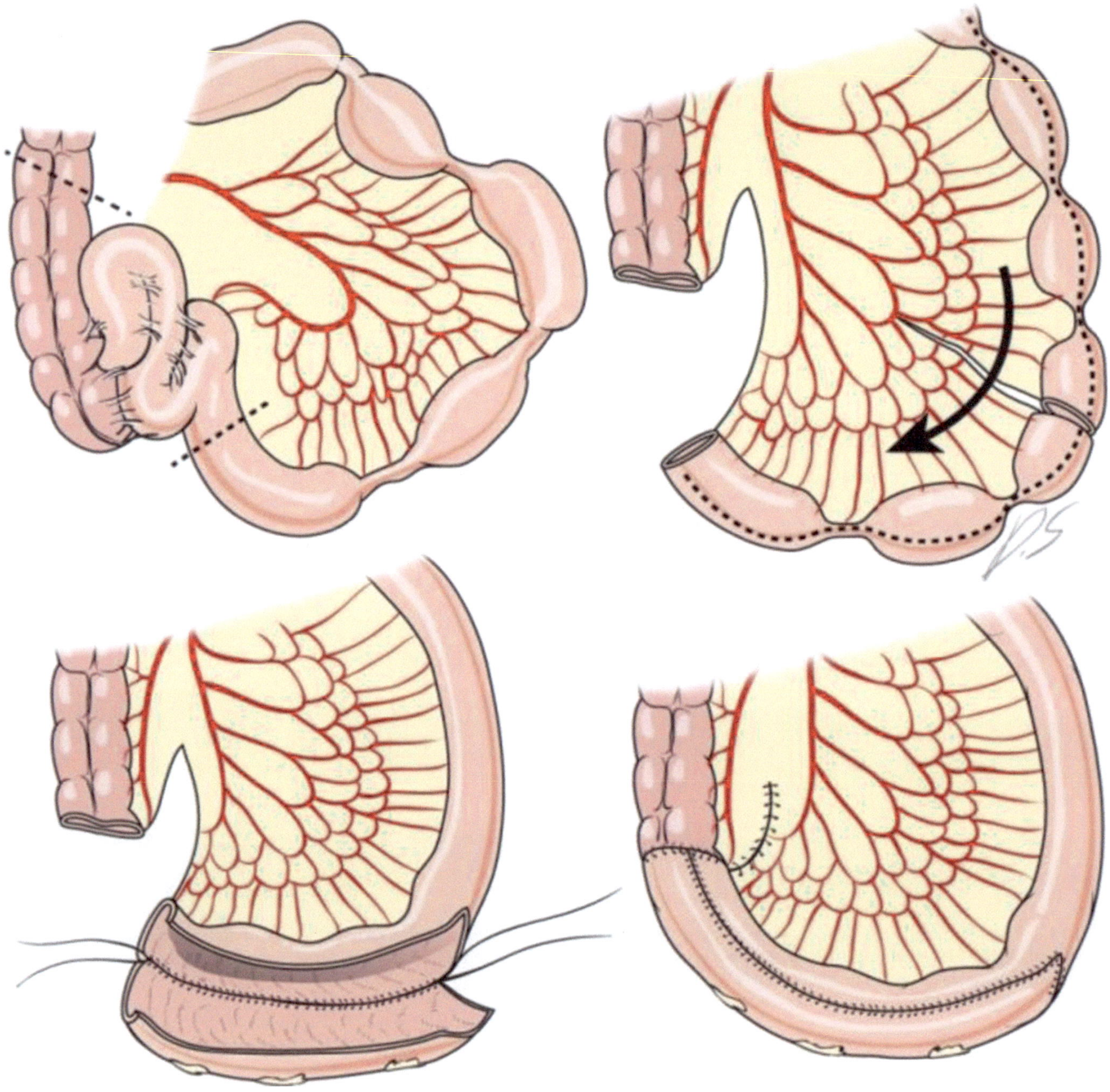

Fig. 14.9 Hotokezaka strictureplasty (side-to-side-to-end strictureplasty)

14.1.3 Resection of Involved Bowel Segment

Resection of a diseased bowel segment is the most frequently performed operation for patients with Crohn's disease. This is a surgical procedure when strictureplasty is not feasible or indicated. Preoperative evaluation to make an accurate diagnosis of the involved bowel segment is difficult. This is because patients with Crohn's disease experience transmural inflammatory bowel change with a thickened mesentery and fat wrapping (Fig. 14.10). Both the location and the extent of the diseased bowel are important to determine proper surgical procedures.

14.1.3.1 Surgical Indications

Resection of the involved bowel segment for Crohn's disease is performed in patients with bowel perforation, hemorrhage, intestinal fistula, toxic megacolon, bowel obstruction, and/or failure of medical therapy. In the situation of urgent surgery as well as elective surgery, bowel resection is usually done with a certain risk of short bowel syndrome. Stone et al. reported that chronic obstruction is the most common indication of bowel resection among patients when the small bowel is involved in Crohn's disease [36].

14.1.3.2 Surgical Techniques

The main gastrointestinal lesions of Crohn's disease are the small bowel, the ileocolonic, and the large bowel. Due to the inflammatory change of bowel segments, a thickened mesentery and fat wrapping are occasionally obstacles in identifying the vessels using clamps. Therefore, the finger fracture technique can be used (Fig. 14.11). After transillumination of the mesentery, the structure of the blood supply is identified in small bowel resection. Then the intestine and mesentery are divided by clamps, and an anastomosis is performed using a stapler or by the hand-sewn method (Fig. 14.12).

A prospective study for long-term results of stapled and hand-sewn anastomoses in patients with Crohn's disease reported that the postoperative recurrence rate of the stapled anastomosis group was lower than the hand-sewn group [14]. These results assume that a wider lumen of stapled anastomosis can bring out the lower rate of stasis and bacterial overgrowth, which can cause disease recurrence after resection [2] (Fig. 14.13).

14.1.3.3 Postoperative Outcomes

The advantage of resectional surgery is to get healthy disease-free margins for anastomosis and macroscopically clear margins. However, it was reported that the presence of diseased or disease-free margins does not influence postoperative recurrence [4, 8, 30]. There is controversy with the association of recurrence between limited resection (Fig. 14.14) and en bloc wide radical resection.

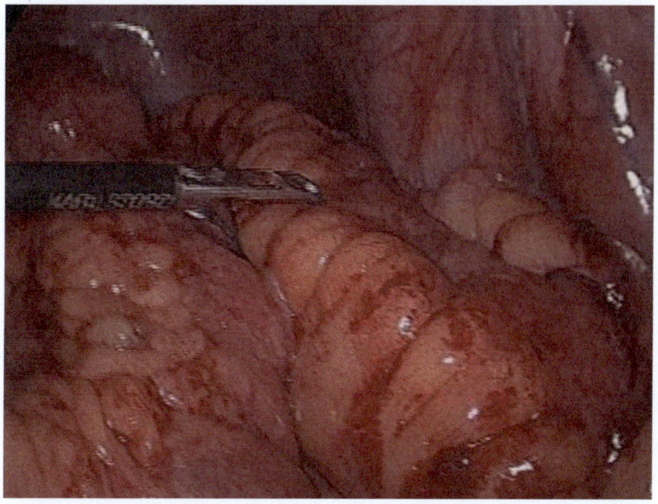

Fig. 14.10 Thickened mesentery and fat wrapping of the bowel in a patient with Crohn's disease

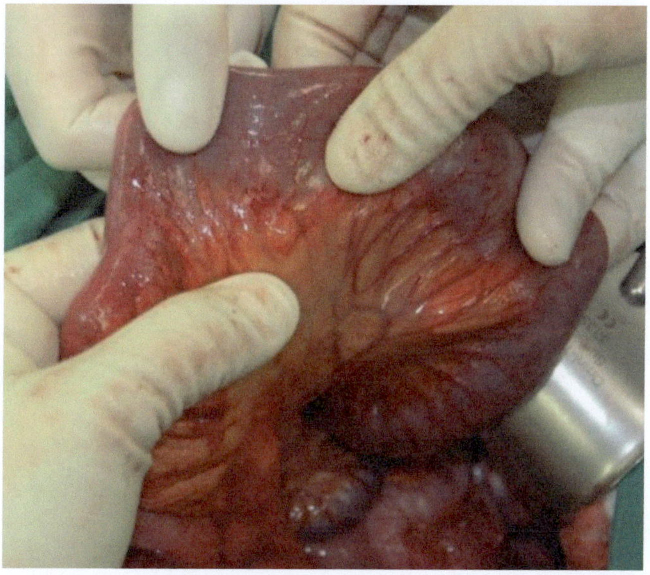

Fig. 14.11 Finger fracture technique

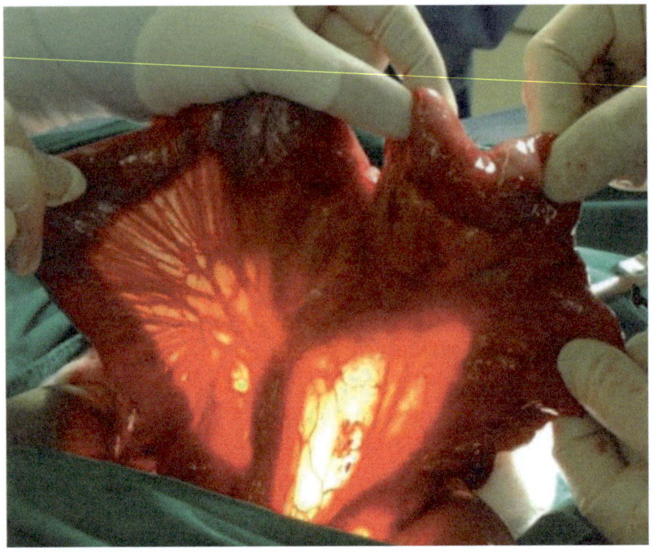

Fig. 14.12 Transillumination of the mesentery in identifying the blood supply

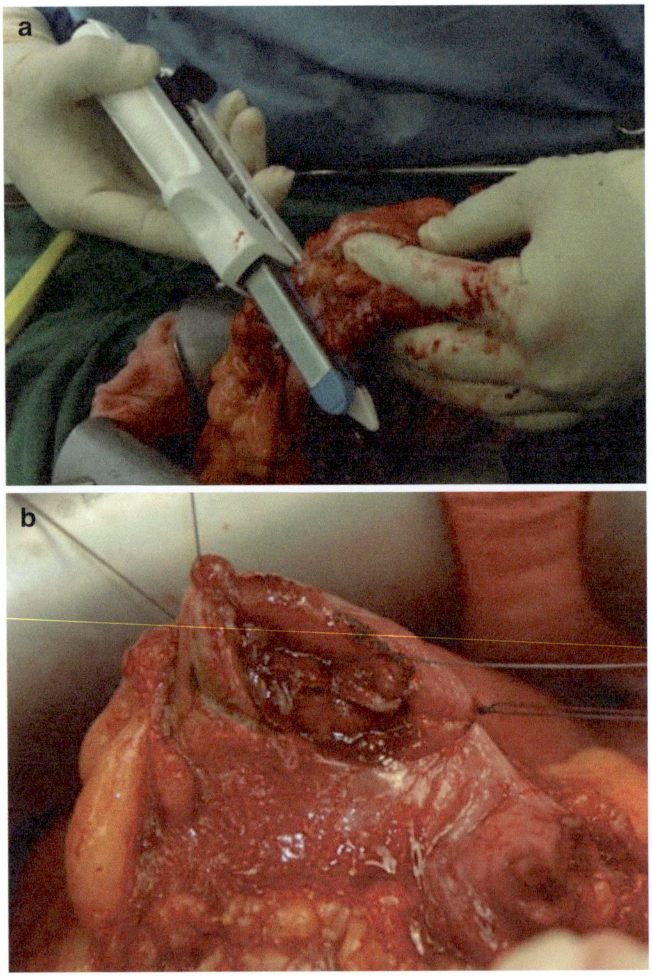

Fig. 14.13 The anastomotic technique: (**a**) stapled anastomosis vs. (**b**) Hand-sewn anastomosis

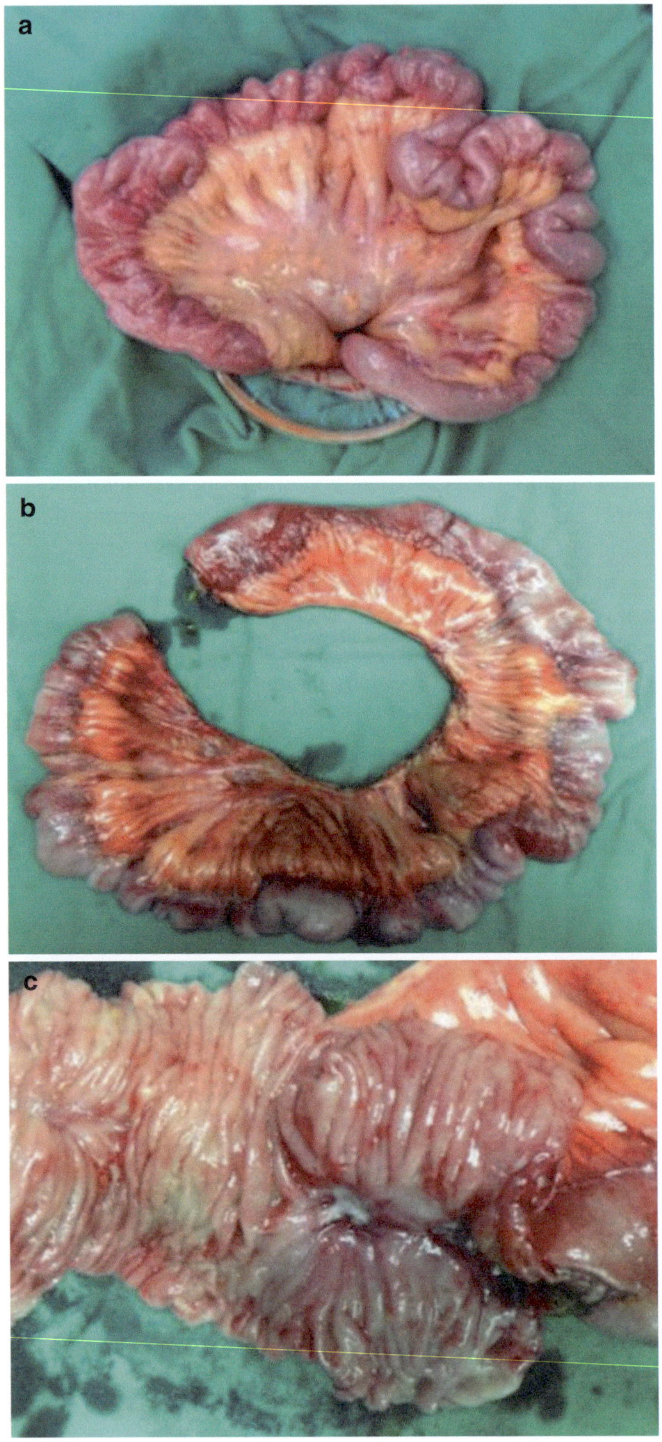

Fig. 14.14 Limited resection of the small bowel involving multiple strictures. (**a**) Extracted specimen through minilaparotomy. (**b**) Resected specimen. (**c**) Luminal feature of the small bowel involving stricture

14.1.4 Surgery for Perianal Crohn's Disease

Perianal manifestations of Crohn's disease are divided into primary and secondary lesions. Primary lesions include anal fissures and perianal ulcers. Secondary lesions are combined perianal lesions with fistulas, strictures, or perianal abscess. The principle of surgery is to achieve adequate drainage of sepsis and to preserve sphincter function without damage [33].

14.1.4.1 Surgical Indications

Crohn's perianal diseases, including skin tags, hemorrhoids, anal fissures, anorectal strictures, perianal abscesses, anorectal strictures, rectovaginal fistulas, and cancer, are potential indications for surgical management [31]. There are four categories for surgical indications: emergency treatment, "bridge" surgery, definitive treatment, and resection of proximal intestinal resection. Emergency treatment includes incision and drainage of an abscess [33]. "Bridge" surgery is managing and treating active inflammatory lesions after stabilization of the disease. Fistulotomy and flap repair of a fistula and internal sphincterotomy are indications for definitive surgery. Intestinal resection, including a proctocolectomy or a proximal bowel resection, is performed as an invasive procedure of perianal surgical treatment.

14.1.4.2 Surgical Techniques

Incision and Drainage

The main principle of incision and drainage of perianal disease is to make adequate elimination of septic conditions and to avoid sphincter damage. It is used in the acute phase and when treatment is needed immediately. Combined surgical treatments with broad-spectrum antibiotics are recommended (Fig. 14.15).

Lateral Internal Sphincterotomy

Acute and painless anal fissures are responsive to conservative therapy, which is known to be effective in the majority of patients. However, if the patients have pain due to the fissure itself, without macroscopically rectal inflammation, a lateral internal sphincterotomy can be indicated [31]. The incision of this procedure is made across the intersphincteric groove with separation of the internal sphincter from the anal mucosa (Fig. 14.16).

Fistulotomy and Fistulectomy

The surgical management of perianal fistulas in patients with Crohn's disease is decided by the presence or absence of inflammatory change of the rectum and the type and location of the fistulas. Perianal fistulas can be classified as superficial, intersphincteric, trans-sphincteric, supra-sphincteric, and extra-sphincteric fistula by Park's anatomical classification, which regards the external anal sphincter as the central reference point [26] (Fig. 14.17). The disease activity and severity of perianal Crohn's disease can be assessed by the Perianal Crohn's Disease Activity Index (PCDAI) [16] (Table 14.2).

A simple fistula is a low superficial type such as low inter- or intra-sphincteric lesions with a single external opening, which are not connected to adjacent organs such as the vagina or bladder. A complex fistula is a high type as high inter- or intra-sphincteric, supra-sphincteric, and extra-sphincteric lesions, which have several external openings [37]. Patients who have low fistulas may be treated by a one- or two-stage fistulotomy (Fig. 14.18).

Seton Procedure

The seton procedure is a surgical technique for Crohn's fistula to maintain proper pus drainage continuously and to avoid perianal abscess formation by using a seton drain. There are two kinds of seton procedures: the noncutting (loose) seton (Fig. 14.19) and the cutting seton (Fig. 14.20). The noncutting seton procedure is performed by a drain insertion through the fistula tract. According to the noncutting seton procedure, the drain is threaded into the cutaneous opening of a perianal fistula across the mucosal orifice of the fistula tract in the rectum. Then after the drain moves to the anal canal, the two ends of the drain are loosely tied. The cutting seton procedure is performed by tying the ends of the noncutting seton tightly, which can result in a slow fistulotomy by pressure necrosis [31].

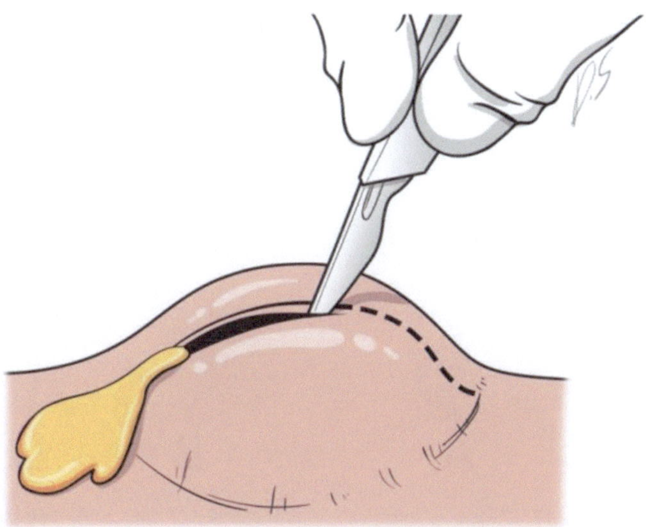

Fig. 14.15 Incision and drainage for perianal abscess

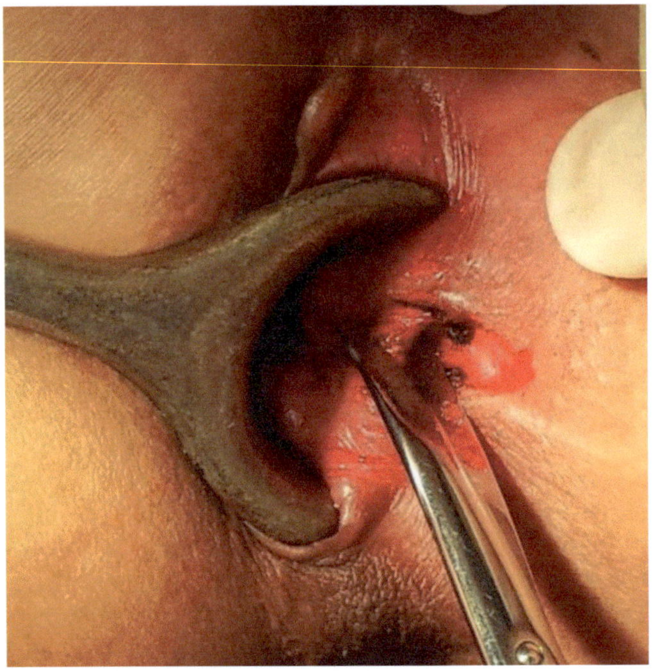

Fig. 14.16 Lateral internal sphincterotomy

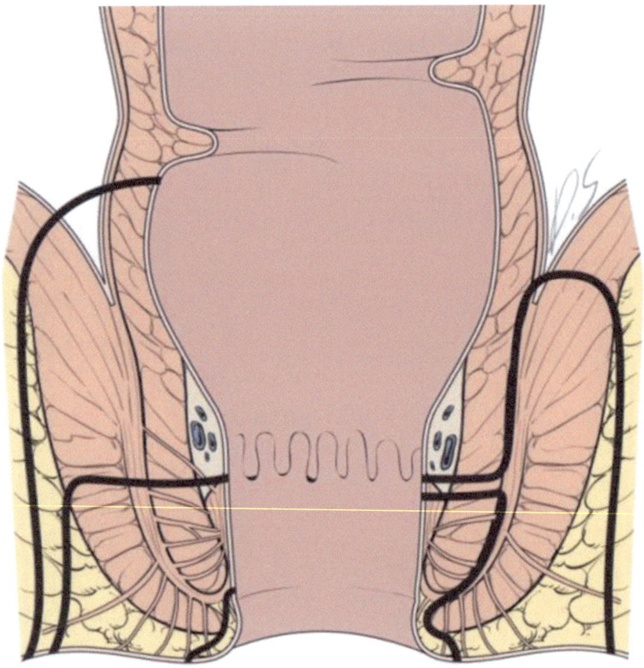

Fig. 14.17 Park's anatomical classification of perianal fistula. *A* Superficial fistula, *B* intersphincteric fistula, *C* transsphincteric fistula, *D* supra-sphincteric fistula, *E* extra-sphincteric fistula

Table 14.2 Perianal Crohn's Disease Activity Index

Perianal disease activity
Discharge
0 No discharge
1 Minimal mucous discharge
2 Moderate mucous or purulent discharge
3 Substantial discharge
4 Gross fecal soiling
Pain/restriction of activities
0 No activity restriction
1 Mild discomfort, no restriction
2 Mod. discomfort, some limitation activities
3 Marked discomfort, marked limitation
4 Severe pain, severe limitation
Restriction of sexual activity
0 No restriction sexual activity
1 Slight restriction sexual activity
2 Mod. limitation sexual activity
3 Marked limitation sexual activity
4 Unable to engage in sexual activity
Type of perianal disease
0 No perianal disease/skin tags
1 Anal fissure or mucosal tear
2 <3 Perianal fistulas
3 ≥3 Perianal fistulas
4 Anal sphincter ulceration or fistulas with significant undermining of skin
Degree of induration
0 No induration
1 Minimal induration
2 Moderate induration
3 Substantial induration
4 Gross fluctuance/abscess
Total score

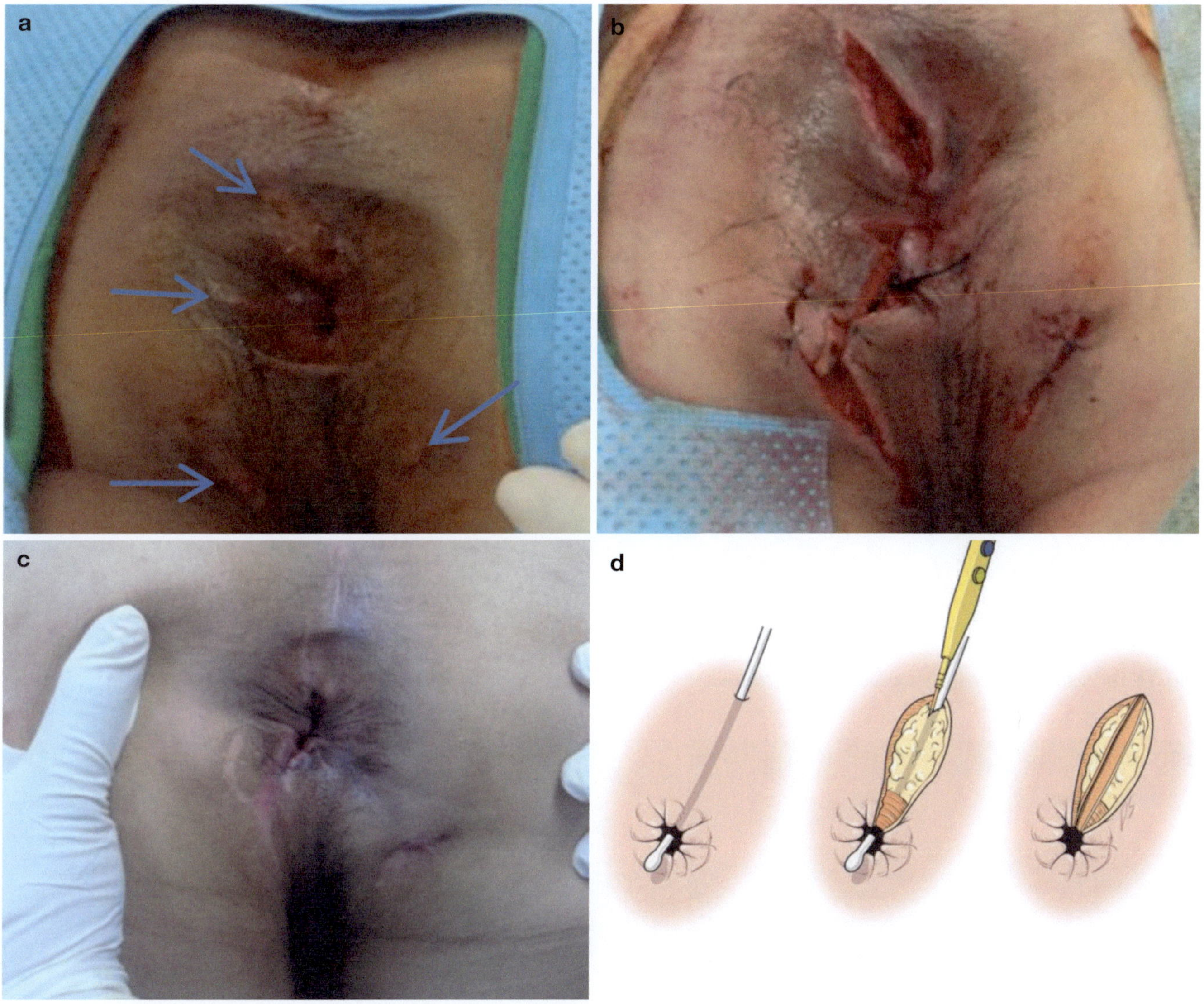

Fig. 14.18 Fistulotomy with the seton procedure. (**a**) Preoperative finding. (**b**) Immediate postoperative finding. (**c**) Postoperative finding after 6 months (*arrow*; external opening, fistula at 5 o'clock was treated by coring-out fistulectomy). (**d**) Schematic figure of fistulotomy for intersphincteric fistula

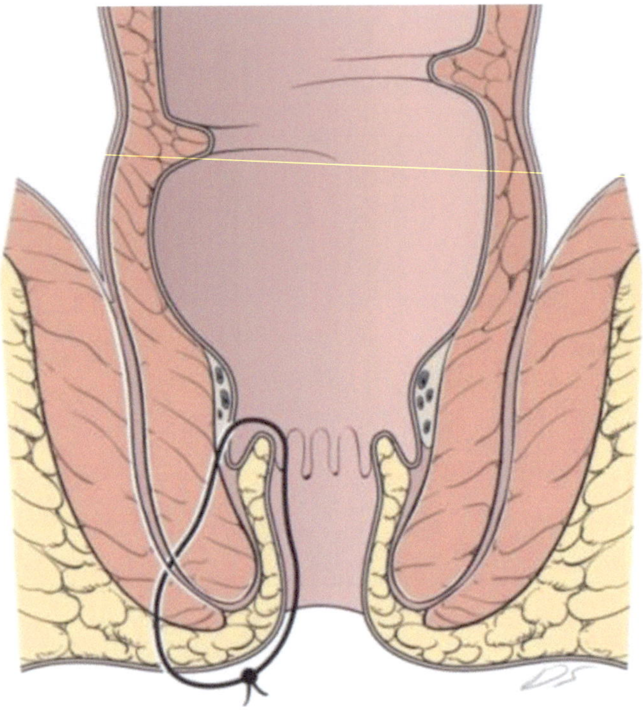

Fig. 14.19 Seton procedure: the noncutting (loose) seton

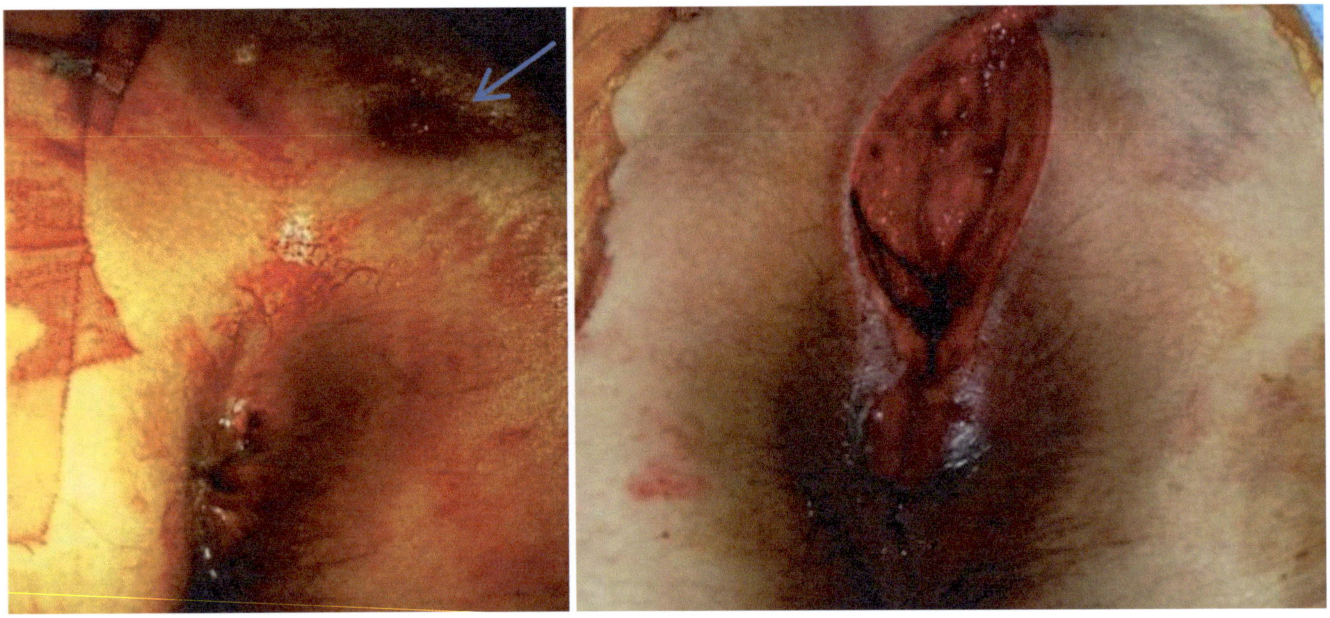

Fig. 14.20 Combined the cutting seton procedure with a fistulotomy (*arrow*; external opening)

Endorectal Mucosal Advancement Flaps

High fistulas have a higher incidence of incontinence and recurrence of fistulas. Therefore, a technique to fulfill the fistula tract by using an endorectal mucosal flap was developed (Fig. 14.21). The advantages of endorectal advancement flaps are that the open wounds are avoided and several problems are prevented by dividing the sphincteric strictures, which can cause incontinence after surgery.

Fibrin Glue Treatment of Complex Perianal Fistulas

Fibrin glue has been used as a sphincter-preserving approach for anal fistulas. This technique begins by evaluating internal and external fistulous openings. After tracing the fistula tract, instilled fibrin glue is filled into the tract [10]. The efficacy is still controversial due to the different results according to the fistula types.

Adipose-Derived Stem Cell Transplantation

Autologous adipose-derived stem cell transplantation in patients with refractory Crohn's disease has been developed since Crohn's disease is an immunologically mediated inflammatory disease. This procedure is delivered by injection of adipose-derived stem cells around the fistula opening and directly into the fistula tract.

14.1.4.3 Postoperative Outcomes

The healing rates of complex fistulas are reported as 47–67 % from the results of the seton procedure and maintenance therapy [34]. Patients who have low fistulas are treated by a one- or two-stage fistulotomy and high fistulas by a more conservative surgical therapy to reduce the risk of incontinence. The rate of incontinence after a fistulotomy is known to be about 50 % of the cases. The seton procedure is useful for continuous pus drainage and reducing the risk of perianal abscess formation.

The results of endorectal mucosal advancement flap were reported as an initial healing rate of 64–89 % and the recurrence rate of up to 50 % [23, 34]. The flap failure was associated with Crohn's colitis, active small bowel Crohn's disease, and proctitis [18]. Active perianal fistulas and long-standing duration of chronic fistulas are associated with the development of anorectal carcinoma in Crohn's disease [15, 31]. The malignancy of Crohn's perianal disease is reported as squamous cell carcinoma, basal cell carcinoma, and adenocarcinoma. Ky et al. reported the incidence of malignancy was 0.7 %, when 1,000 patients with perianal Crohn's disease were evaluated during 14 years [20].

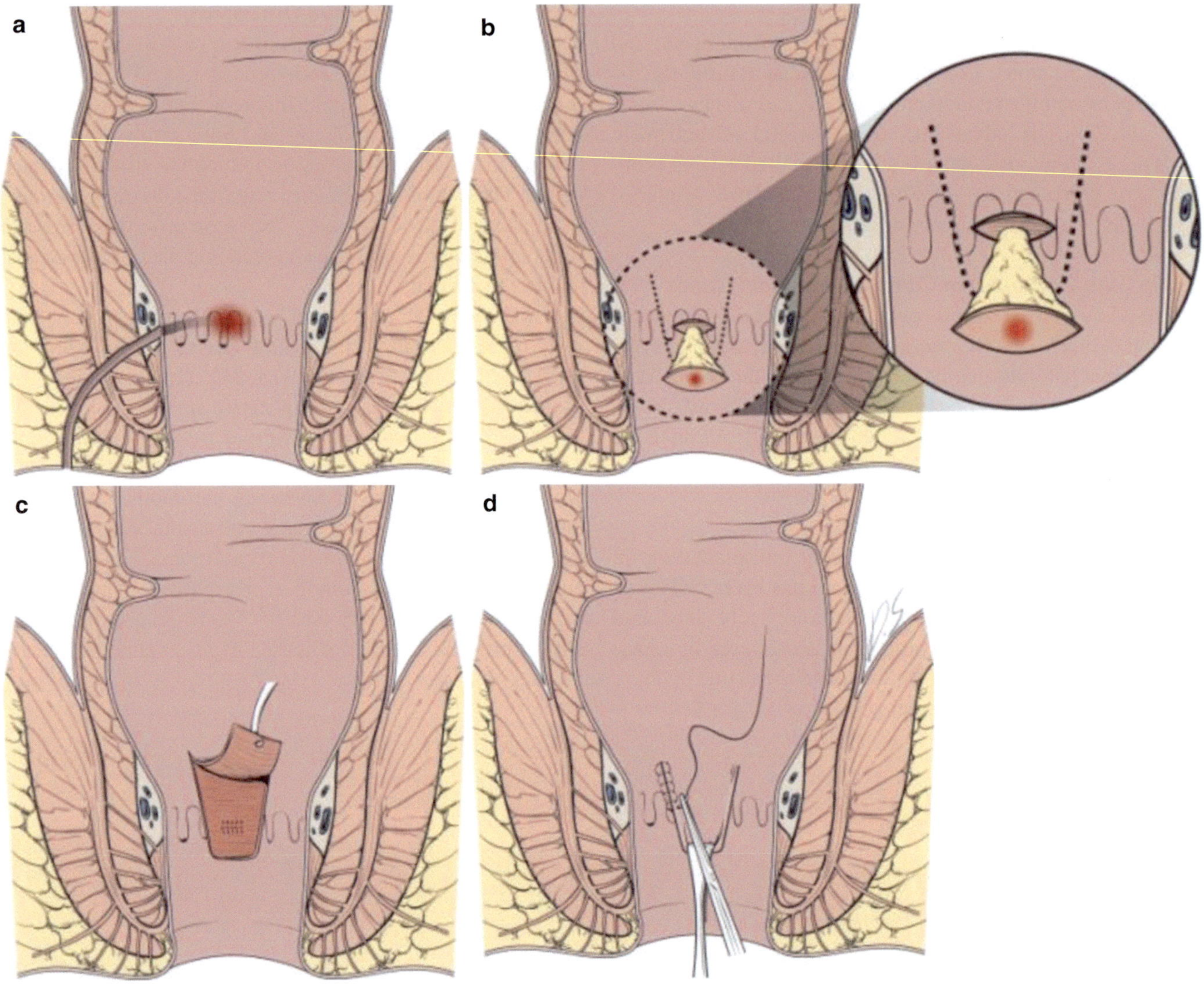

Fig. 14.21 Endorectal mucosal advancement flaps. (**a**) Identifying of the internal fistula opening. (**b**) Coring out the fistula tract. (**c**) The advancement flap and the internal opening are closed by sutures. (**d**) The advancement flap is pulled down to cover the internal opening of the fistula

14.2 Ulcerative Colitis

14.2.1 Introduction

Although medical therapy can ameliorate the inflammatory process and control most symptomatic flares of ulcerative colitis, it provides no definitive treatment for the disease yet. Proctocolectomy or total removal of the colon and rectum can be considered as one of complete treatments. Surgical management of ulcerative colitis requires a comprehensive understanding of all the surgical options. Surgical approaches in UC can be divided into emergency and elective indications (Table 14.3) [52].

A total proctocolectomy (TPC) is the gold-standard surgical procedure to cure ulcerative colitis (UC) because it removes the entire colonic mucosa. After TPC, there are several reconstruction methods. The safest method is an ileostomy, and the functional outcomes related to the sphincter-saving procedure do not matter in this procedure. However, a permanent ileostomy is psychologically difficult to be accepted by patients and to be managed effectively. Other reconstruction methods are the continent ileostomy (Kock's pouch) and a pouch-anal anastomosis. A pouch-anal anastomosis allows patients to use their anal sphincter, and then patients can return to a normal life after a TPC with ileal pouch-anal anastomosis.

14.2.2 TPC with a Brooke Ileostomy

14.2.2.1 Surgical Indications

The indications for elective surgery in patients with UC are (1) failure of medical management to control symptoms, (2) complications associated with side effects of medications, (3) stricture formation, (4) epithelial dysplasia, dysplasia-associated lesion or mass or malignancy, (5) uncontrollable extraintestinal manifestations of UC, and (6) growth retardation in children [96]. TPC with a Brooke ileostomy is a safe and feasible surgical option in terms of not only postoperative surgical complications but also postoperative quality of life [48].

14.2.2.2 Surgical Techniques

The procedure of the TPC contains the right hemicolectomy, transverse colectomy, left hemicolectomy, anterior resection, and low anterior resection, which removes the whole rectum to the dentate line. A characteristic of the Brooke ileostomy is primary maturation of the ileostomy. Primary maturation protects the serositis of the exposed ileum and facilitates healing of the ileostomy. The site of the ileostomy is in the right lower quadrant of the abdomen and the lateral one third of the rectus abdominis muscle. The skin around the ileostomy should be flat, and there must be no scars. Secure attachment of an ostomy plate is very important to maintain the quality of life of a patient with an ileostomy or a colostomy (Fig. 14.22).

14.2.2.3 Postoperative Outcomes

Complications can occur including wound infection or dehiscence, intraluminal or extraluminal bleeding, intestinal obstruction, intra-abdominal infection or abscess, and other medically related postoperative complications such as pneumonia and pulmonary and cardiovascular diseases. Postoperative sexual and voiding dysfunctions are complications after a proctectomy. Permanent retrograde ejaculation or impotence in male and dyspareunia in female can occur as a result of nerve injuries with proctectomy. The superior hypogastric nerve, inferior hypogastric nerve, and both lateral pelvic plexuses should be well preserved to protect postoperative sexual and voiding dysfunctions [51, 73, 85]. Complications related to an ileostomy are ileal necrosis and parastomal skin irritation, stenosis, hernia, and prolapse [49]. A common cause of ileal necrosis is torsion of the mesentery. If ileal necrosis occurs, resection and a new ileostomy formation are necessary.

Table 14.3 General indications for surgical treatment for UC

Elective surgery
Intractability to medical treatment
Colorectal cancer
Continuous uncontrolled hemorrhage
Uncontrolled extracolonic manifestations
Arthritis, uveitis, iritis
Emergency surgery
Toxic megacolon
Toxic colitis
Bowel perforation

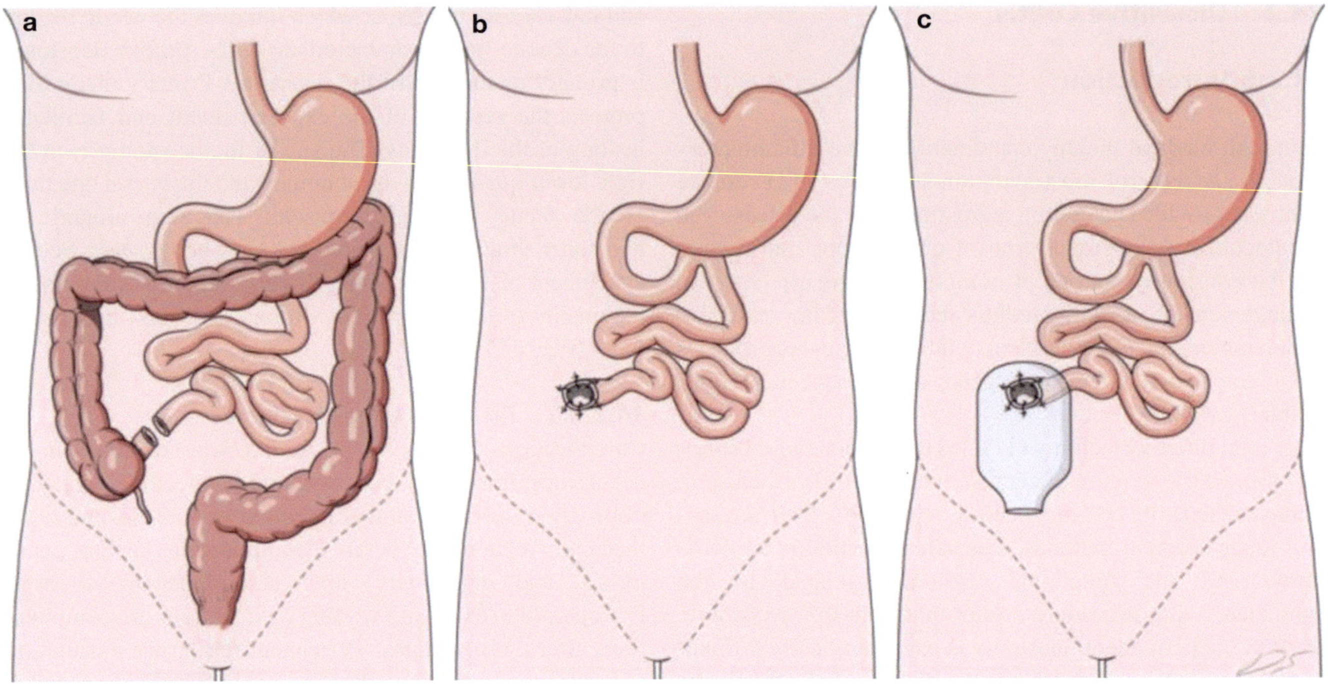

Fig. 14.22 Technique for a total proctocolectomy with a Brooke ileostomy. (**a**) Range of resection. Total colon and rectum are resected, (**b**) Brooke ileostomy, (**c**) ostomy appliances

14.2.3 TPC with an Ileal J-Pouch and Anastomosis (IPAA)

14.2.3.1 Surgical Indications

This procedure is performed electively and contraindicated in an emergency situation and attractive surgical option in terms of complete removal of the whole colorectal mucosa and preservation of the defecation function. TPC with IPAA is also indicated in familial adenomatous polyposis. However, Crohn's disease is a contraindication due to remarkable postoperative complications and poor long-term outcomes [77, 79].

14.2.3.2 Surgical Techniques

After TPC, the whole rectal mucosa is removed, and the end point of the rectal mucosa is the dentate line. The ileal J-pouch is reconstructed, and the terminal ileum is used for formation of the J-pouch (Figs. 14.23 and 14.24). Anastomosis is performed using an absorbable suture by a whole layer stitch of the ileal J-pouch, internal anal sphincter, and anal mucosa. A diverting loop ileostomy is necessary to protect the ileal J-pouch-anal anastomosis. A diverting loop ileostomy closure is usually performed 6–8 weeks later after confirming the intact ileal J-pouch-anal anastomosis. Evaluation of the ileal J-pouch is performed by a rectal examination or colonoscopy. An imaging study using contrast can be used to detect anastomosis leakage.

14.2.3.3 Postoperative Outcomes

The mortality rate is 0–1 % [70]. Anastomotic stricture after an IPAA occurs between 5 and 38 % [64, 68, 78, 80]. Anastomotic stricture can be treated by repeated dilation using a finger or dilator. Postoperative small bowel obstruction occurred in approximately 20 % of the patients. These patients eventually needed operative treatment [67].

Pouch-vaginal fistula is a problematic complication of IPAA with a 3–16 % of overall prevalence rate [54, 55, 74] (Fig. 14.25). The etiologies of a pouch-vaginal fistula are iatrogenic injury of the vaginal wall or pouch-anal anastomotic failure. The correction is divided into two methods according to the level of the pouch-anal fistula. If the location of the fistula is from the anastomosis or above the anorectal junction, the transabdominal approach is preferred. Dissection between the posterior vaginal wall and ileal pouch is divided. Then the posterior vaginal wall and ileal pouch fistula site are repaired. A new ileoanal anastomosis is performed. If the fistula is located below the anastomosis, through the anal canal, transanal or transvaginal approaches are preferred, and the advancement flap procedure is generally used. A gracilis muscle interposition can be used [83].

Pouchitis is a nonspecific inflammation and the most frequent long-term complication [72, 82, 87]. The etiology of pouchitis is unclear. However, overgrowth of anaerobic bacteria is one of the reasons for pouchitis. The main symptoms of pouchitis are abdominal cramping pain, pelvic pain, fever, malaise, anorexia, and increasing stool frequency [66, 81]. The treatment is conservative by using antibiotics such as metronidazole and ciprofloxacin.

Pelvic sepsis occurs in 5–24 % of the patients [56, 76, 84]. It is related to long-term use of steroids and malnutrition. Pelvic sepsis is the reason for early excision of the pouch to treat pelvic sepsis [86]. Overall pouch failure is 5–8 %, which leads to excision of the pouch.

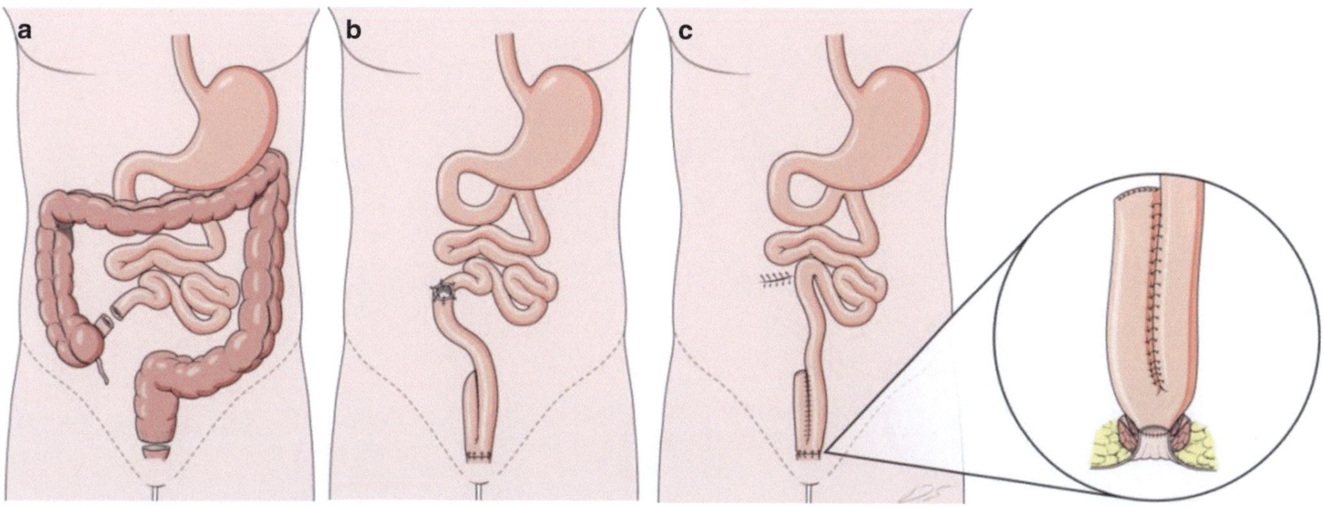

Fig. 14.23 Technique for total proctocolectomy with ileal J-pouch-anal anastomosis. (**a**) Range of resection. Total colon and rectum are resected. (**b**) Diverting loop ileostomy, (**c**) ileal J-pouch-anal anastomosis

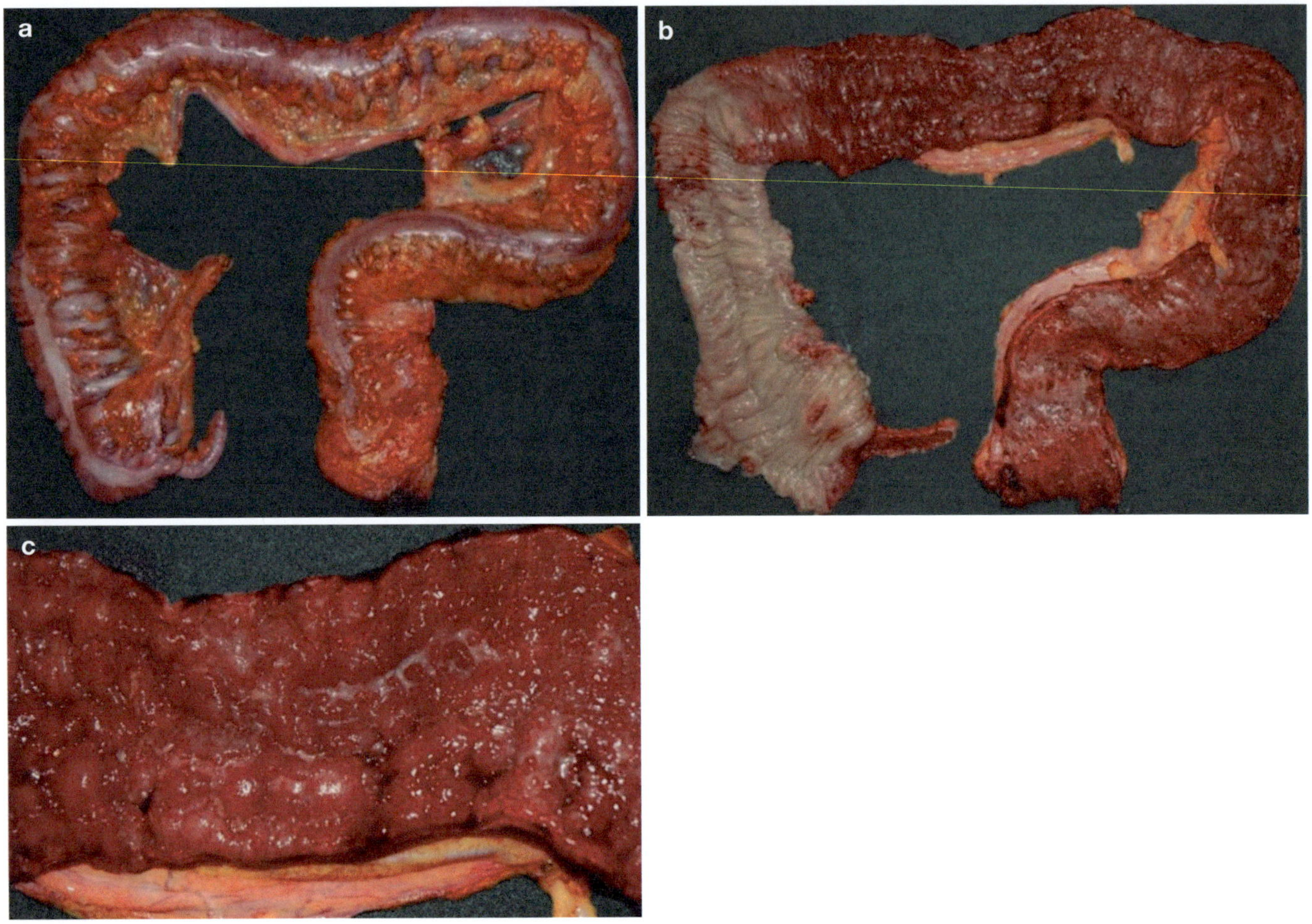

Fig. 14.24 Resected specimen after total proctocolectomy. (**a**) Resected whole specimen. (**b**) Intraluminal feature (opened specimen). (**c**) Transverse colon intraluminal feature

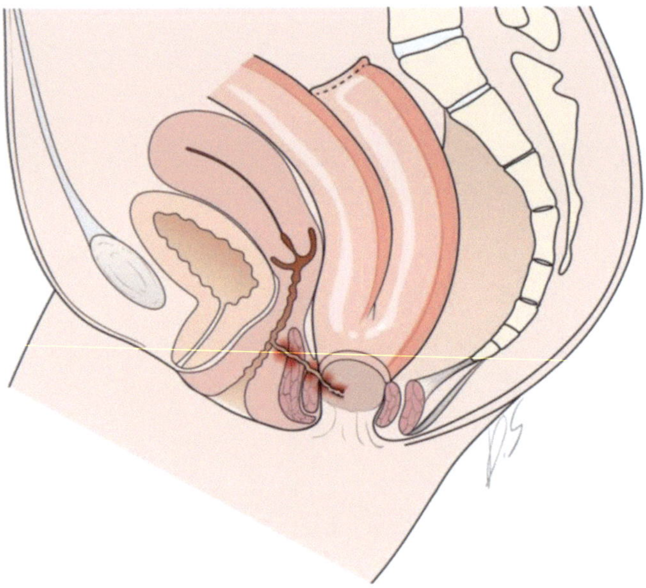

Fig. 14.25 Pouch-vaginal fistula

14.2.4 Abdominal Colectomy with an Ileorectal Anastomosis

14.2.4.1 Surgical Indications

The postoperative functional outcome of this procedure is better than a proctocolectomy because it preserves the rectum [46]. So it can be used in an elective situation. However, about 25 % of UC patients need an eventual proctectomy due to inflammation of the remnant rectum. Thus, the use of this procedure is with caution and should be decided on the patient's specific situation. Old age or high-risk patients can select this procedure. Moreover, female patients who need to preserve fertility can use ileorectal anastomosis after an abdominal colectomy.

14.2.4.2 Surgical Techniques

The resection procedures of the right colon, transverse colon, left colon, and sigmoid colon are the same as TPC except for a proctectomy. In this procedure, the rectum is preserved. Anastomosis is performed between the terminal ileum and the upper rectum (Fig. 14.26).

14.2.4.3 Postoperative Outcomes

IRA is relatively safer procedure compared to IPAA. The anastomotic leakage rate is less than 10 %, and postoperative sexual and voiding dysfunctions are uncommon [57, 62]. A major concern is the fate of the remnant rectal stump. Usually with a remaining rectum, the chance of getting cancer is high. The cumulative risk was 6 % at 20 years and 15 % at 30 years [46]. Proctitis occurs in 20–45 % of patients, and 25 % of these patients eventually need a proctectomy due to severe refractory proctitis [46, 62].

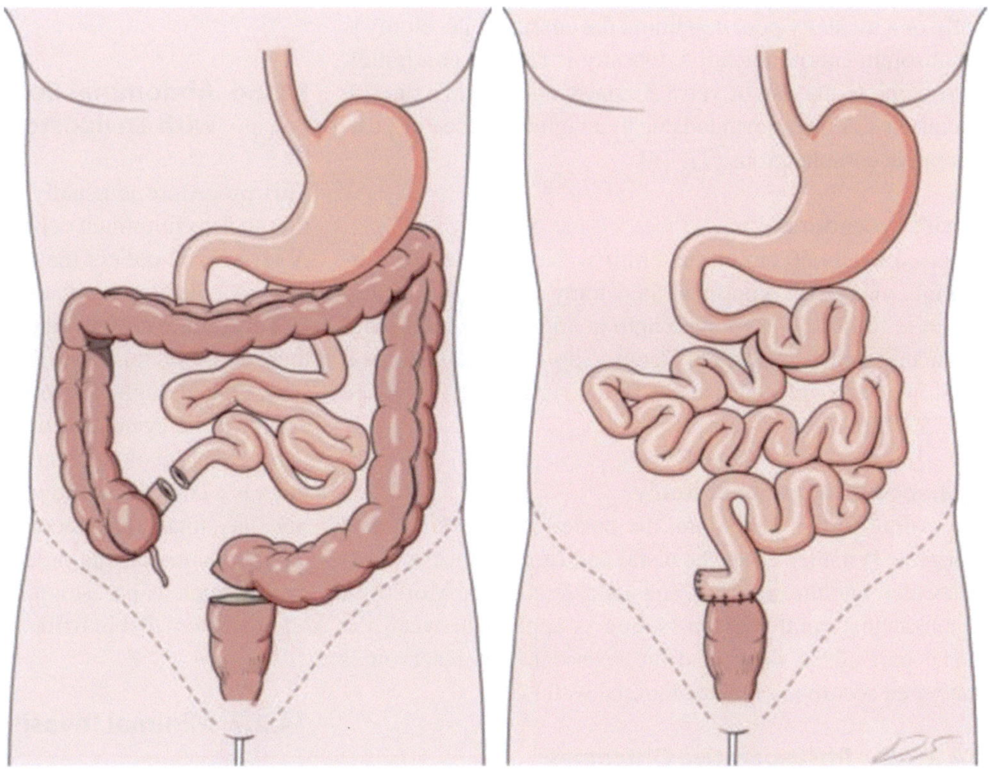

Fig. 14.26 Technique for a colectomy with an ileorectal anastomosis

14.2.5 TPC with a Continent Ileostomy

14.2.5.1 Surgical Indications

A continent ileostomy is now infrequently used because of high postoperative complications and another good alternative surgical option (IPAA). However, there is a still reasonable indication for a continent ileostomy. General indications are failed pelvic pouch, conventional ileostomy malfunction, and the patient's preference. When an IPAA fails, the continent ileostomy can be a proper option instead of a conventional ileostomy. The patient's condition, which is not an indication of IPAA, such as poor anal sphincter function or anal cancer, can be indications for a continent ileostomy.

General contraindications include desmoid disease, obesity, or a situation which anticipates short bowel syndrome after formation of a continent ileostomy and Crohn's disease. The continent ileostomy needs intermittent intubation to evacuate the contents of the reservoir. Thus, if a patient cannot perform this procedure properly due to either a physically or a mentally poor condition, the continent ileostomy is an absolute contraindication. Obesity is relative contraindication due to the risk of valve slippage, and Crohn's disease usually is not recommended due to a high incidence of postoperative complications [77, 79].

Kock's Procedure

Approximately 50 cm of the terminal ileum is used for formation of Kock's continent ileostomy (Fig. 14.27). The ileum is folded with 15 cm length at 15 cm proximal point from the resected terminal ileum. The distal tubular ileal end opening is placed usually in the right lower quadrant [58, 59, 60].

S-Shaped Continent Ileostomy

According to this procedure, the posterior part of the ileal reservoir is made. Then, the distal part of the ileum is intussuscepted into the reservoir, and a nipple is made. Moreover, seromuscular reinforcement suture is applied between the distal part of the ileum and the reservoir. The reservoir is anchored securely on the abdominal wall [75].

14.2.5.2 Postoperative Outcomes

Nipple valve slippage is the most frequent postoperative complication of a continent ileostomy with a prevalence rate about 30 % [53, 63, 65]. Symptoms are outlet obstruction, difficult pouch catheterization, and incontinence. A diagnosis can be made according to clinical symptoms. The confirmation of nipple valve slippage can be done by an imaging study such as a barium enema. Normal radiographic finding of a continent ileostomy is an inverted nipple protruding into the pouch [71]. Conservative treatment can be used initially; repair or a new formation of a nipple can be considered as a surgical option.

A second frequent complication is pouchitis (7–43 %) [47, 53, 63, 65]. Common symptoms of pouchitis are fever, diarrhea, bleeding, and abdominal pain. Bowel contents, stasis, and overgrowth of anaerobic bacteria are considered as the etiology of pouchitis. Diagnosis can be done by clinical symptoms and endoscopic findings. Typical endoscopic findings are contact bleeding, friability, and ulcerative-erythematous mucosa. Treatment is conservative with proper antibiotics [69]. An effective continuous drainage of the reservoir is necessary.

In a rare case, excision of the reservoir is necessary. Intestinal obstruction after a continent ileostomy is usually due to the problem of the nipple valve and kinking of the conduit. The incident rate of intestinal obstruction is about 5 %.

14.2.6 Abdominal Colectomy with an Ileostomy

This procedure is usually indicated in an emergency situation such as fulminant colitis or toxic megacolon (Fig. 14.28). A severely ill patient may also be a candidate for this procedure. A colectomy with an ileostomy is a relatively safe and fast procedure compared to a TPC with anastomosis because there is no rectal dissection and an anastomosis procedure [48]. Even though there is an emergency situation, if a preoperative rectal evaluation using a proctoscopy shows that there is no rectal involvement of UC, the choice of surgical treatment is a colectomy. However, if there is severe rectal bleeding, a total proctocolectomy is necessary. Specific complications of this procedure are ostomy related complications such as parastomal hernia, stoma prolapse, stenosis, and parastomal skin irritation.

14.2.7 Minimal Invasive Surgery

Laparoscopic surgery can be used, and it can be beneficial in decreasing postoperative adhesion and preserve fertility in female patients. However, the operation time is longer than open surgery, and the benefits of minimal invasive surgery for ulcerative colitis are not conclusive [44, 50, 61].

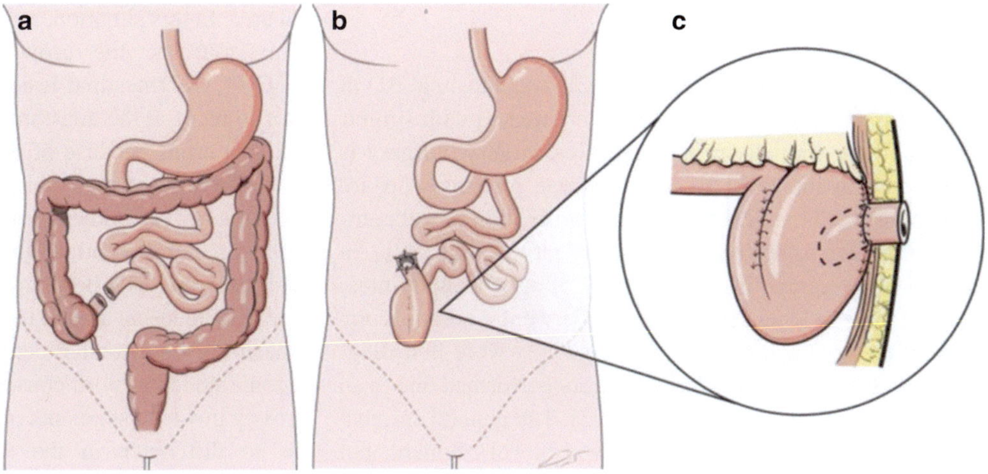

Fig. 14.27 Technique of a total proctocolectomy with a Kock's pouch. (**a**) Range of resection. Total colon and rectum are resected, (**b**) a Kock's pouch front view, (**c**) a Kock's pouch side view

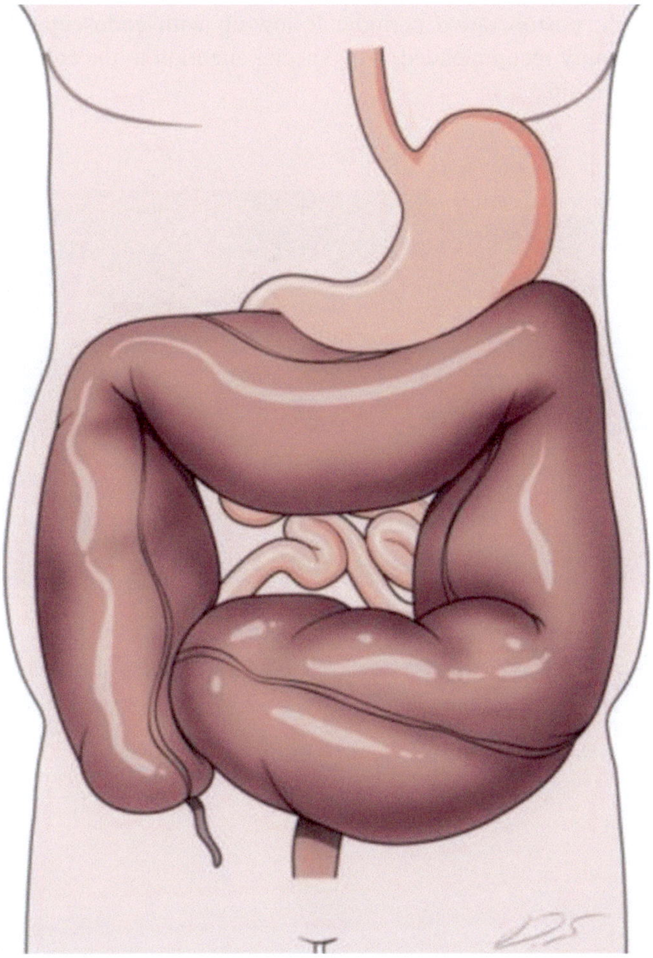

Fig. 14.28 Toxic megacolon

14.3 Behçet's Disease

There are many similarities between CD and intestinal BD in medical treatment and surgery. Both are treated with similar drugs and occasionally require repeated surgery. Surgery is considered in intestinal Behçet's disease patients who are unresponsive to medical treatment or those with bowel complications such as perforation or persistent bleeding [99]. An operation is required in about 5–10 % of patients with intestinal BD [89]. Generally, patients underwent a colonoscopy at the time of diagnosis, but some patients were first diagnosed with intestinal BD during surgery performed due to an acute or complicated presentation [93]. The general surgical treatment is resection of the involved bowel segment, but optimal surgical procedures and the length of normal bowel to be resected are still controversial.

14.3.1 Surgical Indications

The indications of surgical treatment are same with Crohn's disease. Surgery should be selected in patients with intestinal bowel perforation, intractability with medical treatment, intestinal bleeding, intestinal obstruction, presence of an abdominal mass, and enterocutaneous fistula formation. Partial intestinal obstruction, which does not respond to medical treatment, is usually elective surgery. Regarding indications for surgery between CD and intestinal BD, intestinal fistula, obstruction, and abscess were more common in patients with CD, whereas intractability with medical treatment and intestinal bleeding were more frequent in patients with intestinal BD. Early surgery is associated with a longer postoperative course free of clinical recurrence and reoperation compared with surgery performed during the course of the disease, at least in the subset of the patients with acute symptoms. Therefore, surgery should not be delayed in cases of unresponsiveness despite an appropriate effective medical treatment.

14.3.2 Surgical Techniques

The general surgical treatment is resection of the involved bowel segment. The most common involved site is the ileocecal area. In this situation, a right hemicolectomy or ileocecectomy may be the proper surgical option ([88], [97]) (Fig. 14.29). Intestinal lesions, usually at the ileocecal area, tend to recur at the anastomosis site and often require multiple operations because of perforations and fistula formation [94]. Because of mechanical trauma-induced inflammation, the pathergy phenomenon might be important here [90]. The resection margins and range are not established yet in patients with intestinal BD. If the involved colon segment is extensive from the ileocecal area to the sigmoid colon or rectum, a total colectomy or a total proctocolectomy is necessary. Others recommended a more conservative approach, resecting only grossly involved segments of bowel [91], since there seems to be no difference in the rate of recurrences after either modality.

The usual practice is to examine the bowel thoroughly during surgery, and bowel resection should include a generous normal resection margin as well as skip lesions. Since preoperative diagnosis is difficult and the recurrence rate is high, postoperative periodic follow-up with endoscopy is strongly recommended, with special attention to the anastomosis site.

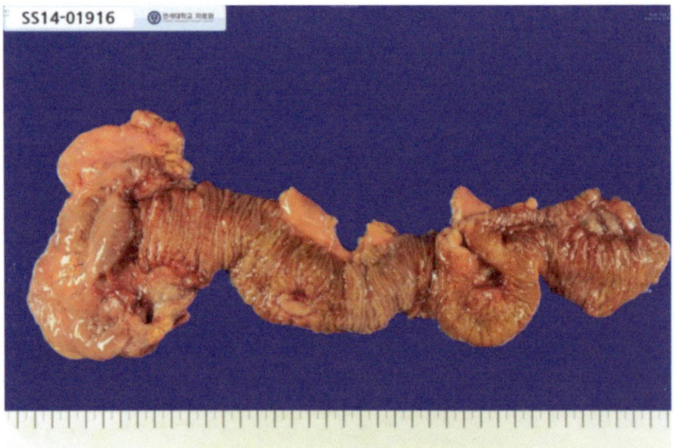

Fig. 14.29 A surgical specimen after ileocecectomy in an intestinal BD patient

14.3.3 Postoperative Outcomes

Operation should be considered early in intestinal BD as complications are common and may be fatal. Recurrent ulceration is a well-recognized complication [89]. The recurrence rate of intestinal lesions was approximately 50 % at 2 years postoperatively [95]. Several types of postoperative recurrence exist, with the most common type being one or two new deep ulcers, followed by multiple aphthous ulcers and enterocutaneous fistulas. Lesions are found at or near the anastomotic site in 80 % of recurrent cases. In point of view in recurrence, repeated resections make massive intra-abdominal adhesion (Fig. 14.30), and dissection is very difficult and technically demanding.

Regarding postoperative outcomes in intestinal BD, the cumulative recurrence rates of intestinal lesions are 28 % at 1 year, 49 % at 2 years, and 75 % at 5 years. Most recurrences occurred at the anastomotic site or within the vicinity of the site as determined by endoscopy [91] (Fig. 14.31). Among the clinical variables studied, previous surgery for perforation or fistula was the only significant factor associated with postoperative endoscopic recurrence. More recently, it is identified volcano-shaped ulcers, higher CRP level (>4.4 mg/dL), and intestinal perforation on surgical pathology as independent predictors of recurrence [92]. Patients who received postoperative azathioprine had lower reoperation rates than those that did not.

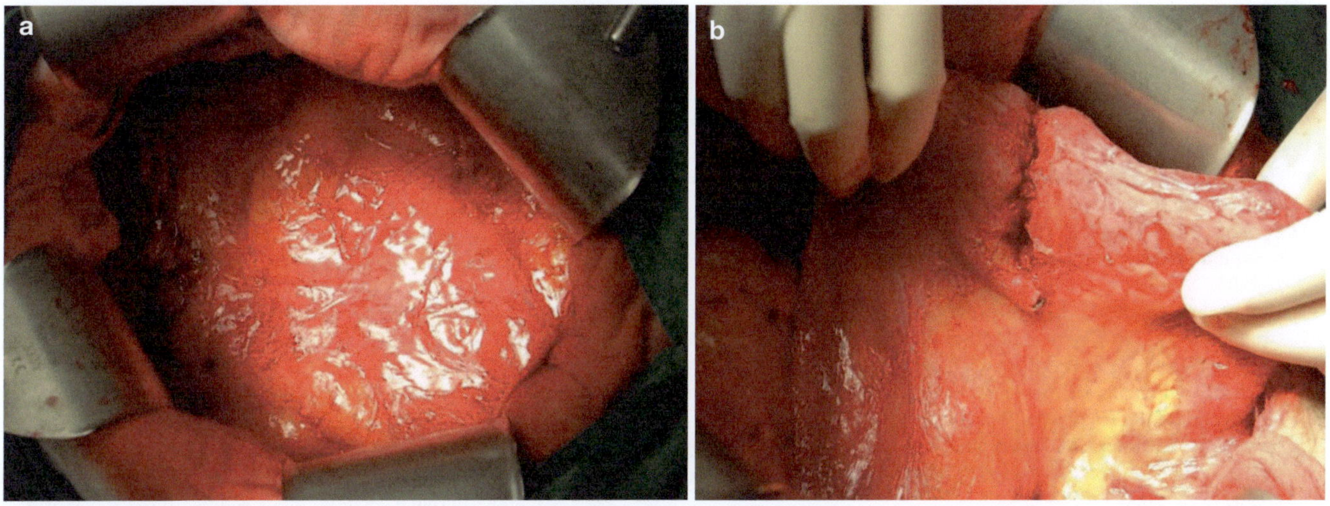

Fig. 14.30 Surgical finding in a Behçet's patient who underwent an operation three times due to recurrence. (**a**) Massive adhesion is observed. (**b**) Segmental resection of involved small bowel and end-to-end anastomosis was performed

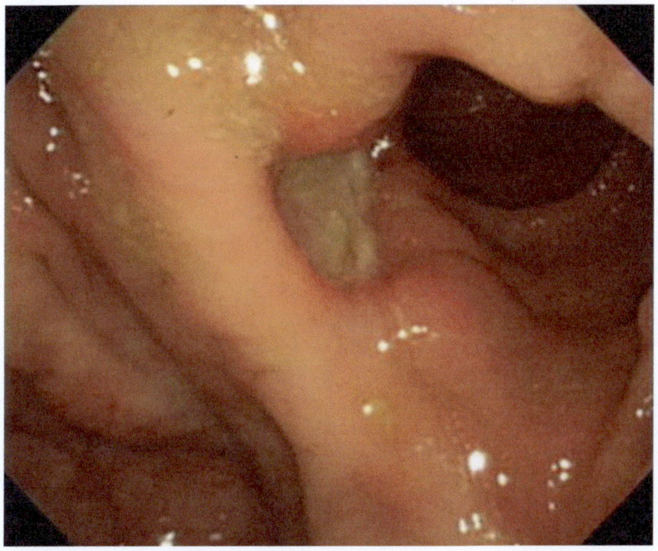

Fig. 14.31 A recurred ulcer at the anastomotic site after surgery in a patient with intestinal Behçet's disease

References

1. Alexander-Williams J, Fielding JF, Cooke WT. A comparison of results of excision and bypass for ileal Crohn's disease. Gut. 1972;13(12):973–5.
2. Borley NR, Mortensen NJ, Jewell DP. Preventing postoperative recurrence of Crohn's disease. Brit J Surg. 1997;84(11):1493–502.
3. Campbell L, Ambe R, Weaver J, et al. Comparison of conventional and nonconventional strictureplasties in Crohn's disease: a systematic review and meta-analysis. Dis Colon Rectum. 2012;55(6):714–26.
4. Cooper JC, Williams NS. The influence of microscopic disease at the margin of resection on recurrence rates in Crohn's disease. Ann Roy Coll Surg. 1986;68(1):23–6.
5. Fazio VW, Tjandra JJ, Lavery IC, et al. Long-term follow-up of strictureplasty in Crohn's disease. Dis Colon Rectum. 1993; 36(4):355–61.
6. Fazio VW, Marchetti F. Recurrent Crohn's disease and resection margins: bigger is not better. Adv Surg. 1999;32:135–68.
7. Futami K, Arima S. Role of strictureplasty in surgical treatment of Crohn's disease. J Gastroenterol. 2005;40 Suppl 16:35–9.
8. Juillerat P, Mottet C, Froehlich F et al. Extraintestinal manifestations of Crohn's disease. Digestion. 2005;71(1):31–36.
9. Hamilton SR. Colorectal carcinoma in patients with Crohn's disease. Gastroenterology. 1985;89(2):398–407.
10. Hammond TM, Grahn MF, Lunniss PJ. Fibrin glue in the management of anal fistulae. Color Dis. 2004;6(5):308–19.
11. Hawker PC, Gyde SN, Thompson H, et al. Adenocarcinoma of the small intestine complicating Crohn's disease. Gut. 1982;23(3): 188–93.
12. Hotokezaka M, Ikeda T, Uchiyama S, et al. Side-to-side-to-end strictureplasty for Crohn's disease. Dis Colon Rectum. 2009; 52(11):1882–6.
13. Hurst RD, Michelassi F. Strictureplasty for Crohn's disease: techniques and long-term results. World J Surg. 1998;22(4):359–63.
14. Ikeuchi H, Kusunoki M, Yamamura T. Long-term results of stapled and hand-sewn anastomoses in patients with Crohn's disease. Digest Surg. 2000;17(5):493–6.
15. Ingle SB, Loftus Jr EV. The natural history of perianal Crohn's disease. Dig Liver Dis. 2007;39(10):963–9.
16. Irvine EJ. Usual therapy improves perianal Crohn's disease as measured by a new disease activity index. McMaster IBD Study Group. J Clin Gastroenterol. 1995;20(1):27–32.
17. Jaskowiak NT, Michelassi F. Adenocarcinoma at a strictureplasty site in Crohn's disease: report of a case. Dis Colon Rectum. 2001;44(2):284–7.
18. Jones IT, Fazio VW, Jagelman DG. The use of transanal rectal advancement flaps in the management of fistulas involving the anorectum. Dis Colon Rectum. 1987;30(12):919–23.
19. Katariya RN, Sood S, Rao PG, et al. Stricture-plasty for tubercular strictures of the gastro-intestinal tract. Brit J Surg. 1977;64(7): 496–8.
20. Ky A, Sohn N, Weinstein MA, et al. Carcinoma arising in anorectal fistulas of Crohn's disease. Dis Colon Rectum. 1998;41(8): 992–6.
21. Lee EC, Papaioannou N. Minimal surgery for chronic obstruction in patients with extensive or universal Crohn's disease. Ann Roy Coll Surg. 1982;64(4):229–33.
22. Lock MR, Farmer RG, Fazio VW, et al. Recurrence and reoperation for Crohn's disease: the role of disease location in prognosis. New Engl J Med. 1981;304(26):1586–8.
23. Makowiec F, Jehle EC, Becker HD, et al. Clinical course after transanal advancement flap repair of perianal fistula in patients with Crohn's disease. Brit J Surg. 1995;82(5):603–6.
24. Marchetti F, Fazio VW, Ozuner G. Adenocarcinoma arising from a strictureplasty site in Crohn's disease. Report of a case. Dis Colon Rectum. 1996;39(11):1315–21.
25. Michelassi F. Side-to-side isoperistaltic strictureplasty for multiple Crohn's strictures. Dis Colon Rectum. 1996;39(3):345–9.
26. Parks AG, Gordon PH, Hardcastle JD. A classification of fistula-in-ano. Brit J Surg. 1976;63(1):1–12.
27. Poggioli G, Laureti S, Pierangeli F. A new model of strictureplasty for multiple and long stenoses in Crohn's ileitis: side-to-side diseased to disease-free anastomosis. Dis Colon Rectum. 2003;46(1): 127–30.
28. Rojas-Feria M, Castro M, Suarez E et al. Hepatobiliary manifestations in inflammatory bowel disease: the gut, the drugs and the liver. World J Gastroenterol. 2013;WJG 19(42):7327–40.
29. Roy P, Kumar D. Strictureplasty. Brit J Surg. 2004;91(11): 1428–37.
30. Sampietro GM, Cristaldi M, Porretta T, et al. Early perioperative results and surgical recurrence after strictureplasty and miniresection for complicated Crohn's disease. Dig Surg. 2000;17(3): 261–7.
31. Sandborn WJ, Fazio VW, Feagan BG, et al. AGA technical review on perianal Crohn's disease. Gastroenterology. 2003;125(5): 1508–30.
32. Sasaki I, Shibata C, Funayama Y, et al. New reconstructive procedure after intestinal resection for Crohn's disease: modified side-to-side isoperistaltic anastomosis with double Heineke-Mikulicz procedure. Dis Colon Rectum. 2004;47(6):940–3.
33. Singh B, Ge Singh B, Mc CMNJ, Jewell DP, George B. Perianal Crohn's disease. Brit J Surg. 2004;91(7):801–14.
34. Singh B, George BD, Mortensen NJ. Surgical therapy of perianal Crohn's disease. Dig Liver Dis. 2007;39(10):988–92.
35. Stebbing JF, Jewell DP, Kettlewell MG, et al. Recurrence and reoperation after strictureplasty for obstructive Crohn's disease: long-term results [corrected]. Brit J Surg. 1995;82(11):1471–4.
36. Stone W, Veidenheimer MC, Corman ML, et al. The dilemma of Crohn's disease: long-term follow-up of Crohn's disease of the small intestine. Dis Colon Rectum. 1977;20(5):372–6.
37. Taxonera C, Schwartz DA, Garcia-Olmo D. Emerging treatments for complex perianal fistula in Crohn's disease. World J Gastroenterol. 2009;15(34):4263–72.
38. Trnka YM, Glotzer DJ, Kasdon EJ, et al. The long-term outcome of restorative operation in Crohn's disease: influence of location, prognostic factors and surgical guidelines. Ann Surg. 1982;196(3): 345–55.
39. Van Bodegraven AA, Pena AS. Treatment of extraintestinal manifestations in inflammatory bowel diseases. Curr Treat Options Gastroenterol. 2003;6(3):201–12.
40. Yamamoto T, Bain IM, Allan RN, et al. An audit of strictureplasty for small-bowel Crohn's disease. Dis Colon Rectum. 1999;42(6): 797–803.
41. Yamamoto T, Keighley MR. Factors affecting the incidence of postoperative septic complications and recurrence after strictureplasty for jejunoileal Crohn's disease. Am J Surg. 1999;178(3): 240–5.
42. Yamamoto T. Factors affecting recurrence after surgery for Crohn's disease. World J Gasteroenterol. 2005;11(26):3971–9.
43. Yamamoto T, Fazio VW, Tekkis PP. Safety and efficacy of strictureplasty for Crohn's disease: a systematic review and meta-analysis. Dis Colon Rectum. 2007;50(11):1968–86.
44. Ahmed Ali U, Keus F, Heikens JT et al. Open versus laparoscopic (assisted) ileo pouch anal anastomosis for ulcerative colitis and familial adenomatous polyposis. Cochrane Database Syst Rev. 2009;(1):CD006267.
45. Alves A, Panis Y, Bouhnik Y, et al. Subtotal colectomy for severe acute colitis: a 20-year experience of a tertiary care center with an

aggressive and early surgical policy. J Am Coll Surg. 2003;197: 379–85.
46. Baker WNW, Glass RE, Richie JK, et al. Cancer of the rectum following colectomy and ileorectal anastomosis for ulcerative colitis. Br J Surg. 1978;65:862–8.
47. Bonello JC, Thow GB, Manson RR. Mucosal enteritis: a complication of the continent ileostomy. Dis Colon Rectum. 1981;24:37.
48. Camilleri-Brennan J, Steele RJ. Objective assessment of quality of life following panproctocolectomy and ileostomy for ulcerative colitis. Ann R Coll Surg Engl. 2001;83(5):321–4.
49. Carlsen E, Bergan A. Technical aspects and complications of end ileostomies. World J Surg. 1995;19:632–6.
50. Chambers WM, Bicsak M, Lamparelli M, et al. Single-incision laparoscopic surgery (SILS) in complex colorectal surgery: a technique offering potential and not just cosmesis. Color Dis. 2011;13: 393–8.
51. Damgaard B, Wettergren A, Kirkegaard P. Social and sexual function following ileal pouch-anal anastomosis. Dis Colon Rectum. 1995;38:286–9.
52. Parray FQ, Wani ML, et al. Ulcerative colitis: a challenge to surgeons. Int J Prev Med. 2012;3(11):749–63.
53. Fizio VW, Church JM. Complications and function of the continent ileostomy at the Cleveland clinic. World J Surg. 1988;12: 148–54.
54. Groom JS, Nicholls RJ, Hawley PR, et al. Pouch-vaginal fistula. Br J Surg. 1993;80(7):936–40.
55. Keighley MR, Grobler SP. Fistula complicating restorative proctocolectomy. Br J Surg. 1993;80:1065–7.
56. Kelly KA. Anal sphincter-saving operations for chronic ulcerative colitis. Am J Surg. 1992;163:5–11.
57. Khubchandani IT, Kontostolis SB. Outcome of ileorectal anastomosis in an inflammatory bowel disease surgery experience of three decades. Arch Surg. 1994;129:866–9.
58. Kock NG. Intra-abdominal "reservoir" in patients with permanent ileostomy: preliminary observations on a procedure resulting in fecal "continence" in five ileostomy patients. Arch Surg. 1969;99:223.
59. Kock NG, Darle N, Kewenter J, et al. The quality of life after proctocolectomy and ileostomy: a study of patients with conventional ileostomies converted to continent ileostomies. Dis Colon Rectum. 1974;17:287.
60. Kock NG, Darle N, Hultén L, et al. Ileostomy. Curr Probl Surg. 1977;14:1–52.
61. Lefevre JH, Bretagnol F, Ouaissi M, et al. Total laparoscopic ileal pouch-anal anastomosis: prospective series of 82 patients. Surg Endosc. 2009;23(1):166–73.
62. Leijonmarck CE, Lofberg R, Hellers G. Long-term results of ileorectal anastomosis in ulcerative colitis in Stockholm County. Dis Colon Rectum. 1990;33:195–200.
63. Lepisto AH, Jarvinen HJ. Durability of Kock continent ileostomy. Dis Colon Rectum. 2003;46(7):925–8.
64. Lewis WG, Kuzu A, Sagar PM, et al. Stricture at the pouch-anal anastomosis after restorative proctocolectomy. Dis Colon Rectum. 1994;35:120–5.
65. Litle VR, Barbour S, Schrock TR, et al. The continent ileostomy: long-term durability and patient satisfaction. J Gastrointest Surg. 1999;3:625–32.
66. Lohmuller JL, Pemberton JH, Dozois RR, et al. Pouchitis and extraintestinal manifestations of inflammatory bowel disease after ileal pouch–anal anastomosis. Ann Surg. 1990;211:622–7.
67. MacLean AR, Cohen Z, MacRae HM, et al. Risk of small bowel obstruction after the ileal pouch-anal anastomosis. Ann Surg. 2002;235:200–6.
68. Marcello PW, Roberts PL, Schoëtz Jr DJ, et al. Long-term results of the ileoanal pouch procedure. Arch Surg. 1993;128:500–3.
69. McLeod RS, Taylor DW, Cohen Z, et al. Single patient randomized clinical trial: use in determining optimum treatment for patient with inflammation of Kock continent ileostomy reservoir. Lancet. 1986;1:726.
70. Michelassi F, Lee J, Rubin M, et al. Long-term functional results after ileal pouch anal restorative proctocolectomy for ulcerative colitis: a prospective observational study. Ann Surg. 2003;238:433–41.
71. Montagne JP, Kressel HY, Moss AA, et al. Radiologic evaluation of the continent (Kock) ileostomy. Radiology. 1978;127:325.
72. Nasmyth DG, Johnston D, Godwin PG, et al. Factors influencing bowel function after ileal pouch–anal anastomosis. Br J Surg. 1986;73:469–73.
73. Oresland T, Fasth S, Nordgren S, et al. The clinical and functional outcome after restorative proctocolectomy. A prospective study in 100 patients. Int J Color Dis. 1989;4:50–6.
74. Ozuner G, Hull T, Lee P, et al. What happens to a pelvic pouch when a fistula develops? Dis Colon Rectum. 1997;40:543–7.
75. Parks AG, Nicholls RJ. Proctocolectomy without ileostomy for ulcerative colitis. Br Med J. 1978;2:85.
76. Pemberton JH, Kelly KA, Beart Jr RW, et al. Ileal pouch–anal anastomosis for chronic ulcerative colitis. Long-term results. Ann Surg. 1987;206:504–13.
77. Peyregne V, Francois Y, Gilly FN, et al. Outcome of ileal pouch after secondary diagnosis of Crohn's disease. Int J Color Dis. 2000;15:49–53.
78. Prudhomme M, Dozois RR, Godlewski G, et al. Anal canal strictures after ileal pouch-anal anastomosis. Dis Colon Rectum. 2003;46:20–3.
79. Sagar PM, Dozois RR, Wolff BG. Long-term results of ileal pouch–anal anastomosis in patients with Crohn's disease. Dis Colon Rectum. 1996;39:893–8.
80. Senapati A, Tibbs CJ, Ritchie JK, et al. Stenosis of the pouch anal anastomosis following restorative proctocolectomy. Int J Color Dis. 1996;11:57–9.
81. Shepherd NA. The pelvic ileal reservoir: pathology and pouchitis. Neth J Med. 1990;37 Suppl 1:S57–64.
82. Shepherd NA, Jass JR, Duval I, et al. Restorative proctocolectomy with ileal reservoir: pathological and histochemical study of mucosal biopsy specimens. J Clin Pathol. 1987;40:601–7.
83. Wexner SD, Ruiz DE, Genua J, et al. Gracilis muscle interposition for the treatment of rectourethral, rectovaginal, and pouch-vaginal fistulas; results in 53 patients. Ann Surg. 2008;248:39–43.
84. Wexner SD, Wong WD, Rothenberger DA, et al. The ileoanal reservoir. Am J Surg. 1990;159:178–83.
85. Wickland M, Jansson I, Asztely M, et al. Gynaecological problems related to anatomical changes after conventional proctocolectomy and ileostomy. Int J Color Dis. 1990;5:49–52.
86. Ziv Y, Church JM, Fazio VW, et al. Effect of systemic steroids on ileal pouch–anal anastomosis in patients with ulcerative colitis. Dis Colon Rectum. 1996;39:504–8.
87. Zuccaro Jr G, Fazio VW, Church JM, et al. Pouch ileitis. Dig Dis Sci. 1989;34:1505–10.
88. Abdullah AN, Keczkes K. Behcet's syndrome with gastrointestinal tract involvement mimicking carcinoma of the caecum – a case report. Clin Exp Dermatol. 1989;14:459–61.
89. Bardbury AW, Milne AA, Murie JA. Surgical aspects of Behcet's disease. British J Surg. 1994;81:1712–21.
90. Bozkurt M, Torin G, Aksakal B, Ataoglu O. Behcet's disease and surgical intervention. Int J Dermatol. 1992;31(8):571–3.
91. Choi IJ, Kim JS, Cha SD, Jung HC, Park JG, Song IS, et al. Long-term clinical course and prognostic factors in intestinal Behçet's disease. Dis Colon Rectum. 2000;43:692–700.
92. Jung YS, Yoon JY, Lee JH, Jeon SM, Hong SP, Kim TI, et al. Prognostic factors and long-term clinical outcomes for surgical patients with intestinal Behçet's disease. Inflamm Bowel Dis. 2011;17:1594–602.

93. Jung YS, et al. Clinical Course of Intestinal Behcet's disease during the first five years. Dig Dis Sci. 2013;58:497–503.
94. Lee KS, Kim SJ, Lee BC, Yoon DS, Lee WJ, Chi HS. Surgical treatment of intestinal Behcet's disease. Yonsei Med J. 1997;38(6): 455–60.
95. Naganuma M, Iwao Y, Inoue N, Hisamatsu T, Imaeda H, Ishii H, et al. Analysis of clinical course and long-term prognosis of surgical and nonsurgical patients with intestinal Behcet's disease. Am J Gastroenterol. 2000;95(10):2848–51.
96. Robert, Cima, Jon H, Pemberton. Medical and Surgical Management of Chronic Ulcerative Colitis. Arch Surg. 2005;140(3):300–10.
97. Suh YL, Sung RH, Chi JG, et al. Intestinal Behcet's disease in a child –a case report. J Korean Med Sci. 1987;2:129–32.
98. Williams JG, Wong WD, Rothenberger DA, et al. Recurrence of Crohn's disease after resection. Brit J Surg. 1991;78(1):10–19.
99. Yurdakul S, Tuzuner N, Yurdakul I, Hamuryudan V, Yazici H. Gastrointestinal involvement in Behcet's syndrome: a controlled study. Ann Rheum Dis. 1996;55(3):208–10.